PRAISE FOR

Natural Choices
for Women's Health

"Dr. Steelsmith has done the remarkable: an interesting book full of accurate information that is not widely available. What a triumph for all health professionals who seek to promote health or whose practice focuses on the preventive, wholistic, integrative, comprehensive, eclectic, and/or leading edge. This book is equally valuable for all lay people who want to participate actively in the decisions about their lifestyle choices that determine much of our healthfulness or suffering as our life progresses."   —Russ Jaffe, M.D., Ph.D., CCN and the IBC
International Scientist 2003

"This book is a must read for every woman who is interested in being proactive about her own health and wellness. Dr. Steelsmith artfully weaves the principles and philosophies of Eastern and Western medicine into a harmonious whole. *Natural Choices for Women's Health* is interesting, easy to read, and an extremely usable guide for women on their personal path to health and wellness."

—Jane Guiltinan, N.D., Clinical Professor and
Director, Bastyr Center for Women's Wellness

Natural Choices
for Women's Health

HOW THE SECRETS OF NATURAL AND
CHINESE MEDICINE CAN CREATE
A LIFETIME OF WELLNESS

Dr. Laurie Steelsmith

with Alex Steelsmith

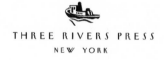

THREE RIVERS PRESS
NEW YORK

Grateful acknowledgment is made to the following for permission to reprint previously published
material: **Dr. Russell Jaffe:** Excerpt from The Alkaline Way: Your Health Restoration by
Dr. Russell Jaffe. Reprinted by permission of the author; and **Marlow & Company:** Specific chart
from The New Glucose Revolution by Jennie Brand Miller, Ph.D., Thomas M.S. Wolever, M.D.,
Ph.D., Kaye Foster-Powell, M. Nutr & Diet, Stephen Colagiuri, M.D. Text copyright © 1996, 1998,
1999, 2002, 2003 by Dr. Jennie Brand Miller, Kaye Foster-Powell, Dr. Stephen Colagiuri,
Dr. Thomas M. S. Wolever. Reprinted by permission of Marlowe & Company, a division of
Avalon Publishing Group.

Published in the United States by Three Rivers Press, an imprint of the Crown Publishing Group,
a division of Random House, Inc., New York.
www.crownpublishing.com

THREE RIVERS PRESS and the Tugboat design are registered trademarks of Random House, Inc.

Library of Congress Cataloging-in-Publication Data
Steelsmith, Laurie.
Natural choices for women's health : How the secrets of natural and Chinese medicine
can create a lifetime of wellness
Laurie Steelsmith.— 1st ed.
Includes bibliographical references and index.
1. Self-care, Health.   2. Medicine, Popular.   3. Medicine, Chinese.   4. Mind and body.
I. Title.
RA776.5.S765   2005
613'.04244—dc22   2004020336

ISBN 1-4000-4796-X

Printed in the United States of America

Design by Meryl Sussman Levavi

10   9   8   7   6   5   4

To my mother,

whose strength, courage, and love for life

touch everyone she meets

Contents

Natural Choices
for Women's Health

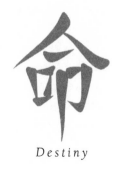

Destiny

Introduction

"A long journey begins with a single step."
—PAMELA METZ AND JACQUELINE TOBIN, *The Tao of Women*

EVERY DAY and in every aspect of your life, you make choices that profoundly affect your capacity to be healthy. Your health is the embodiment of thousands, perhaps millions, of these choices. Each one is like a drop of water; when all of them are added together, they have the power to transform the landscape of your life. We all have to battle genetic predispositions toward disease, of course, but in my years of practicing natural medicine I have become convinced that ultimately the decision to create a lifetime of optimal health lies with you. The choice is yours.

I would like to share with you a little about my own story, because it will shed light on why I so firmly believe that you can create optimal health in your own life. I was born into a family with a strong genetic history of breast cancer and alcoholism. Not only my mother but my grandmother, my first cousin, my great-aunt, and my great-great-aunt, all on the maternal side of my family, were diagnosed with breast cancer. Not all of them have overcome it.

Given this history, it became painfully clear to me early in life that I had a choice. I couldn't change my genetic makeup, but I could assist my body in its fight against disease. I could choose a life of vitality and joy over a life plagued with fear and illness and the consequences of unhealthy choices. I could choose to be optimally healthy.

The long, circuitous path that led me to naturopathic medical school in my early twenties began when I was sixteen years old and had the opportunity to live as an exchange student in rural Norway for the summer. During my stay my host family introduced me to a healthier, more natural lifestyle than I had experienced as an American teenager. My exchange parents, both in their early forties, jogged seven miles a day and never smoked or drank alcohol. They ate healthy food, baked their own bread, and made their own jam. We picked fresh mushrooms in the forest for dinner and flowers off the linden trees for tea. I had been raised on the standard American diet and from an early age suffered from chronic sinusitis and allergies, but that summer in Norway I was amazed to watch these problems disappear. Simply by making changes in my eating habits and lifestyle, I was able to cure my sinusitis and eliminate my allergic reactions. I began to learn the benefits of a new way of life, one that factored in the importance of nutrition to good health, and one that I would use as a model in the years to come.

After my eye-opening visit I returned to my hometown in Connecticut, motivated to educate myself as much as I possibly could about natural health and nutrition. I found an after-school job at the local health food store (an extreme contrast to my previous job in a cheese shop). I learned the meaning of the term *whole foods* and about the benefits of natural foods like tofu and herbs like echinacea. As I devoured every book on the shelf in that store, Adelle Davis, author of the classic *Let's Eat Right to Keep Fit,* and Dr. Henry Bieler, author of *Food Is Your Best Medicine,* became my heroes.

One day while working in the store, I met my first naturopathic physician, who had a reputation for treating cancer patients with whole foods. He explained that he had attended a naturopathic medical college in the Northwest that emphasized the use of natural, nontoxic means of achieving optimal health. I remember telling him, "I want to learn everything that you know!" Little did I realize then what a great impact this conversation would have on my future. Before long I would spend six years studying nutrition, naturopathic medicine, acupuncture, and Chinese medicine at Bastyr University in Seattle, Washington.

During my second year at Bastyr I experienced a personal health crisis that affected my studies and forever altered my comprehension of what it means to be healthy. While working as a licensed massage therapist to support my education, I began to experience chronic pain in my hands and forearms. Over a year's time my symptoms worsened to the point that I was unable to do everyday tasks like drive a car, prepare meals, or even braid my hair—and barely able to take notes in my classes. I consulted various doctors, but none were able to figure out what the problem was.

Eventually, after taking a blood test, I was diagnosed with borderline lupus, a potentially crippling autoimmune disorder. As my condition continued to deteriorate and I was faced with the frightening prospect of losing the use of my hands and having to drop out of medical school, I focused all my attention on finding the underlying cause of my disability. I refused to take drugs with potentially toxic effects that I knew would merely mask my symptoms—even though they might alleviate my discomfort—because I wanted to get to the true root of the problem before attempting treatment.

Finally, after months of research, self-diagnosis, painstaking trial and error, and intensive collaborations with the naturopathic physicians at the Bastyr University clinic, I discovered that the underlying cause of my condition was food allergies resulting from digestive imbalances. Acting on the tenets of natural medicine (in this case, a combination of detoxification, dietary changes, nutritional supplementation, and aspects of Chinese medicine), I was able to heal my condition. Had I not been at the world's leading school of naturopathic medicine and surrounded by such a wealth of resources, it would have been unimaginably more difficult to cure myself. I knew that I had come to the right place and that I had found my life's work. I went on to graduate from Bastyr with a B.S. in natural health sciences (with an emphasis in nutrition), an N.D. (Doctor of Naturopathic Medicine) degree, and an M.S. in acupuncture.

My story has a happy ending. In the fifteen years since my health crisis, the symptoms of lupus have never returned, and I've continued to do massage and participate in a wide range of other activities, from mountain climbing to springboard diving. Thanks to my training and experience, I've been able to use the principles of natural medicine to make a difference in the lives of thousands of women on their own journeys to achieving maximum health. I hope this book will enable me to make a difference in thousands more.

What Is Natural Medicine?

In my practice, and in this book, I use the umbrella term *natural medicine* to include both Western naturopathic and Chinese medicine. Both systems offer natural alternatives to conventional Western medicine for maintaining well-being, preventing illness, and restoring health. Both emphasize stimulating, rather than interfering with, your body's innate ability to heal itself.

WESTERN NATUROPATHIC MEDICINE

Western naturopathic medicine differs from conventional Western medicine in many ways. It focuses primarily on creating health rather than on eradicating disease. If you experience an illness, the goal of naturopathic medicine is to address the underlying cause of your problem rather than simply to suppress your symptoms with drugs or other methods that may have unhealthy side effects. Naturopathic medicine diagnoses your problem by considering every facet of your health. Mental, emotional, nutritional, genetic, environmental, and lifestyle factors are all taken into account, as well as any physical causes of your illness.

The foundation of naturopathic medicine is built on the following principles:

- Respect the healing power of nature.
- Remove the obstacles to the cure.
- Identify and treat the cause of illness.
- First do no harm. (Use the least invasive treatment.)
- Treat the whole person.
- Emphasize wellness.
- Remember that prevention is the best cure.
- Stress the role of the physician as a teacher.

With roots in the nineteenth century, naturopathic medicine preserves age-old knowledge of herbal treatments, homeopathic medicine, and many other natural therapies. It offers health care that is truly comprehensive; more than any other type of medicine, it blends, balances, and integrates the conventional Western sciences with alternative approaches to health. As a naturopathic student, my academic requirements in the basic biological sciences, including all methods of modern physical, clinical, and laboratory diagnosis, were the same as those in other medical schools. In addition, I was required to study in depth a wide range of alternative techniques and natural, nontoxic therapies that are seldom taught in other medical programs, including herbal medicine, homeopathy, nutritional therapy, counseling, massage therapy, and hydrotherapy (treatment using hot and cold water).

The differences between the education of naturopathic and conventional physicians reflect very different philosophies of health and disease. My naturopathic training placed a much greater emphasis, for example, on the science of nutrition and *the impact of nutrition on human health*. (At Bastyr I fulfilled 138 total credit hours of therapeutic nutritional sciences, whereas conventional medical schools typically require none.)

CHINESE MEDICINE

Like Western naturopathic medicine, Chinese medicine is a natural healing tradition that provides a wonderful alternative to pharmaceutical drugs and other approaches that have potentially harmful long-term effects. With deep roots in Taoist philosophy and Chinese culture dating back more than five thousand years, it is based on an "energetic" model of health and illness rather than the biochemical model that is predominant in Western medicine.

For a Westerner accustomed to the straightforward analytical science of conventional medicine, exploring the ancient wisdom of Chinese medicine can be one of life's most transforming experiences. It offers a way of thinking outside the box of cause-and-effect relationships that you are accustomed to, challenging you to think about your body, mind, and spirit in delightfully new, nonlinear ways. It invites you to approach your health through elegant poetic images that are often quite beautiful and rich in metaphor.

Perhaps the single most important tenet in Chinese medicine is the concept of Qi (pronounced *chee*). Qi is your body's vital energy—not merely the energy of your physical body but the life force that is the essence of your being. Chinese medicine uses a systematic approach for maintaining and promoting health based on the premise that Qi is responsible for health and disease. Yin and yang, which are forms of Qi, are the opposites that exist everywhere in the universe and in your body; when your yin and yang are in harmony, you will be in perfect health.

Another concept, one of the most helpful, is the Five Elements. These are the five basic properties that are said to be present throughout the natural world: Wood, Fire, Earth, Metal, and Water. Like Qi, yin, and yang, according to Chinese medicine each of the Five Elements is also found in your body. Each is associated with particular traits and tendencies—you can think of them as metaphors for qualities, or capacities, present in your body and expressed in your physiology, your emotions, and your spirit. One of the Five Elements usually dominates your personality.

Conventional medicine in the West has become a very left-brained process, but when you open your mind to medical traditions from both the Eastern and Western hemispheres, you more fully engage both hemispheres of your brain—the logical, rational left brain and the imaginative, intuitive right brain. As you explore Chinese medicine in this book, you might find, for instance, that you have a "wind cold invasion" in your channels, or "excess fire," or that your "Three Treasures" are well preserved. These notions may seem abstract and foreign at first, but they will become easy to understand. And you can take comfort in the knowledge that they are based on an elaborate system of healing and time-honored techniques that have evolved over thousands of years. (This book necessarily provides only an overview of the very detailed tapestry of Chinese medicine.)

Although some aspects of Chinese medicine remain mysterious to Western science, the discipline is becoming more commonly accepted throughout the conventional Western medical establishment. Many of the treatments used in Chinese medicine have been confirmed with modern diagnostic techniques, and some therapies have been studied and found to be efficacious by the National Institutes of Health. Chinese medicine has proven to be consistently effective in helping people from all over the world who seek out gentle, nontoxic therapies for maintaining and restoring health.

CREATING NATURAL HEALTH

In more than ten years of integrating Western naturopathic and Chinese medical perspectives in my practice in Honolulu, I've seen many striking parallels between these two great traditions of natural medicine. Often the poetic metaphors of the Eastern tradition wonderfully illustrate similar notions that we in the West have discovered through very different means. With my training in both fields, I quite often feel that I'm situated somewhere between them philosophically—much as I am geographically, being smack in the middle of the Pacific Ocean.

Although Western naturopathic and Chinese medicine evolved separately on different continents over the ages, each has arrived at an extremely holistic approach to health care. In very different ways both systems consider the whole person—including diet, environment, and behavior—casting as wide a net as possible in thinking about health and illness. In both systems every aspect of your physiology and personality is taken into account *before* you are diagnosed and treated. Both systems place a great deal of emphasis on the prevention of disease through lifestyle and diet. At the same time both reflect the belief that health is much more than merely the absence of disease; it is a heightened state of awareness and well-being, a dynamic balance of body, mind, spirit, and environment.

In treating illness, both Western naturopathic and Chinese medicine view the body's expression of symptoms as attempts to achieve harmony, homeostasis, or equilibrium. As a practitioner of natural medicine, my job involves helping patients find the underlying cause of illness in order to bring their bodies back into balance. Naturopathic and Chinese medicine both support my view that illness doesn't just materialize overnight: it is the result of a breakdown of the body's natural protections, an imbalance of Qi, and in some cases a clash between environmental forces and genetic susceptibility. Our bodies give us many signs before disease manifests itself. All too often people seek medical attention only when they become ill. Wouldn't it make more sense to seek advice on staying healthy? As you will discover, both naturopathic and Chinese medicine offer many ways to continually maintain great health.

Naturopathic and Chinese medicine also, in different ways, both support my belief that the least toxic, least invasive methods of healing should always be used first. I place the highest priority on using health-affirming medicines and therapies that won't compromise your body's ability to heal, especially when you need it the most. The pharmaceutical drugs that are so often prescribed to suppress symptoms in conventional Western medicine may help patients feel better in the short run, but they seldom address the underlying cause of illness, and this practice can lead to much greater problems in the long run. If you have a headache, I guarantee that the underlying cause is not a deficiency of aspirin.

There is a time and a place for drugs; like surgery, they can be extremely useful, even life-saving, when other possibilities have been thoroughly explored and exhausted. But drugs should not be used to maintain health, and they cannot create great health. If pharmaceutical medications or surgery become necessary, you should use them in conjunction with natural therapies and medicines to ameliorate side effects and expedite healing. Both naturopathic and Chinese medicine offer many options for preserving health and preventing disease with natural, nontoxic methods.

In my daily practice, as I blend both kinds of medicine to diagnose and treat patients, the results can be remarkable. By incorporating specific naturopathic principles and techniques with ancient methods of balancing Qi, yin, and yang and of using the Five Elements, many of my patients have been able to maintain and restore their health and change their lives in ways they never expected. The combined effect of these two time-tested traditions is often more powerful than either would be if applied separately; a synergistic effect happens when they are carefully woven together to create health.

In this book I describe a way of life that I call the Naturally Healthy Lifestyle. It brings together key components of naturopathic and Chinese medicine to keep your body strong, your Qi balanced, and your immunity in peak condition. In the event that you do become ill, it promotes the use of natural methods to restore your vitality and bring you back to abundant health. These methods include dietary changes, exercise, stress management, hydrotherapy, cleansing and detoxification, herbal medicines, nutritional supplements, aromatherapy, flower essences, natural hormones, homeopathy, and many others, including the Five Element system. (I will help you discover which Five Element type you tend to personify and therefore how each element affects your health; this will allow you to make better choices to maintain balance in your lifestyle.) Some of these methods reflect ancient wisdom that has been passed down for many generations, while others incorporate new scientific discoveries. Some are practiced throughout the world, while others have not been made widely known.

Using This Book to Maximize Your Health

In many ways, the book I have written is the book I wanted to read. *Natural Choices for Women's Health* came into existence largely because, in all my research during the past fifteen years, I have not been able to find a single book that adequately combines Western and Chinese medicine into a guide for women's natural health. My goal has been to merge fundamental elements from these two traditions into one practical guide that gives you all the essential tools you need to achieve a lifetime of optimal wellness *naturally.*

This book offers you ten "keys" to unlock your potential for achieving the fullest possible expression of your health. These keys pertain to the ten organs, systems, or areas in your body that I believe to be the crucial components of a woman's health: the immune system, kidneys, liver, heart, digestive system, hormones, bones, breasts, pelvis, and brain. I have found, after working with thousands of patients, that if you use natural methods from both the West and the East to ensure that these ten components of the body are working together as an integrated whole, great health will naturally follow.

For each key, I've pulled together a "best of" list of the tools and techniques that are most likely to maximize health. The medicines and methods I recommend were garnered from the experiences of all of the women I've worked with over the years in my daily practice, selected on the basis of what they have responded to most successfully. My approach to each key varies somewhat, because natural medicine is often eclectic by nature. For me, the art of medicine involves continually making decisions about which combination of therapies will be most beneficial in a specific situation. As a Westerner addressing Western readers, I speak from a primarily naturopathic perspective but weave in Chinese principles and treatments when they may be particularly helpful or revealing. With some of the ten keys, the wisdom of Chinese medicine plays a greater role than with others.

In the pages that follow, I will describe common symptom patterns seen from both a naturopathic and a Chinese medicine perspective. Because the practice of natural medicine is very complex, however, I will limit my discussion mainly to problems common to many women and to remedies that you can easily administer at home. There is a lot of information in this book, but creating health doesn't have to be a full-time job or a daunting task. You won't need to act on every suggestion included here. Leading a Naturally Healthy Lifestyle that supports all the elements of your body can be simple, once you know the essentials.

If your goal is to maximize every aspect of your health, you can read straight through the book, gathering benefits that build on one another as you learn to incorporate these principles into your Naturally Healthy Lifestyle. If you're concerned about a particular area of your health, however, you may want to consult that chapter first; you can pick and choose what works for you in any given area. The chart on pages 10 to 14 will direct you to the chapters that best meet your physical and emotional needs.

Whatever your health concerns, I highly recommend that you begin with the first chapter because it will give you a basic understanding of the principles referred to throughout the book. This chapter will also present the Naturally Healthy Lifestyle and Naturally Healthy Diet, including a detailed discussion of quality proteins, fats, carbohydrates, and the glycemic index—information that will be useful to you as you move through the other chapters in this book. All of the dietary suggestions that you will find in later chapters are modifications of the Naturally Healthy Diet outlined in Chapter 1.

In Chapter 2 you will explore the health of the first key, the immune system. A strong immune system enables you to walk through the world of microbes and disease and yet stay healthy and able to pursue your life goals. You can't accomplish what you want if you're always sick, have no energy, or feel burned out. This chapter will show you how you can keep your immunity functioning at peak level. It will also show you how, according to Chinese medicine, your immune system has a special connection to the Metal element.

Chapters 3 and 4 focus on the kidneys and the liver respectively. These are your primary organs of detoxification, and from a Chinese medicine perspective they are also major players in maintaining your vitality. As you will discover, your kidneys have an intimate relationship with your libido and the Water element, while your liver is uniquely connected with the Wood element.

Diseases of the heart are the leading cause of death for women in the United States, and Chapter 5 focuses on making your heart health a priority every day of your life. This chapter highlights the element of Fire in Chinese medicine and shows you that by balancing the Fire element, you can nurture both your heart and your emotions.

The digestive system, covered in Chapter 6, is an essential key to health, allowing you to assimilate your food properly. Numerous problems can arise if your intestines are plagued with parasites, yeast, and abnormal bacteria. If you are digesting and detoxifying optimally, however, you are already well on your way to great health. In this chapter, you will discover how to optimize the health of your digestive organs, which are closely linked to the Earth element.

Hormones, another important key to overall health, are our focus in Chapter 7. Hormonal changes can powerfully affect the way you feel, how you behave, and how you look. In this chapter you will discover how to balance your hormones from both a Western and an Eastern perspective.

In Chapter 8, you will explore ways to maintain the integrity of your bones, an essential key to health and vigor in your senior years. You will discover how to create and maintain strong, flexible bones and avoid osteoporosis and other bone ailments.

There are numerous health concerns unique to women regarding their breasts and pelvic organs. Chapter 9 will show you how to optimize your breast health and increase your body's own ability to prevent breast cancer and other breast diseases. In Chapter 10, you will delve into the mysteries of the most intimate region of your body, the pelvis. By making your pelvis less mysterious, this chapter will provide you with key information for maximizing your pelvic health.

Since mental health is a critical key in determining overall wellness, Chapter 11 will focus on how you can boost your mental and emotional health and improve your odds of preventing dementia, Alzheimer's disease, and other ills. By improving your mental and emotional health, you will enhance your entire well-being in countless ways.

This book is about empowering you, so that you can make healthy choices and live a fuller and more vital life. It is about teaching you to make the most informed decisions concerning your health, and inspiring you to take control of your health rather than let ill health take control of you. In these pages you will read stories about many patients who experienced health problems that you may recognize. You will meet many women who have achieved a more abundant life by taking an active role in creating their own health. As they share their stories with you, remember that you too can experience this transformation with the tools in this book. The choice is yours.

Which Chapters Are Most Useful for Your Conditions and Symptoms?

The first chapter of this book, "Creating Health," pertains to practically every condition and symptom listed below, so it is not included on this chart. Chapter 1 is recommended for everyone to read, in order to discover the fundamentals of how to manifest and maintain great health.

	2 IMMUNE HEALTH	3 KIDNEY HEALTH	4 LIVER HEALTH	5 HEART HEALTH	6 DIGESTIVE HEALTH	7 HORMONE HEALTH	8 BONE HEALTH	9 BREAST HEALTH	10 PELVIC HEALTH	11 MENTAL HEALTH
Acne					√	√				
Anxiety				√		√				√
Arthritis		√			√	√	√			
Asthma	√		√		√					
Atherosclerosis				√						
Bad breath			√		√					
Bladder pain		√							√	
Blocked sexual energy		√				√			√	
Body odor			√		√	√				
Breast cancer	√		√		√	√		√		
Breast cyst			√			√		√		
Breast swelling or tenderness			√			√		√		
Brittle fingernails					√					
Candida					√				√	
Canker sores	√				√					
Cervical atypia or dysplasia (abnormal Pap smear)	√		√		√				√	
Chronic fatigue syndrome	√	√	√		√	√				√
Colitis					√					
Constipation			√		√					
Depression	√	√	√	√	√	√				√
Diabetes				√	√	√				
Digestive problems	√		√		√					
Eczema	√				√					
Emotional exhaustion	√	√	√	√	√	√				√
Endometriosis			√			√			√	
Excessively driven or aggressive tendencies			√							√
Fatigue	√	√	√	√	√	√				√
Feelings of being overwhelmed	√			√		√				√
Feelings that you are in a fog			√		√	√				√

	2 IMMUNE HEALTH	3 KIDNEY HEALTH	4 LIVER HEALTH	5 HEART HEALTH	6 DIGESTIVE HEALTH	7 HORMONE HEALTH	8 BONE HEALTH	9 BREAST HEALTH	10 PELVIC HEALTH	11 MENTAL HEALTH
Feelings that you are stuck in your life			√							√
Fibroadenoma			√			√		√		
Fibrocystic breasts			√			√		√		
Fibromyalgia	√	√	√		√	√				√
Fluid retention		√	√		√	√				
Food allergies	√		√		√					
Frequent infections	√		√							
Frustration and anger			√							√
Gallstones			√			√				
Hair loss		√				√				
Hay fever	√		√		√					
Headaches			√		√	√				
Heart disease				√		√				
Heart palpitations				√						
Heartburn				√	√					
Heavy periods			√			√			√	
Hepatitis	√		√							
High cholesterol				√		√				
High triglycerides				√		√				
Hives	√		√		√					
Hot flashes						√				
Hypersensitivities to scents, pollution, and smoke	√		√		√					
Hypertension (high blood pressure)		√		√						√
Hyperthyroidism	√					√				
Hypoglycemia						√				
Hypotension (low blood pressure)				√		√				
Hypothyroidism			√			√				
Impatience			√	√						√
Inability to achieve orgasm		√				√			√	
Inability to let go of fear		√								√

	2 IMMUNE HEALTH	3 KIDNEY HEALTH	4 LIVER HEALTH	5 HEART HEALTH	6 DIGESTIVE HEALTH	7 HORMONE HEALTH	8 BONE HEALTH	9 BREAST HEALTH	10 PELVIC HEALTH	11 MENTAL HEALTH
Inability to let go of grief	√			√						√
Inability to stop worrying					√					√
Incontinence		√				√			√	
Increased urinary frequency		√				√			√	
Infertility		√				√			√	
Insomnia		√		√		√				√
Insufficient lactation								√		
Intestinal gas					√					
Irregular periods			√			√			√	
Irritability and moodiness			√			√				√
Irritable bowel syndrome					√					√
Lack of a strong vision for your future			√							√
Loose stools					√					
Low libido		√				√				
Mastitis	√							√		
Menopause		√	√	√		√	√	√	√	√
Migraines		√			√	√				
Multiple chemical sensitivities	√	√	√		√	√				
Osteoarthritis		√					√			
Osteopenia		√					√			
Osteoporosis		√					√			
Ovarian cysts			√			√			√	
Painful periods			√			√				
Parasites					√					
Perfectionism	√									√
Perimenopause		√	√	√		√	√	√	√	√
PMS (premenstrual syndrome)			√			√				
Poor memory			√			√				√

	2 IMMUNE HEALTH	3 KIDNEY HEALTH	4 LIVER HEALTH	5 HEART HEALTH	6 DIGESTIVE HEALTH	7 HORMONE HEALTH	8 BONE HEALTH	9 BREAST HEALTH	10 PELVIC HEALTH	11 MENTAL HEALTH
Psoriasis	√				√					
Puffy eyes					√					
Red eyes			√							
Sinus congestion	√				√					
Skin irritations and rashes	√		√		√					
STDs (sexually transmitted diseases)									√	
Sugar cravings	√				√	√				
Swollen lymph glands	√		√		√					
Ulcers					√					
Unsatisfying relationships				√	√					√
Urinary tract infections		√							√	
Uterine fibroids			√						√	
Vaginal burning and irritation					√				√	
Vulvar pain					√				√	
Warts	√								√	
Weight gain						√				
White spots on your fingernails					√					

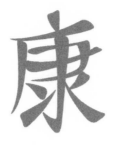

Chapter 1

Health

Creating Health

"What you can do, or dream you can do, begin it;
Boldness has genius, power and magic in it."
—GOETHE, *Faust*

WHEN I first saw Ellen as a patient, she was experiencing fatigue, headaches, and exercise-induced dizziness. Her medical doctors had put her on a slew of drugs in hopes of alleviating her discomfort, but her symptoms had only gotten worse. After learning of her lifestyle and diet habits, I wasn't at all surprised that she was feeling ill. Ellen had been pushing herself too hard, both at work and at home, and eating the all-too-typical local Hawaii diet, which includes lots of sugar, Spam, Portuguese sausage, white rice, soft drinks, and coffee. Once she made up her mind to turn her life around, the results were astonishing. By adopting a healthy diet, eating regular meals, drinking adequate water, and getting enough sleep, she soon discovered that she had vastly more energy, fewer headaches, and symptom-free exercise routines. Ellen now says that she feels like a new person, and much healthier at forty than she did at thirty-five!

The Naturally Healthy Lifestyle

Creating great health means making the right choices, but all too frequently my patients aren't aware of what the right choices are. To help point the way toward optimal health, in this chapter I have outlined a way of life that I call the Naturally Healthy Lifestyle. A lifestyle that I have personally chosen to practice for many years, it has enriched my life and deeply influenced my destiny.

The Naturally Healthy Lifestyle combines elements of both Western naturopathic medicine and ancient Chinese medicine. It consists of an abundantly healthy diet, regular exercise, herbal and nutritional supplementation, and many other approaches. It is about creating a healthy emotional life with loving, fulfilling relationships, enhancing your mental health, and knowing yourself. It means developing a heightened awareness of your health and a conscientious willingness to persevere when it comes to making healthy choices. It entails a level of self-esteem that allows you to make your health your top priority, to commit to taking care of yourself, and to know that you are worthy of your vigilance.

The Naturally Healthy Lifestyle is all of this and much more. If you make healthy choices in every aspect of your life, blending the tools of natural Western and Chinese medicine, the cumulative effect of all of your choices can be extraordinary. I've seen people dramatically improve the quality of their lives in countless ways simply by learning how to make the right choices. Often they had been held back for years by physical and emotional imbalances, their potential so blocked by the fog of poor health that they did not know what they were missing. By adopting the principles and practices of the Naturally Healthy Lifestyle, many of my patients have described achieving states of personal empowerment and well-being that they had never known, a new sense of "health" they had scarcely imagined.

The elements of the Naturally Healthy Lifestyle are outlined in this chapter and are further explored throughout the book. For a brief checklist summarizing some of the essentials you need to get started, see Appendix F.

The View from the West

From the viewpoint of Western natural medicine, practicing the Naturally Healthy Lifestyle means nurturing your body, mind, and spirit to continually regenerate your health and prevent disease. It means choosing healthy relationships with food, people, exercise, therapies, and just about everything else in your life. It means taking the right supplements to maximize your health and to ensure that you are getting everything you need nutritionally. It includes detoxifying your body and managing stress.

The Naturally Healthy Lifestyle is rooted in both common sense and scientific fact. We know, for instance, that eating an abundance of healthy foods and getting regular exercise can vastly reduce your risks for many chronic degenerative diseases, including heart disease, diabetes, and osteoporosis. We also know that decompressing from the stresses in your life on a daily basis can benefit the function of every organ and system in your body. But other, commonly overlooked aspects of your health are important as well. The Naturally Healthy Lifestyle also means making choices about the chemicals you come into contact with in your everyday life. It means minimizing your exposure to environmental toxins and, whenever you can, choosing natural, nontoxic products (for example, makeup, hair color, soap, and household cleaning agents). It means avoiding many items that can compromise your ability to create health.

In the event that you do become ill, the Naturally Healthy Lifestyle includes using natural medicines whenever possible to restore your health and bring your body back into balance. It's a matter of limiting or eliminating the use of many commonly prescribed drugs such as antibiotics, steroids, and antihistamines. The Naturally Healthy Lifestyle also entails being savvy about your options for professional health care guidance and knowing how to find the most qualified natural medicine practitioner. (See Appendix D.)

Simply put, following the Naturally Healthy Lifestyle means asking yourself, whenever you are considering any dietary option, activity, or form of medicine, how natural it is—and how closely it aligns with your body's innate ability to generate your health. In essence, it's about knowing, with each choice you make, whether it will serve your natural capacity to create great health in the long term.

When you create great health, your body sends signals to your brain that can alter your consciousness and have profound effects on your psyche and your sense of self. As you will discover, the Naturally Healthy Lifestyle may also allow you to more fully express your genetic potential, quite literally helping you become who you are. One of my patients has described this feeling as "becoming the me that I always knew was sleeping inside, just waiting to be set free."

The View from the East

From the perspective of Chinese medicine, as from that of Western medicine, the Naturally Healthy Lifestyle incorporates the use of exercise and diet. But the Chinese tradition also includes the ancient principles of Qi, yin and yang, and the Five Elements.

Qi, or vital energy, is critical to the body's innate ability to manifest great health. According to Chinese medicine, we inherit Qi in our physical makeup from our parents, and we also absorb it from the food we eat and the air we breathe. Qi causes

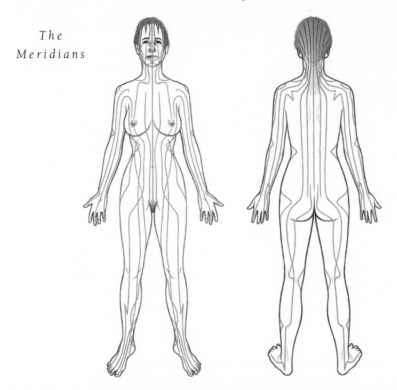

The Meridians

growth and transformation, regulates body temperature, defends the body from foreign invaders such as toxins and bacteria, and governs the movement of fluids throughout the body. (Qi courses through the body in channels of energy called meridians.) You can think of Qi as a deep river of energy, a life-giving force that brings you vitality and well-being. When your Qi is strong and constantly flowing, you exhibit optimal health; but when it is stagnant or weak, you can experience pain, poor immunity, impaired digestion, and many other symptoms. Following the Naturally Healthy Lifestyle will help keep your Qi moving in a healthy, balanced way. As you will see throughout this book, achieving balanced Qi is not a static process but a dynamic one, continually affected by fluctuations in your body, mind, emotions, relationships, and environment.

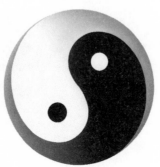

The traditional Tai Chi symbol

The principle of yin and yang is another vital aspect of the Naturally Healthy Lifestyle. Yin and yang, the opposites that exist everywhere in the universe, constantly intermingle in nature: all yin contains some yang, and all yang contains some yin. Yin and yang qualities are eternally conjoined; as the scholar Robert Ballou writes, "Out of the chaos which pervaded the primordial universe came Yang, the bright, the warm, the effusive, the heavenly, and Yin, the dark, the secretive, the silent, the deep, the earthly." The traditional Tai Chi symbol represents yin and yang in perfect harmony; some classic examples of yin and yang counterparts appear below.

YIN	YANG
Darkness	Light
Water	Fire
Nighttime	Daytime
Feminine	Masculine
Cold	Hot
Inward	Outward
Passive	Active
Quiet	Noisy
Receptive	Projective
Downward	Upward
Moon	Sun
Contracting	Expanding

Understanding the principle of yin and yang is important because, like everything else in the universe, your body contains both energies. Following the Naturally Healthy Lifestyle will help you keep them in equilibrium. When they are not, your body will attempt to restore harmony, and you will manifest symptoms of this struggle. For instance, if your yang energy is low, perhaps from too much stress, you will feel fatigue; this is your body's way of crying out for you to nourish your yang by keeping quiet, still, and passive. Or if you are a menopausal woman and your yang energy is in excess of your yin energy, you will experience hot flashes because yang is "hot" and yin is "cold."

Another essential component of the Naturally Healthy Lifestyle is knowing how to use the Five Elements in your life. Discovering your personality type in the Five Element system is vital to your health—once you understand your body's unique relationship to the Elements, you can use the system to help balance your emotional and spiritual life and become more conscious of who you are. The Five Elements are Wood, Fire, Earth, Metal, and Water. According to Chinese medicine, these basic properties are found throughout the natural world—and in your body. Each is associated with particular physiological tendencies, emotional needs, psychological traits, and spiritual qualities. You have each of the Five Elements within you, but your personality is generally dominated by one of them, which is your designated type.

The three "Five Elements" charts give an overview of how each of the elements reflects your personality, connects with your body, and corresponds to qualities in nature. Take a minute to think about which element is dominant in you. The quality of your voice, for example, speaks volumes about your predominant type. Do you sound most like a Wood type, a Fire type, an Earth type, a Metal type, or a Water type? You probably know someone who can walk into a room and demand attention with the tone of her voice: abrupt, forceful, and loud. She is most likely a Wood type. In contrast, the person with a meek, almost mournful voice is typically a Metal type.

The Five Elements in Your Personality

YOUR ELEMENT	WOOD	FIRE	EARTH	METAL	WATER
Your personality type	Determined, aggressive	Loving, passionate	Compassionate, caring	Spiritual, religious	Philosophical, cerebral
How you feel when you are in balance	Motivated, easygoing	Happy, peaceful	Grounded, empathic	Creative, positive	Wise, confident
How you feel when you are not in balance	Frustrated	Anxious	Confused	Pessimistic	Insecure
Your primary emotion	Anger	Joy	Worry	Grief	Fear
The sound of your voice	Shouting, commanding	Laughing, chuckling	Singing, melodious	Mourning, weeping	Groaning, moaning

The Five Elements in Your Body

YOUR ELEMENT	WOOD	FIRE	EARTH	METAL	WATER
Your primary sense organ/action	Eyes/seeing	Tongue/talking	Mouth/tasting	Nose/smelling	Ears/hearing
Your primary tissue	Tendon	Blood vessel	Muscle	Skin	Bone
Your primary taste	Sour	Bitter	Sweet	Pungent	Salty
Your predominant health system	Liver health	Heart health	Digestive health	Immune system health	Kidney health
Your yin organs	Liver	Heart	Spleen	Lungs	Kidneys
Your yang organs	Gallbladder	Small intestine	Stomach	Large intestine	Bladder
Functions of your yin organs include:	Maintaining the flow of Qi	Housing your spirit	Transforming and transporting Qi	Governing and distributing Qi	Storing your "Essence"
Functions of your yang organs include:	Giving you courage for decision-making	Influencing your mental clarity and judgment	Serving as a great source of nourishment and Qi	Receiving food and drink from your small intestine	Removing water from your body by Qi transformation

The Five Elements in Nature

YOUR ELEMENT	WOOD	FIRE	EARTH	METAL	WATER
Color	Green	Red	Yellow	White	Black
Time of day	Morning	Midday	Afternoon	Evening	Night
Season	Spring	Summer	Late summer	Fall	Winter
Climate	Windy	Hot	Damp, humid	Dry	Cold
Direction	East	South	Center	West	North

Once you discover which type you are, this book will speak more directly to you, guiding you in your quest to positively affect your health. (In later chapters, you will discover important ways in which each of the elements connects with specific organs, systems, and areas of your body.) You will learn about the connections between your type and important health and mind-body issues, and you will see how following the Naturally Healthy Lifestyle will help keep your dominant element well balanced. Of course, certain aspects of your Naturally Healthy Lifestyle and diet will be emphasized more than others, depending on your type.

The Naturally Healthy Diet

As former Surgeon General Everett Koop, M.D., has pointed out, "One personal choice seems to influence long-term health prospects more than any other—what we eat."[1] Your diet can protect your health, maintain your weight, and keep your strength, energy, and vitality at peak. Eating in accordance with the Naturally Healthy Lifestyle—what I call the Naturally Healthy Diet—is designed to maximize these benefits.

This all-purpose diet supports every organ and system in your body, from your heart to your hormonal system, drawing from both the Western and the Chinese medical traditions. The two traditions share the idea that your food can be your medicine, allowing you to nourish your body, mind, and spirit, both in sickness and in health.

You are constantly selecting food from your surroundings and putting it into your body, and in this sense your diet is an environmental factor that affects your health. The Naturally Healthy Diet includes ingesting the very best, healthiest food available to you, because every choice you make about what you eat can influence every cell in your body, profoundly changing your biochemistry. Your diet may even play a key role in your ability to tap into your genetic potential. As leading researcher Jeffrey Bland, Ph.D., points out, your food choices can literally "alter the expression of your genes."[2] This idea gives new meaning to the old saying "You are what you eat."

What you eat may allow you to fully express who you are and change your genetic destiny.

Fully expressing who you are means feeling great in your body. Many women find themselves on a weight-gain roller coaster when they follow fad diets or take stimulants purported to help them lose weight. When you follow the Naturally Healthy Diet, along with the rest of the Naturally Healthy Lifestyle, you much more easily shed unwanted pounds, creating a harmonious cycle of beneficial eating habits and a healthy, normal weight. The more you eat quality food, the easier it becomes to choose to eat well because you feel better and your cravings for unhealthy foods virtually disappear. You no longer have a desire for the processed, low-nutrient, sugar-laden foods and the caffeine-laced beverages that tend to put on weight and squander your health. The abundant energy you gain from the Naturally Healthy Diet can help eliminate the need for that extra fix of sugar or caffeine.

By blending dietary principles of natural health from Western and Chinese medicine, the Naturally Healthy Diet can help you maintain both your physiological and your "energetic" equilibrium over the long term. It won't lead to imbalances that could have negative consequences for your health, as seen in many weight-loss diets such as the Atkins diet, which overload you with fat and protein. You can continue to follow the Naturally Healthy Diet throughout your life because it's easy to maintain, you enjoy the food you're eating, and you feel great while eating it. And choosing food from nature's cornucopia in ways that engender your health every day is a fun, creative process.

The View from the West

The Naturally Healthy Diet is a high-nutrient, high-fiber plan that in many ways is the opposite of the standard American diet that many of us were raised on. Instead, it is low in refined sugar, processed foods, and the wrong kind of fats—including saturated and hydrogenated fats—and high in fruits, vegetables, whole grains, beans and legumes, and quality fats such as flax, walnut, and fish oils. It places a premium on eating organic whole foods and other healthy foods.

The term *whole foods* refers to foods in their natural state that have not been altered, processed, fragmented, or mixed with synthetic ingredients. When you eat an apple, for instance, you can see it in its entirety, so you know you are getting all its nutrients. In addition to fruits and vegetables, whole foods include grains, beans and legumes, eggs, and some animal products. Brown rice is a good example of a whole food because its vitamins, minerals, and fiber are intact, whereas white rice is not a whole food because it has been stripped of these ingredients. In some cases, foods that are not whole foods make up part of the Naturally Healthy Diet because they contain original nutrients, fiber, or other benefits from whole foods. Some examples are whole-grain bread, whole-grain pasta, whole-grain cereal, tofu, yogurt, and some oils. Whole-grain bread is one of the best examples of a healthy nonwhole food. (White bread, by contrast, is not as healthy because much of its fiber and nutritional value has been removed, and synthetic vitamins have been added.)

The Naturally Healthy Diet should include three meals and at least two healthy snacks a day. Aim for consistency in your eating habits: your body becomes stressed when you skip meals and allow yourself to feel "starved" for prolonged periods. Skipping meals can also induce low blood sugar, which may include uncomfortable symptoms of light-headedness, weakness, anxiety, and irritability. I recommend that your diet consist of complex carbohydrates, quality protein, healthy fats, an abundance of fruits and vegetables, and plenty of water. Let's look at each of these major categories and see what they can do for you.

CARBOHYDRATES

Carbohydrates are the power sources for energy production in your cells. They fuel your brain and muscles, and when digested slowly they provide you with long-lasting energy. Not all carbohydrates are the same: they range from simple to complex. Simple carbohydrates, which are found in white bread, cakes, cookies, table sugar, and many other products, may be one of the greatest obstacles to a healthy diet. Because they are usually low in fiber, you digest them quickly, which causes a rapid increase in your blood sugar level that can lead to sugar cravings and then weight gain. They are also unhealthy for you because they are almost always low in vitamins and minerals. In contrast, complex carbohydrates, which include whole-grain breads, pasta, and brown rice, are chock full of vitamins and minerals. And because they have a lot of fiber, you digest them slowly, which keeps your blood sugar level on a more even keel.

The glycemic index is a valuable tool for looking at the carbohydrates in your diet. It measures the rate at which your body converts foods into sugar (glucose) in your bloodstream; the higher the glycemic index rating of a food, the more quickly it is converted to sugar. Among carbohydrates, glycemic ratings vary considerably. For example, baked potatoes have a glycemic rating of 85, which is extremely high (pure glucose is rated at 100), whereas steamed brown rice has a rating of 50. As a general rule, simple carbohydrates have higher glycemic ratings and complex carbohydrates have lower glycemic ratings.

Having sugar in your bloodstream is good, up to a point—your cells need it to make energy—but too much all at once can suppress your immune system and put you at higher risk for heart disease and other chronic illnesses.[3] Excessive sugar intake also increases your insulin level, which can induce a pendulum swing effect of rapid removal of sugar from your blood, resulting in low blood sugar symptoms such as headaches, irritability, anxiety, and fatigue. This can lead you to crave sweet foods and more of the same kinds of high-glycemic carbohydrates that may have caused you to have a blood sugar imbalance in the first place. Over time this vicious cycle can cause you to gain weight. When you consistently choose complex carbohydrates with a low glycemic rating, however, not only will your blood sugar level be more steady and your immune system more efficient, you will also curb your sugar cravings, lose weight, have more energy, think more clearly, and feel better.

According to *The New Glucose Revolution,* one of the most informative books on the glycemic index, low-glycemic foods are rated as having a glycemic index of 55 or lower, intermediate-glycemic foods between 55 and 70, and high-glycemic foods 70 or higher. To follow the Naturally Healthy Diet, you should avoid foods above 60 as much as possible, although of course it's okay to indulge in a high-glycemic food every now and then. The following is a list of commonly eaten foods and their glycemic ratings.

The Glycemic Index: Choosing the Right Carbohydrates

GRAINS AND PASTAS	GLYCEMIC RATING	BREADS	GLYCEMIC RATING	CEREALS	GLYCEMIC RATING
Egg fettuccine	32	Pumpernickel rye kernel	41	Oatmeal	42
Noodles (instant)	47	White pita bread	57	Raw oat bran	59
Brown rice (steamed)	50	Croissant	67	Raisin Bran (Kellogg's, USA)	61
Linguine	52	White bread	70	Grape-Nuts (Kraft, USA)	75
Buckwheat (mean of three studies)	54	Waffles	76	Rice Krispies (Kellogg's, Canada)	82
Basmati rice (white, boiled)	58	Middle Eastern flatbread	97	Cornflakes (Kellogg's, USA)	92

BEANS AND LEGUMES	GLYCEMIC RATING	FRUITS	GLYCEMIC RATING	VEGETABLES	GLYCEMIC RATING
Soybeans (canned)	14	Apple	38	Yam (peeled, boiled)	37
Kidney beans (USA)	23	Pear	38	Carrots	47
Lentils	29	Banana	52	Green peas	48
Butter beans (Canada)	36	Cantaloupe	65	Corn (sweet, boiled)	60
Baked beans	38	Pineapple	66	Beets (canned)	64
Chickpeas (canned)	42	Watermelon	72	Baked potato	85

Source: Jennie Brand-Miller et al., *The New Glucose Revolution: The Authoritative Guide to the Glycemic Index* (New York: Avalon, 2004).

PROTEIN

Your body needs protein to regulate thousands of processes that keep you healthy. Protein helps you maintain both the water balance in your body and the cellular balance between acids and bases, which is important for the healthy functioning of all your cells and tissues. Your immune and hormonal systems are also dependent on protein: the antibodies you produce in response to invading viruses or bacteria are made from protein, as are many hormones such as your thyroid hormone and insulin. You also need adequate protein to heal tissue, build bone, and develop muscle.

Healthy sources of protein include beans and legumes, poultry, fish, seafood, and eggs, along with dairy products like nonfat cottage cheese, yogurt, and milk. Contrary to what you may have heard, eggs are a nearly perfect source of protein. They contain all of the essential amino acids, which are the building blocks of protein. Other animal products, such as beef and pork, are loaded with protein also, but I generally recommend that you avoid eating them because they are often riddled with saturated fat. If you choose to consume red meat, I advise you do so in small amounts just a few times a month, eating only lean, free-range organic beef. (Choosing organic meat, incidentally, may help protect you from mad cow disease; according to the Organic Consumers Association, organic beef is safer in this regard than conventional beef in the United States.)

Fish and seafood can be great sources of protein and quality fats. But one of the most toxic heavy metals for humans—mercury—has been found in such foods in increasingly high amounts. Some mercury occurs naturally in the environment, but the increase in mercury in the fish food chain is the direct result of industrial and coal-burning power plants. Mercury is released into the air and accumulates in clouds; when it rains, it ends up in ponds, rivers, the oceans, and eventually the fish we eat. Fish and seafood caught closer to industrial areas are more likely to have higher levels of mercury and other contaminants.

Mercury can take a heavy toll on your health in ways that we are perhaps only beginning to understand. Adults with high levels of mercury in their tissues can experience symptoms of muscle weakness, fatigue, headaches, irritability, hair loss, inability to concentrate, sensations of numbness and tingling (usually around the lips, fingers, and toes), and problems with vision, hearing, speaking, and balance. Researchers have found connections between high levels of mercury in the body and increased risk for heart disease.[4] Other health problems can arise because mercury decreases your level of selenium, an important antioxidant. Selenium is necessary for recycling another antioxidant, glutathione, which is critical to the liver's ability to adequately neutralize many toxins. In extreme cases, when mercury levels are severely elevated, mercury toxicity can lead to tremors, coma, and even death. Let's take a look at how much mercury generally appears in some different types of fish and seafood.

Mercury Levels in Commercial Fish and Seafood
As measured in maximum parts per million (ppm)

Shark 4.54 ppm —
Tilefish (Gulf of Mexico) 3.73 ppm —
Swordfish 3.22 ppm —
King Mackerel 1.67 ppm —
Halibut 1.52 ppm —
Snapper 1.37 ppm —
Lobster 1.31 ppm —
Tuna (Fresh/Frozen) 1.30 ppm —
Grouper 1.21 ppm —
Monkfish 1.02 ppm —
Bass (Saltwater) .96 ppm —
Marlin .92 ppm —
Tuna (Canned) .85 ppm —
Orange Roughy .80 ppm —
Pollock .78 ppm —
Spanish Mackerel (S. Atlantic) .73 ppm —
Bluefish .63 ppm —
Crab .61 ppm —
Tilefish (Atlantic) .53 ppm —
Cod .42 ppm —
White Croaker (Pacific) .41 ppm —
Squid .40 ppm —
Butterfish .36 ppm —
Anchovies .34 ppm —
Perch (Freshwater) .31 ppm —
Whitefish .31 ppm —
Catfish .31 ppm —
Spiny Lobster .27 ppm —
Oysters .25 ppm —
Scallops .22 ppm —
Salmon (Fresh/Frozen) .19 ppm —
Mackerel (N. Atlantic) .16 ppm —
Herring .14 ppm —
Mullet .13 ppm —
Trout (Freshwater) .13 ppm —
Tilapia .07 ppm —
Pickerel .06 ppm —
Shrimp .05 ppm —
Crawfish .05 ppm —
Haddock .04 ppm —
Sardines .04 ppm —
Perch (Ocean) .03 ppm —

Source for ppm levels:
"Mercury Levels in Commercial Fish and Shellfish,"
U.S. Department of Health and Human Services
and U.S. Environmental Protection Agency

You may have noticed that many of the fish containing the highest amounts of mercury are large-sized species. This is because fish absorb mercury from the organisms they feed on. Predator fish generally have more mercury than nonpredator fish, and the older and larger a fish, the more mercury it is apt to have. One commonly eaten large fish to watch out for is tuna—in recent years it has come under the spotlight for mercury contamination.

Unfortunately for fish lovers, mercury-contaminated fish are high in methyl mercury, which is a highly toxic form. And the Food and Drug Administration (FDA) has warned that nearly *all* fish (which presumably includes most seafood) contain *some* mercury. The FDA has issued an advisory to pregnant women, and women of childbearing age who may become pregnant, to avoid eating the four species that they categorize as high-mercury fish: swordfish, shark, tilefish, and king mackerel. Acknowledging that fish and seafood can be an important part of a balanced diet, the FDA has advised that women in these categories "select a variety of other kinds of fish—including shellfish, canned fish, smaller ocean fish, or farm-raised fish . . . these women can safely eat 12 ounces a week of cooked fish." (The size of a serving of fish, the FDA states, is three to six ounces.) In other words, according to the FDA women in these groups can safely eat eight to sixteen servings a month of fish that are not high in mercury.[5] The FDA has also advised that nursing mothers and young children avoid high-mercury fish.

The FDA's recommendations are based on its assessment of what constitutes an acceptable level of mercury in the body. But because of the risks that mercury poses to your health, I believe that a much higher degree of caution is warranted: I recommend that you avoid eating fish and seafood with a mercury content greater than 1.0 part per million (ppm) altogether, regardless of your age or childbearing and pregnancy status. I also recommend that you limit your intake of fish and seafood with a mercury content from 0.5 to 1.0 ppm to two servings a month, and your intake of fish and seafood with a mercury content less than 0.5 ppm to four servings a month.

If you are pregnant, or are expecting to become pregnant, I suggest that you completely avoid fish and seafood. While you are pregnant, your baby is highly sensitive to the toxic effects of mercury in your body. Mercury can easily cross the placenta, where it could potentially disrupt the development of your baby's brain and nervous system. I also recommend that you avoid all fish and seafood if you are a nursing mother. If you are not pregnant (and have no immediate plans to become pregnant) but are of childbearing age, I advise you to eat fish and seafood on the chart on page 26 with a mercury content of less than 0.5 ppm, and not more than twice a month.

If you've been eating a lot of fish and seafood high in mercury, see Chapter 4 to learn how to test for mercury in your body.

THE SKINNY ON FATS

Fats can have a major impact on your health because they play a role in the function of every cell in your body. Some fats are good for you and some are not. "Good" fats are either monounsaturated or unsaturated omega 3 fats. They include nonhydrogenated, cold-pressed oils such as olive, macadamia nut, canola, fish, flax, and walnut oil. Some nuts and seeds are also a source of healthy fats. "Bad" fats are the saturated fats found in most animal products and whole dairy foods, as well as the hydrogenated vegetable oils found in margarines and many processed foods. The unsaturated omega 6 fats found in safflower, sunflower, and soy oils can be "good" fats, but they can also be "bad" fats if you consume them in excess.

Fats affect the whole body by influencing the formation of hormone-like substances known as *eicosanoids,* which regulate the immune system and control inflammation in the tissues. "Good" fats promote the formation of a favorable type of eicosanoids that decrease inflammation. "Bad" fats promote the formation of unfavorable eicosanoids that increase inflammation. When you have too much of these unfavorable eicosanoids in your body, your cells don't receive as much oxygen. High levels of the unfavorable eicosanoids are associated with depressed immunity, increased pain, heart disease, menstrual cramps, headaches, and poor health in general.

Balance is the key when it comes to fats. The typical American diet contains a surplus of omega 6 fats—at a level ten to twenty times higher than it should be—and a deficiency of omega 3 fats. It's critical to keep a balance between these two unsaturated fats. The ideal ratio is four to one: you need to ingest four times as many omega 6 fats as omega 3 fats. To achieve this healthy balance, changing your oil may do the trick: lower your intake of soy, safflower, and sunflower oil (they are often hidden in processed foods) and raise your intake of walnuts, chestnuts, and flax oil. An easy way to do this is to ingest one tablespoon of flax oil a day. If you like the taste, pour it over your salads, steamed vegetables, or pasta dishes. You can also take flax oil in capsule form, but to get the equivalent of one tablespoon of flax oil, or about 6,200 mg of omega 3 fats, you would need to take approximately fourteen average-sized capsules. (Flax oil should always be used cold, so keep it refrigerated, even if you take it in capsule form.)

To help balance your omega 6 and omega 3 fats, you can also choose fish that are relatively low in mercury and high in omega 3 fats, such as salmon, herring, and freshwater trout. In addition, you can take fish oil supplements, which are available at your local health food store. If you use fish oil, look for a product containing two omega 3 fats, EPA and DHA. For general health maintenance take approximately 500 mg of EPA and 300 mg of DHA daily. Make sure that you purchase only high-quality fish oil supplements; poor-quality supplements may contain high levels of lipid peroxides (free radicals) and environmental pollutants, including mercury. As with flax oil supplements, you should keep your fish oil supplements refrigerated. And *never cook with unsaturated omega 3 and omega 6 fats*, because they create very toxic compounds when heated. I recommend that you cook with monounsaturated fats, such as olive oil.

It's important to realize that when it comes to your dietary fats, favorable does not mean unflavorable. Some of my patients were initially reluctant to change the fats in their diet because they didn't want to give up eating the processed foods they craved. They were delighted to discover, however, that foods higher in favorable fats can be every bit as delicious, if not more so. And when you eat the right fats, your good eicosanoids dominate, so you have greater immunity and less potential for inflammation, which means you are more apt to feel better and have optimal health. In the long run, this makes you more able to enjoy the good things in life—including the food you eat!

How to Change Your Oil

Decrease Saturated Fats:
Butter, cocoa butter, palm kernel oil, animal fats from beef, chicken, turkey, lamb, pork, cheese, and whole-milk dairy products

Avoid Hydrogenated Oils (trans-fatty acids):
Fats found in margarines, processed foods, and candy bars

Decrease Unsaturated Omega 6 Fats:
Corn oil, safflower oil, sunflower oil, soy oil, and cottonseed oil

Increase Unsaturated Omega 3 Fats:
Fish oil, flax oil, walnuts, and chestnuts

Use Monounsaturated Fats for Cooking:
Olive oil, macadamia nut oil, and canola oil

FRUITS AND VEGETABLES

Eating an abundance of fruits and vegetables is essential to maximizing your health. The American Cancer Society states that fruits and vegetables are sources of important nutrients that may help prevent disease, and it recommends that you eat at least five servings a day to help prevent cancer. I suggest that you eat at least *ten* servings every day and that you focus on eating *low-glycemic* fruits and vegetables. According to the U.S. Department of Agriculture (USDA), one fruit serving is one medium apple, banana, or orange; half a cup chopped, cooked, or canned fruit; or three-quarters of a cup fruit juice. One vegetable serving is one cup raw, leafy vegetables; half a cup other raw or cooked vegetables, chopped; or three-quarters of a cup vegetable juice.

There are many fruits and vegetables available to choose from, all loaded with nutrients and health-promoting phytochemicals. They are an excellent source of fiber—which is important in your digestive health and also boosts the health of your whole body by escorting many toxins out of your system. Fruits and vegetables are great gifts for your immune system, but they also top the list of foods containing environmental chemicals, which may increase your risks for cancer and immune disorders. Whenever possible, eat organic fruits and vegetables.

WHY ORGANIC?

Eating in accordance with the Naturally Healthy Lifestyle means eating as naturally as you can. The best way you can do this is by choosing organic food. Organic food can be expensive, but it's worth your investment a thousandfold. As I often tell my patients, you either pay for it now or you pay for it later. If you pay later, you will probably pay a much higher price. Your long-term commitment to eating organic food is vital to your Naturally Healthy Diet, because it may be one of the most important ways you can affect your chances of staying healthy.

Thanks to the efforts of many consumers and the National Organic Program, the USDA now requires that to be labeled "organic," any food product sold in the United States, even if it is imported, must meet national organic standards. A food is organic, as defined by the USDA, if it is produced without the use of irradiation, most conventional pesticides, organisms that have been genetically modified (GMOs), or fertilizers that are made with synthetic ingredients or sewage sludge, and (in the case of meat, poultry, eggs, and dairy products) if it comes from animals that are given no antibiotics or growth hormones. By choosing organic foods, you can protect yourself from all of these potential threats to your health in one fell swoop! The cumulative effects on your well-being could be immeasurable.

The organic labeling requirement seems especially valuable when you consider that without it there is often no way of knowing the extent to which any of these potential health risks exist in the food you eat. For example, in the case of GMOs, the FDA does not require any specific labeling to inform you whether they are contained in the foods you purchase.

Genetically Modified Organisms

Genetically modified organisms (GMOs) are organisms that have had genes from other plants, animals, or bacteria transferred into their genetic structure. This may have been done for a variety of reasons: to insert nutrients into foods, for example, or to make plants such as corn and wheat resistant to certain bugs, allowing farmers to use fewer pesticides and chemical fertilizers while producing higher crop yields. These seeming benefits have led some to believe that GMOs will be good for your health and for the environment.

But by altering gene lines and mixing genes across species to produce plants with specific characteristics, biotechnology companies are tampering with nature in ways that are unprecedented. Many GMOs are combinations of genetic material that have never before existed in the natural world and did not evolve at the same pace as other life-forms. GMOs have not been adequately tested for safety: no one knows what the potential risks are to your health or the environment. There are immediate concerns that people could have unusual allergic reactions to genetically modified foods, and more ominous concerns that GMOs could have widespread damaging effects, wreaking havoc in the environment and adversely affecting any number of species in unpredictable ways. Once released into the environment, GMOs may cause unforeseen and irreversible genetic contamination of natural organisms through the drifting of pollen.

Those who argue that GMOs are safe in your food are often concerned with issues of cost-effectiveness in the food industry. While well intentioned, they may be far less concerned with what is best for you, the consumer, and what it could mean for your health over the course of your life.

Science gives us many other indications that eating organic food is good for your health. The Environmental Working Group states that chemical residues found on foods may increase the risk of cancer and other diseases.[6] Research suggests that environmental toxins with hormone-mimicking effects may cause girls to enter puberty at an earlier-than-normal age, which could put them at risk for estrogen-related cancers later in life.[7] If you are a lactating mother, you should be especially vigilant about choosing organic foods: an infant's organs and nervous system are less developed and more vulnerable to the potential harmful effects of pesticides, and studies have confirmed that environmental chemicals are found in breast milk worldwide.

There is good news: a study at the University of California looked at certain organically grown foods and found they had consistently higher levels of phenolic metabolites (which have potent antioxidant and cancer-fighting properties) than conventionally grown foods. The study, which measured phenolic metabolites in corn, strawberries, and marionberries, reported that the plants grown with standard commercial chemical fertilizers and pesticides had significantly fewer of these health-benefiting constituents than the plants grown organically.[8]

If organic fruits and vegetables aren't available, on the whole it's better to eat nonorganic fruits and vegetables than none at all. But be sure to wash all nonorganic fruits and vegetables thoroughly, and avoid those with higher levels of pesticide residues. The Environmental Working Group tested forty-two commonly eaten nonorganic fruits and vegetables for pesticide residues and found that the following twelve had the highest levels: strawberries, bell peppers, spinach, cherries, peaches, cucumbers, celery, apples, apricots, green beans, grapes from Chile, and cantaloupe from Mexico.

Your conscious decision to choose organic, whole foods is an important part of the Naturally Healthy Lifestyle because it is, in a sense, an extension of your immune system: you are safeguarding your health while you are shopping, in the moment you are making the choice on what to buy. Although it may seem as if organic food is a strange step away from the "normal" food on which you were probably raised, it's important to remember that only in the last few generations have we been producing foods with herbicides, insecticides, chemical fertilizers, genetic modification, irradiation, antibiotics, and hormones—and only in our lifetimes has this list grown so long that we need national organic standards to protect us. After all, what we call "organic" food is merely as close as we can get to food in its natural state—what the vast majority of our ancestors ate throughout the ages. Looked at from this perspective, choosing organic food is simply an effort to get back to eating normally.

What to Look for When You Buy Organic Groceries

The key is the way the word *organic* is used on the product. Here's a summary of the USDA requirements.

- If a product is labeled "100% organic" it must contain 100 percent organic ingredients.
- If a product is labeled "organic" the contents must be at least 95 percent organic.
- If a product is labeled "made with organic (ingredients or foods)" it must contain at least 70 percent organic ingredients.
- Products with less than 70 percent organic ingredients cannot make any organic claims on the package, except by listing organically produced ingredients in the ingredient statement on the side panel.

Source: The U.S. Department of Agriculture

WATER, THE SOURCE OF LIFE

Water bathes every cell in your body. It brings nutrients to your tissues, maintains your body temperature, helps your kidneys filter your blood, carries away waste products, and provides lubrication for your joints, eyes, and mucous membranes. Water is vital to your diet, and following the Naturally Healthy Lifestyle means drinking water that is as clean and natural as possible.

To maintain your health, make sure you drink at least forty-eight ounces of pure water every day. Drink extra if you live in a hot climate, if you exercise, or if you consume beverages that dehydrate you such as caffeinated tea, coffee, or beer. Most tap water contains chlorine and fluoride, and some may contain heavy metals, so I highly recommend you drink filtered water as part of your Naturally Healthy Diet. (See Chapter 3 for more information on water filters.)

The View from the East

Nutrition plays a very important role in Chinese medicine, just as it does in Western naturopathic medicine. Chinese nutrition, however, takes into account not only the vitamin and mineral components of the foods you eat but also their "energetic" properties. (The term *energetic* refers to certain qualities of foods and how they affect Qi; as you will discover, the term is also used in both naturopathic and Chinese medicine to describe effects that aren't readily understood in terms of the biochemical model of Western science.) Following the Naturally Healthy Diet, from a Chinese perspective, means balancing Qi and strengthening the health of the entire body using these energetic properties. By understanding how foods affect you energetically, and eating them in the right combinations, you can use your diet both to maintain health and recover from illness.

In Chinese medicine foods, herbs, and spices are categorized according to their energetic properties as "cold," "cooling," "neutral," "warming," or "hot." Everything we eat falls somewhere on this continuum. Foods that are traditionally classified as energetically "cold," such as watermelon and cucumber, build your yin energy. Foods that are "cooling," such as cantaloupe and celery, also build your yin energy, though less strongly. Energetically "neutral" foods, such as carrots and oats, don't affect your yin or yang significantly. "Warming" foods, which include walnuts and chicken, build your yang energy, while foods that are considered "hot," such as trout and ginger, nourish your yang most intensely. Generally speaking, it's best to maintain a daily balance of "cold" and "hot" foods, and of "cooling" and "warming" foods.

As you become familiar with these designations for foods, you will discover that you can use the principles of Chinese medicine to create greater health in very simple, immediate ways. At times you may need to make only the slightest shifts in your diet to reestablish harmony in your body—harmony that can make a huge difference in your health. Many of my patients have used the energetic properties of foods to help treat conditions as different as colds and flus, arthritis, digestive problems, and breast cysts.

In Chinese medicine, conditions are themselves classified as imbalances of either "cold" or "hot" in the body. Once you know if a condition is due to too much or too little cold or heat, you can make dietary changes to help relieve it. In general, "hot" and "warming" foods are recommended if you have a condition with too much cold or too little heat, whereas "cold" and "cooling" foods are recommended if you have a condition with too much heat or too little cold. For example, if you have chronic loose stools, which is usually regarded as a cold condition in Chinese medicine, increasing your intake of "hot" and "warming" foods can help to alleviate the condition (and eating an excess of "cooling" or "cold" foods can aggravate it). But if you have a rash, which is most commonly understood as being related to an excess of heat in the body, you can help your body heal by eating "cooling" or "cold" foods (and avoiding "hot" and "warming" foods).

In this book, you will see how many illnesses and conditions are classified along the energetic continuum, and you will learn how you can use the "energetic" properties of foods to restore and create health by balancing each important organ, system, or area of your body. The extent of the dietary adjustments you may need to make will be unique to your particular health situation; as you explore the energetic properties of foods in Chinese medicine, you will learn to select foods that are most appropriate for your own body and avoid those that cause imbalances. As you read along, you may find it helpful to refer to the following list of common foods and their energetic properties.

"Energetic" Properties of Foods from a Chinese Medicine Perspective

FRUITS

COLD	COOLING	NEUTRAL	WARMING	HOT
Mulberries	Apples	Figs	Cherries	
Persimmons	Bananas	Grapes	Litchi	
Grapefruit	Pears	Red dates	Peaches	
Papayas	Cantaloupe	Pineapple	Raspberries	
Watermelon	Honeydew	Apricots	Guavas	
Tomatoes	Kiwis		Kumquats	
	Loquats		Lemons	
	Oranges		Coconut	
	Plums			
	Pomegranates			
	Pomelos			
	Strawberries			
	Tangerines			

VEGETABLES AND LEAFY GREENS

COLD	COOLING	NEUTRAL	WARMING	HOT
Asparagus	Alfalfa sprouts	Carrots	Cauliflower	
Bamboo shoot	Broccoli	Corn	Chives	
Burdock root	Cabbage	Olives	Mustard greens	
Kelp	Celery	Potatoes	Onions	
Lotus root	Eggplant	Yams	Pumpkin	
Summer squash	Lettuce	Beets	Scallions	
Cucumbers	Mushrooms			

COLD	COOLING	NEUTRAL	WARMING	HOT
Nori	Radishes			
	Soybean sprouts			
	Spinach			
	Sweet potatoes			
	Swiss chard			
	Turnips			
	Watercress			

GRAINS, NUTS, SEEDS, BEANS, AND LEGUMES

COLD	COOLING	NEUTRAL	WARMING	HOT
Barley	Buckwheat	Adzuki beans	Chestnuts	Soybean oil
Tofu	Millet	Almonds	Pine nuts	
Water chestnuts	Mung beans	String beans	Pumpkin seeds	
	Wheat	Hazelnuts	Glutinous rice	
	Gluten	Oats	Walnuts	
	Millet	Peas		
	Sesame oil	Peanuts		
	Tofu	Rice		
	Wheat bran	Sesame seeds		
		Soybeans		
		Sunflower seeds		
		Rye		

DAIRY, MEAT, AND SEAFOOD

COLD	COOLING	NEUTRAL	WARMING	HOT
Clams		Beef	Chicken	Trout
Crab		Eggs	Lobster	
Octopus		Duck	Crayfish	
		Cow's milk	Eel	
		Oysters	Lamb	
		Pork	Goat's milk	
		Shark	Mussels	
		Squid	Shrimp	
		White fish	Venison	
		Sardines	Yogurt	
			Anchovies	
			Butter	

OTHER FOODS, DRINKS, AND SPICES

COLD	COOLING	NEUTRAL	WARMING	HOT
Salt	Marjoram	Honey	Alcohol	Black pepper
Soy sauce	Green tea	White sugar	Anise	Cayenne pepper
			Basil	Cinnamon
			Caraway	Dry ginger
			Cardamom	Sichuan pepper
			Cloves	
			Coffee	
			Coriander	
			Dill	
			Fennel	
			Garlic	
			Uncooked ginger	
			Molasses	
			Nutmeg	
			Rosemary	
			Saffron	
			Brown sugar	
			Thyme	
			Turmeric	
			Vinegar	

Source: Bob Flaws, *The Tao of Healthy Eating* (Boulder, Colo.: Blue Poppy Press, 1999), and Misha Ruth Cohen and Kalia Donner, *The Chinese Way to Healing: Many Paths to Wholeness* (Baltimore, Md.: Perigee Books, 1996).

In essence, following the Naturally Healthy diet in everyday life means eating a balanced diet that promotes good health and keeps you at your optimal weight. The following is a summary of the general guidelines:

The Essence of the Naturally Healthy Diet

- Eat three meals a day, with snacks such as fruits between meals if you're hungry.
- Eat carbohydrates with a low glycemic index, such as brown rice, whole-grain bread, and whole-wheat pasta.
- Eat beans and legumes a few times a week.
- Eat moderate amounts of lean protein, such as low-mercury fish, skinless poultry, or eggs; if you are vegetarian, consume adequate quantities of plant-based protein.
- Unless you are lactose intolerant or allergic to dairy products, eat nonfat organic dairy products.

- Use quality fats in your diet, such as olive oil for cooking and flax oil in salad dressings.
- Eat ten servings of low-glycemic fruits and vegetables each day.
- Eat the highest-quality organic foods whenever possible, and emphasize whole foods in your diet.
- Drink at least forty-eight ounces of pure water every day.
- Keep your Qi strong by eating a balance of hot, cold, warming, and cooling foods.
- Avoid processed foods, fast foods, fried foods, soft drinks, and nonnutritive sugary foods such as cookies, candies, and pastries.

Women in Motion

When I ask many of my older female patients, who are in their eighties and in great condition, how they manage to stay so healthy, their unanimous answer can be summed up in one word: exercise.

Movement is one of the most important ways you can create health. Not only does exercise make you feel and look better, it improves your bone density, increases your oxygen intake, strengthens your heart, stimulates your circulation, moves your lymph, releases stress, helps you eliminate toxins through sweating, enhances the function of all your cells, and boosts your overall vitality. Many people think of exercise only in terms of "depleting" their energy, but exercise can also literally increase your energy by raising the number of mitochondria, the energy-making "factories," in your muscle cells.

Exercise is a major part of the Naturally Healthy Lifestyle. The best formula is a combination of aerobic activity, stretching exercises, and resistance training such as weight lifting. The important thing is consistency: your body needs regular activity to keep it functioning optimally. Exercise can be addictive—in a good way—because when you are getting enough exercise, you feel more alive, your thoughts are clearer, you feel good in your body, and you feel good about yourself. But keep in mind that while exercise can do wonders for your health up to a point, too much exercise can cause wear and tear on your body, reduce your immunity, and have a negative impact on your health.

You can make exercise fun by doing whatever you love to do, rather than trying to fit into someone else's idea of what you ought to do. I once had a patient who was very large and felt uncomfortable moving her body—until she discovered belly dancing. She found an exercise that she looked forward to doing because it celebrated her ample body.

From a Chinese medicine perspective, exercise is a wonderful way to balance and increase the flow of your Qi. In ancient China, of course, people didn't work out at the gym; they worked in the fields and practiced martial arts like Qi Gong. Today our culture offers many other options for strengthening and balancing the circulation of Qi. I've found some physical activities to be inherently yin-supportive, gently nurturing to body, mind, and spirit; I refer to these as *yin exercises.* Other forms of exercise, which I call *yang exercises,* tend to push the body to its limits and are essentially yang-boosting. In general, it's best to practice both types of exercise, building your yin and yang energy while also keeping them balanced with each other.

The following is a list of typical yin and yang exercises and activities. As you can see, just about any exercise that is primarily yin can be made more yang simply by increasing the intensity. Yoga is particularly good for building both yin and yang energy; it can be a quiet exercise that gradually increases your flexibility (the Chinese say your goal should be to have muscles like a cat—long, lean, and supple), or it can be a very intense experience that leaves you gasping and sweating profusely.

Yin and Yang Exercises

YIN	YANG
Tai Chi	Karate
Hula	Tahitian dance
Gentle hatha yoga	Iyengar or Bikram yoga
Stretching	Pilates
Aikido	Kickboxing
Slow ballroom dancing	Fast disco dancing
Leisurely walking	Power walking
Unhurried hiking	Mountain climbing
Weight lifting with light weights	Weight lifting with heavy weights
Low-intensity cross-country skiing	Downhill skiing
Gentle biking	Mountain biking
Surfing small waves	Surfing large waves
Low-impact aerobics	High-impact aerobics

Most fitness programs lend themselves to a balance between yin and yang in an exercise routine. For instance, weight lifting is typically a yang exercise, but it can be done in a way that nourishes your yin. For yin weight lifting, I recommend you use light weights; lift them slowly and methodically for a set of twenty to thirty repetitions or until your muscles feel fatigued. After you finish three sets of repetitions, completely stretch out the muscle group you have exercised. Always take your time, and make sure you breathe deeply.

If you swim, you can balance your yin and yang exercise by starting with a few leisurely laps and slowly building up to a faster pace. Once you're pushing yourself, maintain this level of intensity for a few laps, then slowly decrease the pace to a more comfortable level. Listen to your body: *if you feel any unusual pain while exercising, stop what you're doing.* Remember, you should always feel revitalized from your workouts, and all exercise should be done to enhance your health.

In Chinese medicine as in Western medicine, too much of a good thing can be bad for you: the Chinese say that excessive exercise results in a deficiency of Qi. Again, the key is often how well you balance your exercise routines. If you do too much yang exercise, you are susceptible to overtraining and injury. If you do too much yin exercise, you miss out on the aerobic benefits of pushing your heart rate up to your full potential. And while too much exercise of any kind drains your Qi, too little exercise causes stagnation of Qi and can also lead to deficient Qi.

The Naturally Healthy Lifestyle places particular emphasis on exercise if you are postmenopausal or a senior. If you are an older woman, exercises that maintain your coordination, balance, and strength are especially critical to keeping your vitality high. Dancing, gentle hatha yoga, Qi Gong, swimming, walking, and light weight lifting are excellent ways to sustain your quality of life. Not only do they enhance your overall health, they may also help prevent bone fractures. Frequency and consistency are also important; most of my octogenarian patients exercise every day. In Hawaii many women learn hula when they are young and continue to dance through their senior years. Throughout China people of all ages gather in parks in the early morning to do Tai Chi, an ancient form of exercise that quiets the mind and encourages strength, balance, and flexibility.

Nature's Pharmacy

The natural pharmacy that I recommend draws from both Western and Chinese herbal medicine traditions; it also includes other plant-based forms of natural medicine that have evolved in the West: nutritional supplementation, homeopathy, aromatherapy, and the use of flower essences. In blending Western and Chinese medicine, I sometimes describe Western remedies and techniques in terms of the principles of Chinese medicine. In doing so, in some cases I am following in the footsteps of noted acupuncturist, author, and Chinese medicine researcher Bob Flaws, who first elucidated the Chinese energetic properties of certain Western nutritional supplements. In other cases, I take the liberty of describing Western treatments in Chinese terms, even though (to the best of my knowledge) they have never been traditionally used within the Chinese medicine paradigm. I do this when I feel it will help you make better choices for your health, such as with certain of the energetic actions of herbs, essential oils, and flower essences. The following is a general overview of key aspects of nature's pharmacy that are part of the Naturally Healthy Lifestyle.

For a list of companies that sell herbs, nutritional supplements, homeopathic remedies, essential oils, and flower essences, see Appendix B. (In some cases, the companies listed sell only certain products over the counter. For some products recommended in this book, you will need to consult your licensed naturopathic physician or acupuncturist.)

HERBAL MEDICINE

Herbs are among nature's most delightful gifts. Through the ages they have been used in Western and Chinese cultures to enhance food and flavorings, to maintain physical and emotional health, to boost vitality and energy, or simply to relax. For many thousands of years, herbs were our primary source of medicine; only in the last century in the West did synthetic drugs become the most often prescribed method of treatment for common maladies.

Herbs contain many active constituents that are scientifically proven to have potent effects on the physiology of the body. Their natural medicinal qualities can enhance your immunity, stimulate your digestion, encourage detoxification, and protect your tissues from damage. As you will discover in this book, there are numerous ways to incorporate herbal medicines into your life to create great health. And if you are not well, the healing properties of many herbs can provide you with a safe, gentle, yet powerful means of treating illness without toxic side effects.

Herbal medicines are typically derived from a plant's leaves, stems, or roots. In addition to taking them directly or with food, you can also ingest them as teas, tinctures, or standardized extracts in capsule or tablet form. Herbal tea preparations are generally weaker in their effects than tinctures and extracts; herbal tinctures, which are made by soaking herbs in glycerin or alcohol, have more concentrated active constituents, and standardized herbal extracts are also highly concentrated with active constituents. In modern herbal medicine, the term *standardized* ensures that each pill or capsule contains a specific amount of the principal active constituent of the original plant, obtained directly from the actual plant itself, and standardized extracts often contain other ingredients of the plant as well. In Chinese medicine, herbs are traditionally prescribed in formulas that include many herbs in various quantities, prepared to have specific effects on the flow of Qi.

I recommend using herbs as close to their natural form as possible, because this can result in a *synergistic* effect—which happens when more than one of the components of the plant are working together to benefit health. Many well-known pharmaceutical drugs are made by extracting the active constituent of a plant, usually an herb, and manufacturing a synthetic replication in a laboratory, altering the molecular structure of the plant's active constituent to make it patentable and therefore profitable. (Aspirin, for example, is based on the chemical composition of the herb white willow bark.) Although the process may begin with an actual plant, such drugs represent a marked deviation from the natural world; they contain neither the plant's original active constituents nor any of its other natural ingredients. This explains why some herbal medicines may have strong synergistic effects on your body that cannot be duplicated by synthetic drugs.

In addition to the measurable physical effects that herbs can have, they also have "energetic" properties—much as foods do in Chinese medicine—that may cause immeasurable and powerful effects on your body and your emotions. By using the energetic properties of herbs, you can positively influence the health of your body, mind, and spirit.

NUTRITIONAL SUPPLEMENTATION

Nutritional supplements include vitamins, minerals, amino acids, and other compounds that science has shown can enhance health in countless ways. For instance, vitamins C and E are potent antioxidants that can promote the function of the immune system, while minerals like calcium and magnesium are important for bone health.

As with herbs, I recommend that you choose nutritional supplements that are as close as possible to their source in nature rather than synthetically produced. There are important differences between these two classes of supplements. For example, synthetic vitamins are manufactured in a laboratory rather than extracted directly from their natural origins. (Often other synthetic ingredients, such as colorings, fillers, flavors, and sweeteners, are added.) Natural vitamins, by contrast, are derived from sources such as plants or foods and may include other naturally occurring components, providing synergistic effects. This is why many naturopathic physicians maintain that natural vitamins, like all natural supplements, offer numerous health benefits that their synthetic counterparts do not.

In addition to this physiological advantage, natural supplements may also provide you with gains on an "energetic" level, through their connection with the vital energy of the original plant or food. And according to some modern authorities of Chinese medicine, choosing the right nutritional supplements can also improve your Qi and boost your energy, just as foods and herbs do.

An additional way to evaluate the overall quality of nutritional supplements is to look for the GMP (Good Manufacturing Practices) certification on the product label. The National Nutritional Foods Association has established this certification to ensure that supplements have been tested for quality and screened for contaminants.

HOMEOPATHY

Founded by the German physician Samuel Hahnemann in the late 1700s, homeopathy is based on the principle that "like cures like." This idea dates back to Hippocrates, an ancient Greek physician and a father of Western medicine, who said

"Through the like, disease is produced, and through the application of the like, it is cured." Essentially, this means that a substance that causes adverse symptoms in a healthy person can cure the same symptoms in a sick person. For instance, a healthy person who ingests the toxic herb belladonna, also known as deadly nightshade, will suddenly experience symptoms including a flushed face, high fever, dilated pupils, dry mouth, and a sore throat. An unhealthy person who has many of these same symptoms due to a flu, however, will often recover quickly after taking the homeopathic remedy known as belladonna. Through this core principle, homeopathic medicines are used to treat a wide range of conditions and symptoms, from the common cold to anxiety disorders.

Homeopathic medicine encourages the body to activate its natural defense system and heal itself by stimulating its "vital force." In homeopathy, the vital force is described as the energy in your body, as well as the energy that organizes matter and all of life. In an intriguing parallel between East and West, the concept of the vital force in homeopathy is strikingly similar in some ways to the notion of Qi in Chinese medicine.

Homeopathic remedies are prepared through a series of dilutions, usually in water or alcohol, leaving only an "energetic" imprint of the original substance in the medicine. For recommendations on treating yourself with homeopathic medicines, see Appendix A.

AROMATHERAPY

Aromatic plants have been used for thousands of years in both East and West as perfumes, to promote well-being, and to treat numerous ailments. One of the most effective ways of using the beneficial qualities of aromatic plants is through the natural volatile plant constituents known as essential oils. Some essential oils have strong antimicrobial properties, while others are known for the effects they can have on the emotions.

The term *aromatherapy* is defined as any use of the essential oils of plants to enhance health. Essential oils can be massaged into the skin as ointments, applied with compresses, or smelled after they have been diffused into the air with an atomizer. For a wonderful effect, you can sprinkle them into your bath water—which allows you to smell them at the same time that you are absorbing them into your skin. In some cases, you can drink essential oils as teas. (Use the dried form of the herb for your tea; the highly concentrated liquid extract of the essential oil is not recommended for ingestion.)

Aromatherapy is remarkable because scents can profoundly impact your emotions. Your olfactory nerve, which is responsible for your ability to smell, appears to have direct access to your limbic system, the emotional center in your brain. All your other nerves must go through a "switchboard" in your brain before being connected to your limbic system. This direct access to your brain's emotional center may enhance the power of essential oils to affect your emotions and alter your moods. They can lower your level of anxiety, release nervous tension, calm your mind, and gently soothe your spirit.

FLOWER ESSENCES

Flower essences are botanical medicines made from flowers and preserved in liquid form. The study of flower essences was founded by Edward Bach in the 1930s and has since grown to include hundreds of remedies from all over the world. As with Chinese medicine, flower essences are a type of "energy" medicine, and their effects have not been fully understood by Western science.

Flower essences are gentle in their actions, have no known side effects, and are used to treat a wide variety of emotional imbalances. They may help lift a sad, grief-stricken person out of an emotional quagmire or help an angry person become calm. They are usually taken as drops or pellets under the tongue in specific doses; they can also be added to drinking water or be absorbed through the skin.

Putting Herbal Controversies in Perspective

Herbal medicines are safe and effective, and side effects are extremely rare, when they are prepared and taken correctly. Some ancient herbal remedies have stood the test of time because people have used them with great care and respect for the natural forces they contain. Needless to say, if herbs are not used according to traditional wisdom (particularly those that have potentially toxic properties), they could be deleterious to your health. For instance, kava kava root, which has been traditionally used for thousands of years by the Polynesians, was given bad press around the world after it was discovered that certain producers who were more interested in profits than in safety sold kava kava preparations containing plant parts (other than the root) that can cause toxic reactions. After tragic consequences were reported, kava kava was banned from some countries. A similar reaction prevailed when the herb ma huang, also known as ephedra, was banned in the United States—even though it has been a traditional part of Chinese medicine for millennia—after being improperly used (and abused) by some producers and consumers. To keep such controversies in perspective, it is important to remember that many commonly prescribed Western drugs and even over-the-counter medications (which have never been banned) can cause serious side effects and, when not taken as directed, can have severe consequences for your health.

Creating Health: Final Thoughts

In this chapter, we've seen many ways you can lay the groundwork for your foundation of health. The Naturally Healthy Lifestyle helps build abundant vitality by blending elements of naturopathic and Chinese medicine, including approaches to diet, exercise, and emotional health. All of these, and more, play important roles in your well-being, influencing not only your immune system and every key area of your physiology, but also your Qi, your vital force or energy, which permeates your body, mind, and spirit.

The Essence of Chapter 1

- Adopt the Naturally Healthy Lifestyle as your foundation for creating health.
- Familiarize yourself with the principles of Chinese medicine in order to keep your Qi strong and your yin and yang balanced.
- Explore the Five Elements so that you can discover your type and balance your primary element.

- Follow the Naturally Healthy Diet.
- Choose a form of exercise that you enjoy and can maintain consistently.
- Embrace herbal medicine from both the Western and Chinese traditions to create great health.

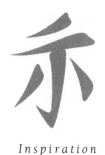

Chapter 2

Your Protective Shield:
Creating Optimal Immunity

*"If we go down into ourselves we find that we possess
exactly what we desire."*

—SIMONE WEIL, *Gravity and Grace*

"MY HEALTH is a mess!" Susan told me when she first came to see me. For too long she had been overworked, pushing herself to the point where she was frequently ill. She had almost daily headaches, suffered from asthma, and experienced frequent urinary tract and yeast infections. Her body was giving her plenty of painful signals that she was out of balance. She knew she had to make a major change in her life in order to feel good again, but she wasn't sure what to do.

Susan had been taking a battery of drugs and medications to gloss over her symptoms, but she just kept getting sicker. Her asthma, for example, continued to worsen despite the numerous inhalers she used every day. And the more drugs and medications she used, the more she seemed to need; she was stuck in a vicious cycle.

By the end of her appointment, after telling me everything that she had been through, Susan was in tears. I explained that her symptoms were not the cause of her problems but rather were the attempts her immune system was making to restore balance in her body.

Trying to remove the symptoms with drugs, I told her, would never get to the bottom of the problem. I assured her that with time and patience she would be able to uncover the root cause of her distress—the underlying imbalance in her body—and find tools to re-create her health. And that's exactly what she did.

Three years later Susan told me, "I knew natural medicine wouldn't be a quick fix, but little by little I started feeling better. Now I've got my energy back, and my headaches are completely gone. I haven't had a single urinary tract or vaginal infection in the last three years. The most remarkable thing that has happened is that I've stopped taking all of my asthma medications—drugs that, for most of my life, had allowed me to breathe. Choosing natural medicine is the best thing I've ever done for myself."

❧⨯☙

Your Immunity

Have you ever wondered why some of us can go for years without being sick, while others seem to come down with every cold that comes along? If ten people are in a crowded elevator and someone with the flu sneezes, why do some people "catch" it while others don't? Much of the answer lies in the strength of our immune systems. A healthy immune system allows you to maintain mental and emotional clarity, preserve your physical well-being, and ultimately achieve your goals and fulfill your dreams. But your immunity is not a given. You make choices, on a daily basis, that either strengthen or weaken your immune system's ability to protect you. If you make the right choices and your immunity is optimal, you have abundant health and energy. If you choose poorly, your whole life suffers—when your immune system is weak, you are less able to handle stress and are more susceptible to sickness, and if your immune system remains depressed for a prolonged period, you are more likely to suffer from a serious disease such as breast cancer, arthritis, or an autoimmune disorder.

Too often people take drugs to mask their symptoms of physical and emotional imbalance. A symptom is a messenger from your immune system, bringing you information about your body. Whether the messenger is gently tugging at your elbow or screaming to get your attention, you will benefit by listening carefully to what it is trying to communicate. Taking drugs can be a way of destroying the messenger and missing the message. In the long run, this can be extremely counterproductive.

I'm always astonished, for instance, when a physician prescribes a decongestant to a patient with a dripping nose who is fighting a cold. A dripping nose is an unmistakable sign that the immune system is doing an excellent job at eliminating a foreign irritant (virus or bacterial infection). If you take a decongestant, it dries up your mucous membranes and prevents your immune system from doing its duty. Through the Naturally Healthy Lifestyle, I emphasize working *with* your immune system, not against it. If you have a cold, it is best to support your body's natural ability to fight the infection by using herbs and nutrients that gently push your immune system into action. Instead of prescribing a decongestant, I recommend that you help your body eliminate the foreign irritant by steaming with eucalyptus, drinking plenty of hot fluids, taking supplements to assist with thinning out mucous secretions, and using other methods that will encourage your ability to effectively fight the cold itself—as opposed to ineffectively fighting the symptom.

As you will find elsewhere in this book, you can use natural medicine to work with your immune system rather than against it in countless other ways. For instance, if you have a fever less than 104 degrees, I recommend that you *don't* suppress it with aspirin (as many conventionally trained Western doctors advise) because the fever is your body's natural way of defending itself against an infection. You will get better much more quickly by supporting your body through the fever, using therapies and medicines that help you fight the infection by stimulating your immune system, than by taking drugs that can hinder your body's innate ability to restore your health.

Your immunity is the protector of your health and vitality, critical to your capacity to feel fully alive—physically, emotionally, and spiritually. Are you protecting your protector?

The View from the West

From the Western viewpoint, taking care of your immune system means taking care of every aspect of your health. The specific treatments and techniques that you'll find in this chapter—from nutritional supplementation to stress management—are the basic tools you need to do so. By using these tools, you can build a strong protective shield to serve you now and in the future.

You are exposed to thousands of bacteria and viruses every day, but your immune system prevents them from occupying your body. It performs so outstandingly well that many aspects of immunity are still a mystery to modern medicine, but we do know that diet, hormones, lifestyle, emotions, and ability to detoxify can all have a powerful effect on maintaining strong immunity. The reason is that your immune system includes millions of white blood cells that destroy both abnormal cells and foreign invaders such as viruses, bacteria, and parasites—and white blood cells function at their best when you take really good care of yourself.

White blood cells emanate from your bone marrow throughout your life, and some of them migrate from there to your thymus gland, where they reach maturity. Your thymus gland, which is located just behind your breastbone, is essential to your immune system. It creates mature white blood cells that can help you fight infections. Some of your other white blood cells make antibodies to foreign invaders. These antibodies have a remarkable memory; you make them when you have an infection, and they protect you if you are ever exposed to the same foreign invader again.

Many of your white blood cells travel in your lymph system, a network of vessels linked together like a drainage system. Along some of the larger vessels are lymph nodes, such as the ones you can feel as small lumps in your armpit or under your jaw. These lymph nodes are packed with white blood cells that fight off foreign invaders. The lymph system, which drains lymph fluids from all over your body back to the bloodstream, relies on your bodily movements to circulate lymph fluids. This is one reason why regular exercise is great for your immunity: it forces your lymph fluid to move through your body. When your lymph fluid becomes stagnant, you feel sluggish and you can experience swelling in your tissues.

Although taking really good care of yourself in general will help boost your white blood cells and therefore your immunity, keeping your skin and tissues healthy is also critical. Your skin and the delicate mucous membranes that line your mouth, sinuses, throat, and genitals are your outermost barriers to foreign invaders; when their integrity is disrupted, you are more vulnerable to infections. Your sinuses, for example, can act as a breeding ground for viruses and bacteria; an irritated urinary tract may make you more prone to a bladder infection.

Hormones also play a unique role in immunity. When you experience stress, your body releases certain hormones, such as cortisol, that can suppress your immune system. In addition, your immune system can be adversely affected by certain changes in your estrogen and progesterone levels and a lowered thyroid gland function.

The View from the East

The power of the body's own natural protection is also essential in the Eastern philosophy. According to Chinese medicine, we have a type of Qi, or vital energy, called Wei Qi (pronounced *way chee*), which acts as a defense against anything that might challenge our health. And in Chinese medicine, disease is not always caused by invading microbes or viruses; it can be brought on by either external or internal factors that create imbalances in Qi. External causes of disease include the "six evils," environmental factors that can contribute to illness if you are exposed to them for a long period of time: wind, heat, fire, cold, dryness, and dampness. (The term *dampness* is used in Chinese medicine to describe both humid weather and a sticky, heavy condition in your body.) For instance, a single windy or rainy day won't make you sick, but if you experience prolonged, unrelenting windy or damp weather, it could adversely affect your Qi and contribute to the development of illness. Other external causes of disease are inactivity, excessive indulgence in sexual activity, trauma, accidents, improper diet, and insect and animal bites.

Internal factors that create disharmony in Qi and can cause disease include imbalances in the "seven emotions": joy, fear, worry, sadness, grief, fright, and anger. An excess of any of these emotional states can damage your Qi, resulting in impaired Wei Qi and deficient immunity. In Western medicine, it is only in recent decades that "mind-body" medicine has begun to be accepted, and even today some conventional Western physicians still resist the notion that emotions can have a tremendous impact on your body. Yet thousands of years ago Chinese physicians clearly recognized and mapped out many ways that emotional excesses can influence health and disease.

Protecting against all these factors is your Wei Qi, distributed throughout your body by your lungs. Therefore when your lungs are healthy, your Wei Qi is strong. Your lungs are said to have a particularly important connection to your skin and mucous membranes—which means that they play a major role in your immunity.

In addition to distributing protective Wei Qi, the lungs have other functions that support overall health and immunity. They regulate the release of fluids, specifically urine and sweat, from the body, and lung Qi works with kidney Qi to ensure that fluids don't accumulate. The lungs also govern the circulation of Qi in the blood vessels and throughout the meridians—the pathways of energy in the body. (You can determine the status of your lung Qi by the temperature of your hands and feet. They will be warm if your lung Qi is strong and cold if your lung Qi is weak.)

Chinese medicine often describes illness in terms of natural phenomena, and a cold is thought of as "wind invading the meridians." If you have a high fever, body aches, and a dry cough, you are said to have a "wind heat invasion," and you are treated with "cold" or "cooling" herbs to purge the wind heat. If you come down with sniffles, a sore throat, and chills, you have a "wind cold invasion," and you are treated with "warming" or "hot" herbs to purge the wind cold. Much as Western medicine holds that stress can increase your susceptibility to illness, Chinese medicine teaches that stress creates an imbalance in your body, which weakens your Wei Qi. You can keep your Wei Qi strong by eating high-quality food, breathing clean air, maintaining a harmonious emotional state, and leading a balanced lifestyle.

The Metal Element

*"The Metal Element represents the special core, the divine spark which fires
the whole process and whose pure and refined essence enhances the body,
mind and spirit."*

—J. R. WORSLEY,
Classical Five Element Acupuncture

*Karen was suffering from chronic bronchial infections and a flare-up of her psoriasis. An
artist and writer, she loved her job but found that her creative energies had come to a stand-
still. She was frustrated with taking antibiotics every time she got ill and had come to my office to see if I could help her change her condition with natural medicine.*

*I learned that Karen had recently experienced a difficult breakup with her boyfriend of
two years, and her health problems had begun shortly thereafter. She felt grief-stricken, depressed, and unable to adjust to her life as a single woman. She had tried to meet new men
but distrusted their motives and found herself feeling "bored to tears" with small talk. She had
withdrawn into her work yet felt that she had lost the heart-and-soul connection she once had
with her career.*

*Karen was a creative, sensitive woman whose primary areas of imbalance suggested
that she was a classic Metal type with an out-of-balance Metal element. I prescribed natural
therapies that included dietary changes and herbs to stimulate her overall immunity, steam
inhalation with essential oils to treat her bronchial infections, flower essences to help her cope
with the grief in her life, and deep-breathing exercise to strengthen her lung Qi and further
balance her Metal element.*

*Within a few weeks Karen's condition was noticeably improved. She was optimistic,
very engaged with her social life, and willing to breathe new life into her creative projects at
work. By supporting her immunity and addressing the issue of her grief—the underlying
cause of her chronic bronchial infections—Karen was able to get her health and vitality back
on track.*

The Metal element plays an especially important role in immunity. As we've seen, the
Five Elements—Wood, Fire, Earth, Metal, and Water—all reside within you, but one
is usually dominant. If you are a "Metal type," you need to pay extra attention to the
issues in this chapter. Even if you are not predominantly a Metal type, what you'll
learn in this chapter can still help you balance your Metal element and strengthen
your immunity.

The Metal element represents the purity, quality, and high ideals symbolized by
gold or polished gems. If you are a Metal type, you are apt to be quiet, intellectually

sharp, spiritually inclined, reverential, and creative. Seeking perfection in everything you do, you are likely to be a talented craftsperson, very detail-oriented, and you are often deeply immersed in a healing meditative state when you are engaged in your craft. You flourish with regular meditation or prayer. As a Metal type, you probably enjoy activities such as hiking and mountain climbing, which require self-discipline, can be done alone, and fulfill your needs for beauty and spiritual growth. In your personal relationships you thrive on consistency and tend to be very committed to a small number of people. You are interested in important issues and are easily bored with trivial matters, and if you believe firmly in a particular cause, you are willing to act on it and challenge authority, despite what others think.

If you are a Metal type, when your life is consistent, ordered, and in balance it is a pleasure for you to be freely creative in an atmosphere of fresh ideas: you are positive and energetic, have high self-esteem, and love to take on new challenges. When your life is not in harmony, you lose your creative spark, wallow in grief, and have a pessimistic outlook. Withdrawing from others, you feel distrustful, jealous, unwilling to form new relationships, judgmental of other people, and deeply sensitive to their judgments of you. Instead of maintaining a balance of work and social engagements, you isolate yourself to an unhealthy extent. And in place of the orderly environment you prefer, your work and home life become disorganized with heaps of papers and unpaid bills.

Your lungs are especially important if you are a Metal type. According to Western medicine, when you breathe your lungs inhale oxygen and exhale carbon dioxide. Chinese medicine says that your lungs receive pure Qi from the air when you inhale, and release the old Qi from your body when you exhale. In this context, the notion of "inspiration" has more than one meaning: you inspire air when you inhale Qi, and you become inspired when you take in new ideas. For a Metal type, it is healthy to be artistically inspired; it is also healthy to seek out spiritual growth—to be inspired in the sense that it means to be "filled with spirit."

Along with your lungs, your large intestine has special significance if you are a Metal type: the lungs and large intestine are considered the primary Metal organs, working together to create harmony and balance in the body. Your large intestine is responsible for making room for new growth and change by removing all of the physical, emotional, and spiritual wastes from your system. If waste products are not readily and efficiently removed, toxins can build up and spill over into your skin, resulting in eczema, psoriasis, and rashes. In fact, in Chinese medicine your skin is often referred to as your "third lung." Later in this chapter, we will explore ways that you can nurture your skin while also detoxifying your body and strengthening your immunity.

As a Metal type you have certain characteristic signs if your Metal element is imbalanced. You tend to have a fast metabolism, and you experience symptoms of low blood sugar if you don't eat frequently and regularly. (Skipping meals may induce headaches, fatigue, and irritability.) You are particularly prone to a depleted immune system. The organs primarily affected are your skin and lungs, so you are most likely to suffer from eczema, psoriasis, hives, asthma, and chronic respiratory infections. (Eating dairy products tends to increase mucus production in your sinuses and set the stage for upper respiratory infections.) You are also prone to intestinal imbalances—constipation, diarrhea, or chronic irritable bowel symptoms—and you crave spicy foods because they can promote elimination through the large intestine. (If you are a Metal type with an intestinal imbalance, see Chapter 6 on how to create balance in this area of your body.)

Are You a Metal Type?

- Are you energetic and creative?
- Are you an intellectual?
- Do you tend to seek out spiritual growth?
- Are you an artist or craftsperson?
- Do you enjoy your time alone?
- Are your primary relationships of utmost importance to you?
- If you believe in something strongly, are you willing to take a stand on it?
- Are you meticulous and detail-oriented?
- When you have a sad experience, are you easily overwhelmed by grief?
- Do you have a lot of self-discipline?
- Do you feel bored by small talk?
- Is autumn your favorite time of year?
- Do you have a fast metabolism?
- Do you tend to be judgmental of others and very sensitive to their judgments of you?
- Are you particular about being well organized?
- Are you especially attracted to beauty, whether in works of art or in people?
- Do you tend to get a lot of respiratory infections?
- Do you have a history of intestinal imbalances—constipation, diarrhea, or chronic irritable bowel symptoms?
- Are you prone to eczema, psoriasis, rashes, or hives?
- Do you crave spicy foods?

If you answered yes to most of these questions, you are probably a Metal type, and it is especially important for you to maintain your immunity and keep your Metal element in balance. Try taking the following measures:

Maintain organization in your home and workplace.
Create time to satisfy your intellect.

Maintain consistent relationships in your personal life.

Seek out spiritual growth with regular meditation or prayer.

Keep a healthy balance between time alone and time spent with other people.

Explore your creativity.

Eat regular meals and avoid dairy products.

Nurture your lungs with regular aerobic and deep-breathing exercises.

Use herbal medicines during difficult emotional periods.

Throughout this chapter you will find tools to support your immunity by keeping your Metal element in balance. Remember that you have each of the Five Elements within you: even if you are not a Metal type, this chapter can help you balance your Metal element and keep your immune system strong and vital.

How's Your Immunity?

In order to take the best possible care of yourself, it is important that you learn to recognize the signals your body sends you when your immunity is compromised. This may mean knowing as well as *feeling* the capacities of your immune system. Some of the signals are obvious, while others may surprise you. You can begin to assess the overall strength of your immunity by asking yourself the following questions:

Do you get a cold or flu more than once a year?

Do you have chronically swollen lymph nodes?

Are you almost always tired?

Do you have a lot of environmental allergies?

Are you allergic to many foods?

Are your allergic symptoms getting worse?

Do you have frequent skin infections such as boils or sties?

Do you often have cold sores or herpes infections?

Does it take you an exceptionally long time to heal from an illness?

Do you get a lot of vaginal yeast infections?

Do you chronically feel overwhelmed by stress?

Have you ever had cancer?

Have you taken antibiotics at least once a year?

Are the mucous membranes of your sinuses and throat chronically irritated?

If your answer to any of these questions is yes, you may want to consider why your immunity may be low and how you can enhance it. Some common stressors that may be interfering with your immunity include imbalances in exercise, diet, work, relationships, yin and yang, and hormones, as well as a lack of sleep, detoxification, quality air, water, and vitamins and minerals. You could also be suffering from too much exposure to environmental chemicals or heavy metals, and too much cigarette, alcohol, and prescription or recreational drug use. You can take a number of tests to further evaluate any underlying causes of weakened immunity, including a complete blood test that assesses your red and white blood count, a serum ferritin test that measures your iron, a thyroid test, a stress test that measures cortisol, a heavy metal test, and a stool test. These tests can be ordered by your naturopathic physician.

ASSESSING YOUR IMMUNITY WITH CHINESE MEDICINE

If your protective Wei Qi is strong and vital, your immunity is high and you are most likely to be free of disease; if your Wei Qi is weakened, your immunity is low and you are more susceptible to disease. In Chinese medicine, assessing your immunity and your Wei Qi involves looking at your tongue. Each part of your tongue relates to a different part of your body and provides information on whether your organs are functioning optimally. The following illustration shows how areas of your tongue correspond to various parts of your body.

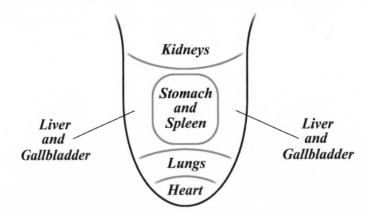

The unique qualities of your tongue—its color, coating, and shape—may indicate that you have imbalances in your Qi that could affect your ability to keep your immunity strong. You are healthiest when your tongue has a moderate pale-red color and a thin white coating that is slightly moist. If your tongue has a color that is unusually pale, red, or purple, or a dry or thick coating that is yellow, white, gray, or black, you are likely to have Qi imbalances, and your Wei Qi may be weakened. The shape of your tongue can further indicate that your Qi is imbalanced if it is excessively swollen; teeth marks caused by swelling, which look like scalloped edges on the sides of your tongue, are a classic sign of deficient Qi.

In Chinese medicine, your pulse is another important means of assessing your Qi and the strength of your immunity, as it varies depending on your fluid intake, menstrual cycle, stress level, and eating habits. A practitioner of Chinese medicine will use three fingers to feel your pulse at both of your wrists in order to gather information about the flow of Qi through your organs and meridians. In Chinese medicine, your pulse may be described in terms such as "floating," "slippery," "wiry," "empty," "thin," "weak," "excessive," or "deficient." To anyone not trained in pulse reading, feeling these subtle qualities can be difficult.

It is also important to evaluate your lifestyle and diet, which are critical to maintaining the health of your Qi and your immunity. Chinese medicine recommends that you avoid overeating or indulging in excessively sweet and fatty foods. It's best to eat regularly, in a stress-free environment. If you find yourself always eating in a hurry, you could be setting the stage for imbalances in your Qi that lead to impaired Wei Qi and lowered immunity. Chinese medicine was probably one of the first systems of medicine to acknowledge that stress and an unhealthy lifestyle can be disruptive. Daily exercise, adequate sleep, and fulfilling work are essential to maintaining the flow of Qi throughout your body.

If the color, coating, or shape of your tongue has unusual qualities, or if your pulse shows signs of Qi imbalance, the first six chapters of this book will be especially helpful in restoring your health and creating a more balanced flow of Qi in your body. I also recommend that you see your Chinese medicine practitioner for further guidance.

Vital Skin = Strong Immunity

The skin is the body's largest organ, so it's no wonder that the health and vitality of your entire body visibly resonates in your skin. A complex, many-layered organ of touch, your skin is crucial to your immunity from a Western as well as a Chinese perspective.

You can do a lot to keep your skin vital, starting with taking care of yourself from both the inside and the outside. To nurture from the inside, eat well, drink clean water, exercise regularly (sweating is your skin's natural way of cleansing), and lead a balanced life—all of which are elements of the Naturally Healthy Lifestyle. Externally, you can help create healthy skin by choosing the right skin care products. Most cleansers, toners, and moisturizers are absorbed directly into your body, so think of them as nutrients for your skin. The best nutrients you can put on your skin, like the ones you put in your mouth, are those that nourish you naturally. Look for soaps, body oils, and other products that don't contain synthetic ingredients and fragrances that might cause skin irritation. For example, to make a simple skin toner at home, mix equal parts of aloe vera juice, witch hazel, and water. For a great natural acne treatment, use honey. Honey has known antibacterial qualities and has been used for facial masks by naturopathic physicians for decades. A honey mask is very simple: apply honey to your face, leave it on for fifteen minutes, then wash it off. Other forms of external skin care include hydrotherapy (your skin will glow with regular hot tub, steaming, or sauna use) and brushing your body with a loofah sponge.

In Chinese medicine, much as in the West, your skin is a reflection of the general state of your health and vitality. By feeling the moisture level, texture, and temperature of your skin, you can learn a lot about your health. If your skin feels moist because you sweat profusely and easily, it means that your Qi is deficient. Excessive swelling in your skin suggests an inability to regulate fluids in your body due to an imbalance in kidney Qi or spleen Qi. As in Western medicine, Chinese medicine views dry, scaly skin as an indication that your body fluids are depleted. Generally, if your skin feels cold, you have too much yin, and if it feels hot, you have too much yang. If you have any of these imbalances, refer to Chapter 1, as well as the chapters that follow, to discover how you can create health and balance your Qi.

Your skin can also help reveal which of the Five Elements tends to dominate your constitution. When you look in the mirror, you will see a delicate tone emanating from your skin. (It may help if you look at the skin near your temples under natural lighting.) Identify the color of your complexion, and refer to the "Five Elements" charts on pages 20–21. Notice that each of the elements has a corresponding color: red, yellow, white, black, or green. To which does your skin tone most closely correspond?

Vitamins, Minerals, and Antioxidants to Boost Immunity

A nutritious diet is one of the foundations of the Naturally Healthy Lifestyle, but by taking the right supplements you can be sure you are getting what you need on a daily basis. While you probably don't need to take handfuls of supplements, taking a good daily multivitamin can be essential to keeping your immunity at peak level.

YOUR DAILY MULTIVITAMIN

Vitamins play a vital role in health—in fact, they were named after this characteristic. Your daily multivitamin should consist of vitamins as well as extra minerals and specific antioxidants. There's a wealth of research validating the many health benefits of vitamins, minerals, and antioxidants. Together they help prevent disease and give your immune system an extra layer of protection from the environmental chemicals you are exposed to on a daily basis. Some help your liver break down toxins for safe removal from your body, and some help support your immune and nervous systems, heart, and bones. Others help you tolerate the stress that you deal with every day.

Handle your vitamins with care; they can become ineffective when exposed to high heat, oxygen, or light. Some vitamins, such as the B vitamins, have to be taken in small, frequent doses because they are not retained by your body. Other vitamins are more readily stored in your tissues, and they can be taken less often and in larger doses. Extra attention is advised when taking vitamins A and D, because if taken in excess they can reach toxic levels in your tissues. This is not likely to be a concern unless you are taking separate doses of these vitamins, in addition to the amounts in your daily multivitamin.

Chemically simpler than vitamins, minerals are virtually indestructible because they retain their chemical composition whether they are exposed to heat, air, or light. Ideally, your diet would give you all the minerals you need, but many of the vegetables and grains you eat may be low in minerals because of depleted mineral stores in the soil they were grown in. Therefore it's especially important to supplement your diet with minerals. Like vitamins, some minerals taken in excess can be toxic, but again, the amounts in most well-rounded daily multivitamins do not reach toxic levels.

Antioxidants can protect your tissues from the damaging effects of compounds known as free radicals, and they play an important role in the prevention of many diseases, such as cancer. They include beta-carotene, vitamin A, vitamin C, vitamin E, and the mineral selenium. You will get many antioxidants from fresh fruits and vegetables, but taking additional antioxidants in supplement form can bolster your immunity.

In Chinese medicine, vitamins, minerals, and antioxidants, like foods, have "energetic" properties. Dr. Bob Flaws, a leading researcher and author on Chinese medicine in the United States, has classified most vitamins and minerals by their traditional Chinese medicine functions in his book *The Tao of Healthy Eating*. For instance, calcium and magnesium support yin and suppress yang, vitamin C clears heat and calms the spirit, and most of the B vitamins help support the liver Qi.

The "What You Need in a Daily Multivitamin" chart gives you a list of the vitamins, minerals, and antioxidants you should have in your daily multivitamin, and brief descriptions of how each supports your body from both a Western and an Eastern standpoint. When choosing a daily multivitamin, look for one derived from natural sources and available in either capsule or powder form for easy absorption by your body. It's a good idea to take multivitamins with food, because some people experience nausea when taking them on an empty stomach.

What You Need in a Daily Multivitamin

VITAMIN, MINERAL, OR ANTIOXIDANT	AMOUNT	WESTERN BIOCHEMICAL PROPERTIES	CHINESE "ENERGETIC" PROPERTIES
Beta-carotene	20,000 i.u.	An antioxidant that can enhance immunity. Beta-carotene converts into vitamin A in the body as needed. (Note: Vitamin A can be toxic when taken as a supplement in high doses, but beta-carotene is not toxic in high doses.)	Clears heat, releases toxins, and moves stagnant Qi
Vitamin C	1,000 mg	An antioxidant important in immune functions and for strengthening blood vessel walls	Clears heat, releases toxins, and quiets the spirit
Vitamin D_2	200 i.u.	Assists with calcium absorption and may have anticancer benefits	Supports kidney Qi and strengthens bones and yang
Vitamin E	400 i.u.	An antioxidant that protects fat cells from damage due to oxidation and that can be important in preventing heart disease and Alzheimer's disease. It is best taken in the form of mixed tocopherols	Nourishes Blood* and strengthens bones and yang
Vitamin B_1	100 mg	Contributes to energy production in cells	Rebalances Qi through its action on the liver
Vitamin B_2	75 mg	Contributes to energy production in cells	Nourishes liver Qi and kidney Qi
Vitamin B_3	150 mg	Contributes to energy production in cells	Harmonizes liver Qi and stomach Qi
Vitamin B_5	150 mg	Supports adrenal gland function	Clears heat, resolves depression, and harmonizes liver Qi
Vitamin B_6	50 mg	Plays an important role in protein and hormone metabolism	Harmonizes liver Qi, stomach Qi, and spleen Qi, and clears heat
Vitamin B_{12}	300 mcg	Is necessary for producing healthy red blood cells and proper functioning of nerves	Nourishes Blood and supports Qi
Biotin	400 mcg	Supports hair and nails	Calms liver Qi, nourishes Blood, and quiets the spirit
Folic acid	800 mcg	Is required for healthy multiplication of cells	Harmonizes liver Qi and nourishes Blood
Calcium	1,000 mg	Strengthens bones and may help prevent cancer	Strengthens yin and bones

VITAMIN, MINERAL, OR ANTIOXIDANT	AMOUNT	WESTERN BIOCHEMICAL PROPERTIES	CHINESE "ENERGETIC" PROPERTIES
Iodine (kelp)	150 mcg	Supports thyroid gland function	Clears heat and harmonizes liver Qi
Magnesium	500 mg	Strengthens bones and is important for the heart	Strengthens yin and quiets the spirit
Zinc	40 mg	Helps keep the immune system healthy and assists in the production of stomach acid	Nourishes liver Qi and kidney Qi
Selenium	200 mcg	An antioxidant that assists the immune system	Strengthens yin and quiets the spirit
Copper	2 mg	Works with many enzyme systems in the body and affects iron absorption, collagen integrity, and the immune system	Strengthens spleen Qi
Manganese	20 mg	Works with many enzyme systems in the body that are involved in blood sugar control and bone health	Nourishes liver Qi and kidney Qi
Chromium	200 mcg	Helps keep blood sugar level normal	Strengthens spleen Qi
Potassium	99 mg	Protects against problems associated with high sodium intake	Strengthens spleen Qi and clears heat
Bioflavonoids	200 mg	Work with vitamin C and can strengthen cell walls	Clear heat from Blood

*In Chinese medicine, the term *Blood* refers not only to the fluid in the veins but also to a form of Qi that nourishes and moistens the body tissues and provides the material foundation for the spirit. Throughout this book, *Blood* used in the context of Chinese medicine includes both these meanings.

The vitamins, minerals, and antioxidants in your daily multivitamin are like an insurance policy that will cover your basic nutritional needs. Elsewhere in this book I recommend higher doses of certain individual vitamins, minerals, or antioxidants for specific health conditions that may concern you. The amount I recommend at any point is always the *total* amount that you should be taking. In other words, if you are taking a daily multivitamin, take that into account if you add on any supplements. For example, if you are taking a daily multivitamin that gives you 1,000 mg of vitamin C, and I recommend that you take up to 3,000 mg of vitamin C a day because you are at high risk for heart disease, you should add on up to 2,000 mg of vitamin C a day.

If you don't take a daily multivitamin regularly, I recommend you fortify your immune system by supplementing your diet on a daily basis with 400 i.u. (international units) of vitamin E and 1000 mg of vitamin C, your two most important antioxidants. Vitamin E should be taken as a supplement because it is very difficult to obtain from your diet in therapeutic amounts. It can thin your blood, however, so it is important that you don't take it—either as part of a daily multivitamin or as a separate supplement—if you are currently on blood-thinning medication or about to go into surgery.

Overcoming Stress

What do you live with every day that in moderation you benefit from but in excess can make you sick? If you answered stress, you would be right. If you had no stress whatsoever in your life, you would probably be bored and lethargic; stress may often be what motivates you to make healthy changes in your life. But too much stress can lead to an exhausted nervous system, a depleted immune system, depression, and illness.

When you experience a high level of stress, your body leaps into action, sending out hormones that cause your heart to race, blood pressure to increase, and pupils to dilate. This is the same response that your ancestors experienced when they ran from lions, tigers, and bears. But in the modern world, you are no longer running from wild beasts; your enemy is the stress caused by frantic efforts to provide for your family, deal with rush-hour traffic, or meet imposing deadlines.

From the viewpoint of Chinese medicine, excessive stress will ultimately deplete your energy, creating a weakness in your Wei Qi. Chinese and Western medicine are in accord in suggesting lifestyle choices that keep your immunity at peak level by overcoming stress in your life. According to *The Yellow Emperor's Classic,* a Chinese medical text written during the third century B.C. or earlier, "When the mind is calm and stable, the vitality of life circulates harmoniously throughout the body. If the body is nourished and protected by this circulation of vitality, how can it possibly become ill?"

SELF-NURTURING FOR YOUR IMMUNITY

As a woman, your biological makeup predisposes you to be a caregiver. I call estrogen the "compassion hormone," and like it or not, you may find that you have a tendency to direct your compassion more toward others than yourself. Over time this tendency can distract you from your own needs, add stress to your life, and place an extra burden on your immune system.

As we've seen, symptoms can be your body's way of demanding that you pay close attention to your needs and take better care of yourself. With a little practice, you can get in touch with your inner wisdom, the intuition that recognizes the signs your body gives you when you need to nurture yourself. Directing some of your compassion inward, toward yourself, can help you release stress, prevent illness, create balance in your life, strengthen your immune system, and reinforce your health in countless ways. Self-nurturing means setting aside some time every day to serve your own body, mind, and spirit. It means taking a close look at whether you are honoring your true values by spending time and energy on what matters most to *you*. It might mean taking a walk, stretching, exercising, meditating, preparing your favorite meal, drawing a warm bath, using aromatherapy and flower essences, or simply luxuriating in anything else you love to do.

AROMATHERAPY

In the previous chapter, we saw that aromatherapy can be a wonderful way to treat yourself. When stress is adversely affecting your immune system, the following essential oils can be used as aromatherapy, together or individually. Although the use of essential oils is not part of traditional Chinese medicine, I include a brief description of each oil's Chinese "energetic" actions as interpreted by Gabriel Mojay, author of *Aromatherapy for Healing the Spirit*. It seems especially appropriate to use aromatherapy to balance Qi; the Chinese character for Qi depicts wind blowing over a rice field, and in Chinese medicine Qi can be perceived as a kind of air, wind, ethereal vapor, or even scent.

Clary Sage. Used to help you feel calm when you are tense and revive you when you are fatigued, this essential oil also has antibacterial properties and can help fight infections, as well as helping with shallow breathing and a constricted chest. It can also act as an expectorant when you are fighting a bronchial infection. From a Chinese medicine point of view, clary sage supports your Metal element and benefits your respiratory system by strengthening your lung Qi.

Cypress. Recommended for helping you move through transitions in your life, especially when you have a great deal of self-doubt, cypress is a good remedy for Metal types, from a Chinese perspective, because they often have trouble coping with change, letting go, and moving on. Cypress also helps to circulate Qi, which is helpful when you are under stress.

Thyme. Used for an exhausted nervous system, thyme can be uplifting and fortifying. Physically, it can be used for any weakness or infection of the lungs, such as bronchitis. From a Chinese medicine perspective, thyme is particularly helpful if your Metal element is out of balance. And if you are a Metal type, it can help if you are lacking in self-confidence. Thyme strengthens the body's yang energy, so it is also useful for treating chronic fatigue.

Flower Essences to Nurture Your Emotions and Immunity

As we've seen, flower essences can gently help keep your emotions balanced. The effects of a remedy are strengthened by taking it with greater frequency rather than by increasing the dose. The usual recommended dosage is four drops or pellets under your tongue four times a day, but you can take flower essences once every two hours until your symptoms are alleviated; if you see no improvement with this dosage within twelve hours, discontinue the treatment or try a different remedy that may better match your symptoms. Flower essences can also be taken in drinking water, massaged into the skin, or added to a bath. The following remedies are recommended for nurturing your immune system and helping you shift your emotions so that you'll feel better able to cope with stress.

- **Pine** is used to help you move past feelings of guilt, regret, and low self-worth, which can ultimately lead to depression and lowered immunity. From a Chinese medicine perspective, this flower essence can help balance your Metal element.
- **Goldenrod** is recommended if you find that you are ignoring your feelings, not living by your values, and excessively seeking approval from others.
- **Dandelion** can be helpful when you feel overwhelmed by a busy schedule and your entire body feels tense and "wound up."
- **Dill** is recommended if you've been under unusual stress, feel totally exhausted at the end of the day, or feel like your nerves are at a breaking point.

BREATHING NEW LIFE INTO YOUR IMMUNITY

According to Chinese wisdom, deep breathing can strengthen Qi, create clarity of mind, and promote inner relaxation. Deep breathing is especially important for keeping your Metal element in balance. It builds up lung Qi and Wei Qi, which protects you against challenges to your immune system.

The ancient Chinese art of Qi Gong, which translates as "energy exercise" or "breathwork," offers many deep-breathing methods that you can use on a regular basis to support your immunity. Once you master the basic techniques, you can tune in to your breath in just about any situation. Some of my patients have told me they practice Qi Gong breathing at bus stops, during movies, and even while waiting for a slow computer to open a big file. Qi Gong breathing has the added benefit of being very calming and stress-relieving, so with a few creative adjustments in technique, it can help you through many a dentist appointment or intense business meeting!

To begin the most basic form of Qi Gong breathing, sit in a straight position in a comfortable chair or on the floor, put your hands at your sides or in your lap, and close your eyes. Pay close attention to your breathing. As you inhale, become aware of how you draw the air downward into your expanding lungs. Next, as you exhale, focus on how the air feels as it moves from your lungs and out of your body. Keep your concentration on the cycle of your breath and the qualities of the air flow; notice how it passes rhythmically in and out of your body. Continue breathing this way for a few minutes, increasing your awareness of your normal breathing process.

There are many other methods of Qi Gong breathing. Books, CDs, and classes are widely available for exploring more advanced techniques. (See Appendix B for more information.)

OTHER STRESS-RELIEVING TIPS

There are a number of other ways to relieve stress and boost immunity. These include following consistent eating habits and doing regular exercise to keep your blood sugar even. Exercise also decreases the hormones that make stress bad for you. When our ancestors fled from wild animals, they were acting out of a "fight-or-flight" response and naturally discharged their stress in the act of running. When you are stressed, you are seldom able to relieve your tension with such immediate physical activity. You are likely to be stuck in traffic, late for an appointment, or having a difficult confrontation during a business meeting. You are trapped in what I call the "neither-fight-nor-flight" response. By incorporating exercise into your life, you can release the pent-up stress from your body—while also gaining all the other benefits of exercise that we've explored thus far.

Some have speculated that girlfriend time helps decrease a woman's stress level. An article published in *Psychological Review* in 2000 suggests that women have an additional response to stress other than "fight or flight," called "tend and befriend." It was hypothesized that this response occurs when women create social networks, including those with other women, and get involved in nurturing activities designed to protect their families and themselves. The writers theorized that the hormone oxytocin, which may have a calming effect on the body (it is released when a woman is lactating, giving birth, or experiencing an orgasm), may play a role in this response and thereby help reduce stress.[1]

Spending time with a loving partner can also be an important part of stress relief. When women have fulfilling relationships, their hormones may be affected in ways that release stress considerably and thereby enhance their overall health and immunity. This is reflected in Chinese medicine by the principle that health is the result of equalized yin and yang; for example, the natural balance of yin and yang is embodied in the harmonious union of female and male.

Getting enough sleep is another great stress reliever. Sleep is one of the most precious healers. While you are dreaming, your body is mending; from the Chinese perspective, you are regenerating your Qi. Without sufficient sleep—at least eight hours a night—your immune system is less able to handle stress, and your health suffers. As we will see in Chapter 11, sleep is important for the health not only of your body but of your mind, emotions, and spirit as well. If you need to improve your sleep, there are a number of herbal and nutritional supplements that can help. Insomnia can result from stress, anxiety, or as the Chinese say, from "too much thinking." Fluctuations in your hormones can also cause insomnia; many women experience changes in their sleep patterns near menstruation, or during perimenopause and menopause. If you have insomnia, see Chapter 7, which addresses the issue of insomnia due to hormonal fluctuations, and Chapter 11, which explores insomnia resulting from other causes.

Finally, you can reduce stress in your life by avoiding caffeine. Although you may feel that it gives you an extra boost—or even wakes you up—in the morning, in reality caffeine adds to your total stress load if you drink it on a daily basis. Caffeine is a stimulant that over time can exhaust your adrenal glands and trick your body into thinking it has lots of energy when in fact it may be running on empty. From the Chinese viewpoint, caffeine ultimately reduces Qi. It can also interfere with your sleep and inhibit your appetite—which can cause further stress by throwing off your regular meal schedule.

Herbal Supertonics for Long-Term Immunity

There are a number of herbs that boost your immune system and your ability to cope with stress, and they are especially useful if your immunity has been chronically deficient for an extended period of time. Generally, these herbs are recommended for shoring up your immune system on a long-term basis rather than simply when you have a cold or flu. Long used in China, they are sometimes referred to as *supertonics*—*tonics* not in the sense that they are drinks but rather because they "tonify" your immune system and other systems in your body, strengthening and balancing your Qi. The following is a description of how you can use three of the most potent of these herbal supertonics on a long-term basis. As you can see, Western research is in complete concurrence with the Chinese tradition on the benefits of these herbs for maintaining immunity.

Siberian Ginseng. A powerful herb for boosting long-term immune and adrenal functions, Siberian ginseng can be used for a variety of immunity-building purposes. From a Chinese medicine perspective, it helps to build Qi and can be used both in a low dose to treat yin deficiency and in a high dose to correct yang deficiency. From a Western perspective, the benefits of Siberian ginseng include the following:

- Increases your ability to cope with stress[2]
- Raises the white blood cell count and promotes antibody formation[3]

- Helps the body cope with both high and low blood sugar[4]
- Boosts energy without leaving you feeling like you're on caffeine
- Elevates your mental alertness and sense of well-being
- Increases the lungs' ability to absorb and efficiently use oxygen[5]
- Helps the body normalize low blood pressure[6]
- Improves the liver's ability to remove harmful toxins
- Enhances athletic performance and decreases recovery time after exercise
- Decreases the frequency, duration, and severity of herpes infections[7]
- Protects the body from free-radical damage by acting as an antioxidant[8]

Recommended dose: two capsules, each containing 200 mg of a standardized extract of 0.5 percent eleutheroside E (the active constituent of Siberian ginseng), taken once or twice a day. Numerous studies have demonstrated that Siberian ginseng can be taken without adverse side effects and is safe for pregnant and lactating women. But if you take the herb too close to bedtime, you may experience insomnia, and if you take it in excess, you may have mild diarrhea. (Note: Do not use Siberian ginseng if you have uncontrolled high blood pressure or are taking barbiturates or the pharmaceutical drug digoxin.)

Astragalus. Long used in China to help to restore Qi and vitality, astragalus can be used to fortify Wei Qi, or protective Qi. It is also recommended if you've experienced frequent colds due to deficient Wei Qi, or if you've had a protracted illness and lack the strength and vitality to restore your health. Chinese medicine specifically recommends that you *not* take astragalus during the acute phase of a cold or flu, though it can be taken afterward, during your recovery.

From the standpoint of Western medicine, astragalus is useful in the treatment of both immune deficiency and excessive immunity, as in autoimmune diseases. It contains compounds that modulate your immune system, including polysaccharides that are strong immunity enhancers. Astragalus has the following benefits:

- Increases white blood cell activity while suppressing excessive immune activity[9]
- Has effective antioxidant properties[10]
- Helps the skin eliminate toxins[11]
- Assists with wound healing

Recommended dose: 3 grams (g) taken three times a day. (Note: Do not use this herb if you are on steroids, beta-blockers, or a blood-thinning drug such as warfarin.)

Reishi. Also known as ganoderma, reishi is a mushroom used in Chinese medicine to build Qi throughout the body. From a Western perspective, it contains many medicinal compounds that are powerful immune system regulators and it helps rebuild the immune system. It is used for conditions associated with low immunity and for autoimmune diseases. Reishi is a powerful antistress herb with a broad range of actions in the body, including the following:

- Activates the immune cells[12]
- Diminishes allergic responses[13]
- Decreases cholesterol and lowers "unfriendly" LDL cholesterol[14]
- Protects your tissues through its antioxidant properties[15]
- Eases tension and calms the mind
- Helps repair liver damage
- Enhances liver detoxification
- Has anti-inflammatory properties
- Is used to enhance memory in old age
- May help prevent Alzheimer's disease
- Has potential anticancer effects[16]
- Helps maintain your white blood cell count and can decrease some adverse side effects of chemotherapy and radiation[17]

Recommended dose: For health maintenance, take 0.5 to 1 g a day; for chronic fatigue, stress, autoimmune disorders, or other chronic health problems, take 2 to 5 g a day; for a serious illness such as cancer, consult your physician. (Note: Some people may experience drowsiness when they begin taking reishi.)

Many varieties of reishi are available. Look for wild red reishi, duanwood reishi, or reishi spores (superior to the black reishi sold at most herb and supplement stores), and buy the highest quality available. (Suppliers are listed in Appendix B).

Hydrotherapy

Hydrotherapy is the use of water in any of its forms—solid, liquid, or vapor—to maintain health, stimulate immunity, or treat disease. Water has been used for centuries by people in many cultures as a detoxifying and therapeutic agent. In the West, the founders of naturopathic medicine passed down the ancient wisdom of hydrotherapy. My naturopathic training included an extensive focus on hydrotherapy because it can be a powerful way to influence health gently and naturally, and it has so many uses and benefits.

Hydrotherapy (or *contrast hydrotherapy*) usually consists of alternating hot and cold water in showers, baths, hot tubs, saunas, steaming, compresses, or wraps. For some purposes your entire body is immersed in water, and for others only specific areas are treated. Hot water draws your blood toward an area of your body and causes dilation of your blood vessels, which allows more oxygen and blood to flow into the area. Conversely, cold water constricts your blood vessels and causes your blood to "retract" toward your heart.

You can do hydrotherapy to increase your blood flow, move your lymph, soothe pain, assist with detoxification, improve digestion, relieve stress, and enhance your overall health and vitality. Hydrotherapy is also useful for sprains, strains, localized infections, fevers, and upper respiratory infections such as a cold or bronchitis. Depending on your regimen, hydrotherapy can be either stimulating or sedating. The Chinese explanation for the benefits of contrast hydrotherapy for immunity is strikingly similar to the Western view: hot water has a yang effect, coaxing the blood outward toward the surface of the body, while cold water has a yin effect, shunting the blood inward, back toward the center. Together these two tendencies represent a perfect balance between your yin and yang energies; by engendering their ebb and flow, contrast hydrotherapy can be a wonderfully effective way of stimulating and strengthening your protective Qi.

How to Do Contrast Hydrotherapy

One of the best ways to do contrast hydrotherapy is to use a facility that has a hot tub (a sauna or steam room may also be used) with a cold tub or shower nearby. The water temperature in a hot tub is typically between 98 and 104 degrees Fahrenheit, but the temperature of your tub should depend on your overall vitality. If your vitality is high, you can probably handle a temperature of 102 to 104 degrees. To get the strongest effect, use the hottest temperature that you are comfortable with, but don't push beyond your comfort level. If your vitality is low, begin with a lower temperature, and stay in the tub for shorter periods. Refrain from doing hydrotherapy if you have high blood pressure.

Do this treatment with a friend, since it may make you feel dizzy. Drink plenty of fluids before and after your treatment.

- Get into a hot tub, and stay for five to ten minutes.
- Get out, and immediately get into a cold tub or shower. The cold water temperature should be between 51 and 65 degrees Fahrenheit.
- Stay in the cold tub or shower for at least one minute, then return to the hot tub. If you need to, rest for a few minutes before returning.
- Repeat the entire sequence three times, always ending with a cold bath or shower.
- Be gentle on yourself: if you feel any dizziness, lie down and discontinue your treatment.

You can boost your immunity every day at home with a few minutes of contrast hydrotherapy at the end of your shower. Before you turn the shower off let the water run down your back for thirty seconds at the hottest temperature that is comfortable, then switch to cold. Allow the cold water to run down your back for about ten seconds, then immediately switch back to hot. Repeat this cycle three times, and always end with cold before you step out of the shower. This can have an invigorating and warming effect on your entire body.

What to Do for a Cold or Flu

So far we've talked about how you can keep your immune system healthy, but there may be times when your immune system becomes compromised and you come down with a cold or flu. Natural medicine can get your immunity back on track. You may have heard people say "There's no cure for the common cold." Don't believe it! Not only is there a cure for both the cold and the flu, there are *many* cures. All of the following methods can help you treat, and cure, a cold or flu—and when combined the results can be extremely effective. Each of these methods is a natural way of approaching a cold or flu, and each can be safely used in conjunction with the others.

Treating a cold or flu with natural methods, rather than synthetic drugs, will benefit your immune system in the long run. Resorting to drugs when you don't need them may itself weaken your natural immunity. In some cases, drugs may actually prolong an illness; in others they may cause side effects with symptoms more damaging to your health than the condition you originally took them for. If you take drugs for every cold and flu you get over the course of your life, the cumulative effects could compromise your immunity in any number of ways. For example, many medical doctors routinely prescribe antibiotics for colds and flus, even those caused by a viral infection—despite the fact that antibiotics do nothing to get rid of a virus. Taking antibiotics for colds and flus, even if only a few times a year, can lead to chronic vaginal infections as well as intestinal overgrowth of both yeast and abnormal bacteria—either of which can in turn lead to food allergies and other immune system imbalances.

HOT AND COLD WINDS

In conventional Western medicine, if you have a cold, you are almost always given medicine that suppresses the symptoms, and just about anyone with a cold who walks into a typical clinic will be treated with the same kinds of medications. In fact, conventionally trained Western physicians tend to see all colds as being more or less the same.

In Chinese medicine, as in natural Western medicine, two cases of the "common" cold may have little in common, and each person is treated according to her unique symptoms. In the Chinese system most colds and flus are categorized as either

Treating a Cold or Flu with Natural Medicine

CONDITION	SYMPTOMS	GOAL OF TREATMENT	TREATMENT
"Wind heat"	A dry cough with a reddish sore throat, yellow-colored mucus, high fever, aches all over, feelings of heat, constipation, and a tongue with a red tip and sides	To help your immune system fight the cold or flu by releasing heat from your body	**Diet:** Avoid sugar; eat immunity-enhancing foods and "cold" or "cooling" foods (see Chapter 1). **Herbs:** Spearmint, chamomile, and coltsfoot **Chinese herbal formula:** Yin Chiao Jie Du Wan **Aromatherapy:** Eucalyptus and spearmint oils **Homeopathy:** Aconite, Belladonna, and Oscillococcinum **Supplements:** Zinc, vitamins A and C, and thymus extracts **Immune support:** Echinacea **Hydrotherapy:** Cold compresses on the forehead to reduce a high fever
"Wind cold"	A runny nose and cough with clear mucus, low-grade fever, achy muscles, chills, sore throat, headache, and a whitish tongue coating	To help your immune system fight the cold or flu by increasing heat and decreasing cold in your body	**Diet:** Avoid sugar; eat immunity-enhancing foods and "warming" or "hot" foods (see Chapter 1). **Herbs:** Cinnamon, ginger, hyssop, and basil **Chinese herbal formula:** Ge Gen Wan **Aromatherapy:** Peppermint, thyme, and ginger oils **Homeopathy:** Oscillococcinum and Gelsemium **Supplements:** Zinc, vitamins A and C, and thymus extracts **Immune support:** Garlic **Hydrotherapy:** Steaming, showers, baths, and hot compresses

"wind heat" or "wind cold" conditions affecting the lungs; generally understood, they are the result of either a "hot wind" or a "cold wind" that is said to "invade" the meridians, or energy channels. The chart on page 69 shows how these two categories are diagnosed from the Chinese viewpoint, and how you can treat them with natural medicine.

DIET THERAPY

One of the great things about the Naturally Healthy Diet is that what you eat every day is so good for you that, if you ever become sick, your food will be your medicine. If you find yourself coming down with a cold or flu, your immune system will already be well situated to fight off the infection. And by making a few small shifts in your diet when you are not well, you can further enhance its medicinal powers. Simply by increasing your intake of foods that are especially immunity-enhancing and nutrient-rich, you can help restore your health more quickly. These foods include garlic, onions, leeks, squash, zucchini, cauliflower, broccoli, cabbage, yams, carrots, green beans, peas, cooked spinach, chard, kale, shiitake mushrooms, and seaweeds.

When you have a cold or flu, eat easily digestible foods and drink plenty of fluids to moisten the mucous membranes of your lungs, throat, and sinuses; warm soups and herbal teas can be very comforting. When you have a fever, ingest clear broths made from miso, vegetables, or organic chicken. Be especially careful to avoid sugary foods, because sugar can depress the function of your immune cells. Even fruit juice, including orange juice, is high in fruit sugar and can be detrimental to your immunity. You should also avoid rich, fatty foods that are hard on your digestive system, and dairy products, which can create mucus and congestion.

STEAM INHALATION, ESSENTIAL OILS, AND HERBS

Steam inhalation is one of the best ways to get the healing benefits of essential oils and herbs directly into your throat and lungs. It is easy to do and very soothing to irritated mucous membranes, and it can help you with many cold or flu conditions. It can decrease a spasmodic cough, loosen up phlegm, and open up your sinuses and bronchial passages. In addition, some essential oils also have direct antibacterial and antiviral actions. And steam inhalation has an extra bonus: it will leave you feeling like you've had a wonderful facial.

From a Chinese medicine perspective, you can treat yourself with a steam inhalation whether your diagnosis is a "wind heat" or a "wind cold" condition. For "wind heat," mix the dried herbs spearmint, chamomile, and coltsfoot in a large clean bowl, and add a few drops of eucalyptus oil. Pour boiling water over the herbs, and with your face directly above the bowl of steam, create a miniature "steam tent" by draping a towel over your head and shoulders. If the steam is too hot to breathe, let a waft escape, or leave a small gap in the towel to circulate fresh air until you can inhale comfortably. Breathe in the steam for five minutes; do this up to three times a day. For a "wind cold" condition, follow the same procedure but instead mix the herbs hyssop and basil in the bowl, and shake in a few drops of peppermint and thyme oil.

You can also use essential oils by applying them directly to your skin. To help ease a dry cough, I recommend that you massage eucalyptus, peppermint, spearmint, or thyme oils onto your chest and neck at night. (If you have sensitive skin, dilute essential oils in olive or almond oil before applying.) While you sleep, the therapeutic qualities of these oils will permeate your skin, soothe your throat and lungs, and alleviate your cough—and you might even have more pleasant dreams.

Herbal teas can help you relieve a sore throat through their gentle actions on your mucous membranes; they can also relieve sinus and lung congestion and help your immune system fight a cold or flu infection. From a Chinese medicine perspective, herbal teas can ameliorate the effects of hot and cold winds. For a "wind heat" condition, make a tea using equal parts of spearmint, chamomile, and coltsfoot: add a teaspoon of each herb to three cups of boiling water, cover tightly, and remove from heat. Let the tea steep for ten minutes, strain, store it in the refrigerator, and drink a few cups a day. (Rewarm it before you drink it.) For a "wind cold" condition, make a strong ginger tea: slice up two or three inches of ginger root and simmer it in four cups of boiling water for ten minutes. Add a pinch of cinnamon, grate in a clove of garlic, strain, and sip slowly.

Chinese herbal formulas are extremely effective at treating the onset of a cold or flu due to either a "wind heat" or a "wind cold" invasion. Yin Chiao Jie Du Wan, known in English as "Honeysuckle and Forsythia Clear Toxins Pills," is a classic Chinese herbal formula for a common cold caused by "wind heat." It consists of herbs that not only cool heat but also have antibacterial properties. Some of the herbs help to strengthen lung Qi, which fortifies Wei Qi.

The Chinese formula Ge Gen Wan, also known as "Kudzu Formula Pills," is used to treat the common cold due to "wind cold." It contains herbs that have warming and antibiotic properties, and fresh ginger root, which helps to break up phlegm. Ma huang, or ephedra, has also been traditionally used in this formula in minute doses to help open the air passages of the lungs and induce sweating. (In the future, due to recent FDA legislation, Ge Gen Wan may be sold without ma huang, or its use may be limited to licensed acupuncturists.)

The typical recommended dose of both Yin Chiao Jie Du Wan and Ge Gen Wan is eight pills three times a day, depending on what type of pill or pellet is used, taken at the earliest stage of symptoms. You can purchase most Chinese herbal formulas from a practitioner of Chinese medicine.

HOMEOPATHIC TREATMENTS

Homeopathic medicines can be helpful when you have a cold or flu, and they can be used along with any other immunity-supporting treatments recommended here. (If, however, you are taking a homeopathic remedy, you should refrain from using essential oils such as peppermint and eucalyptus, because they may render the remedy less effective.) For more information on using homeopathic medicines, see Appendix A.

The following chart shows how you can use common homeopathic remedies to help fight five different manifestations of colds and flus. You can use these remedies even if your symptoms don't exactly match the ones shown on the chart; as long as you have some of the symptoms listed, a remedy may be effective.

Homeopathic Remedies for a Cold or Flu

ACONITE	BELLADONNA	OSCILLOCOCCINUM	PULSATILLA	GELSEMIUM
Use with these symptoms: Rapid onset of high fever (brought on by exposure to cold, dry wind), anxiety, dry cough, feelings of heat, bursting headache **Dose:** 30c, 3 pills under your tongue every 2 to 3 hours at the onset of symptoms	**Use with these symptoms:** Rapid onset of high fever, restlessness, flushed face, runny nose, sore throat, throbbing headache **Dose:** 30c, 3 pills under your tongue every 2 to 3 hours at the onset of symptoms	**Use with these symptoms:** Sneezing, thick mucus from sinuses, dry irritating cough, ear pain, chills with shivers, anxiety, pale complexion **Dose:** 1 tablet under your tongue at the onset of symptoms, and every 6 hours afterward	**Use with these symptoms:** Thick yellow-green mucus from sinuses and lungs, coughing, chills but with an aversion to heat, headache, weepiness, desire for fresh air **Dose:** 30c, 3 pills under your tongue every 2 to 3 hours at the onset of symptoms	**Use with these symptoms:** Dull headache, drowsiness, drooping eyelids, dizziness, sneezing, dripping nose, sore throat, dry cough, trembling, apathy, muscular weakness **Dose:** 30c, 3 pills under your tongue every 2 to 3 hours at the onset of symptoms

SUPPLEMENTS

There are a number of nutrients you can take to give your immune cells an extra helping hand when you need it the most. Vitamins A and C, zinc, and thymus extracts are the most essential supplements you can use to boost your ability to fight off a cold or flu. From a Chinese medicine viewpoint, these supplements can be used whether you have a "wind heat" or a "wind cold" condition.

Vitamin A was not recommended in the "What You Need in a Daily Multivitamin" chart on pages 58 and 59 because if taken in high enough amounts over the long term (at doses of 100,000 i.u. a day for three months), it can accumulate in your liver and be toxic. But short-term use of vitamin A is safe and can be beneficial when you have a cold or flu: it has antiviral and immunity-enhancing actions and can help restore the integrity of your mucous membranes.[18] Vitamin C is well known for its immunity-supportive properties; much data support its positive effects on many aspects of the immune system, including white blood cells, antibodies, and the thymus gland.

Studies have shown that zinc has antiviral properties and can shorten the duration of a cold or flu by improving the ability of your white blood cells to fight the infection. Supplements containing thymus extract can also augment the function of your immune system when you have a cold or flu by supporting your thymus gland, which helps to mature your white blood cells.

I recommend that at the onset of a cold or flu you begin taking the following:

- Vitamin A: 10,000 i.u. three to five times a day, for up to one week. (If you're pregnant or think you might be pregnant, take no more than 10,000 i.u. a day.)
- Vitamin C: 1,000 mg three to five times a day, for up to five days. (Larger doses of vitamin C can sometimes cause loose stools. It is recommended that you increase your dose until you reach a level of "bowel tolerance." This means taking increasing amounts until you experience loose stools, then reducing your dose to the next lower amount that does not give you loose stools. Your digestive system will much more easily tolerate vitamin C if you take it in a buffered rather than a nonbuffered form.)
- Zinc: 40 mg a day. You may already be taking a multivitamin that gives you this amount; if not, when you have a cold or flu, make sure that you are getting at least 40 mg a day by taking a zinc lozenge.
- Thymus extract: 750 mg twice a day. Thymus extract can be found at your health food store.

Extra Immunity Support

In the 1980s, when I began the doctoral program at Bastyr University in Seattle, it seemed as if no one outside the naturopathic community had ever heard of a native American herb called echinacea. Within a decade the herb had achieved such superstar status that it was a household word; by the late 1990s it was even being mentioned in popular movies like *You've Got Mail*. Echinacea's rise in popularity is a tribute to its effectiveness as an immunity-boosting agent. It contains polysaccharides, which are beneficial sugars that mobilize your immune cells to go into action when you have a viral, bacterial, or parasitic infection.[19] Echinacea can be safely taken on a continuous basis for up to eight weeks at a time. But it's best used in the treatment of an acute infection, such as a cold or flu, and I don't recommend using it on an extended basis.

Although echinacea has not been traditionally used in Chinese medicine, it can be helpful if you are diagnosed with a "wind heat" condition because it can be considered a "cooling" herb.

Echinacea can be taken during pregnancy and lactation, or given to children, but it should not be used if you have rheumatoid arthritis, lupus, or any other autoimmune disease. To take echinacea as a tea, simmer four tablespoons of dried echinacea root in four cups of water for ten minutes, strain, and drink one cup every hour. (You need to drink a lot to get the full benefits of the herb.) If you take echinacea as a tincture, choose one made by a reputable company in Appendix B, and take one teaspoon three to six times a day. If you prefer taking echinacea as a pill, I suggest 300 mg, taken three times a day, of a standardized extract containing 3.5 percent echinacosides.

When you have a cold or flu, it is especially easy to make food your medicine if you love garlic. I can't say enough good things about garlic. From a Western perspective, it is a potent immunity-promoting food that is antimicrobial, antiviral, and antiparasitic. From a Chinese point of view, if you are diagnosed with a "wind cold" condition, garlic will help you get over it more quickly because of its strong "warming" qualities.

At the very first sign that you have a cold or flu, I recommend that you chop up one or two medium-sized cloves of raw garlic, mix the pieces into a spread or nut butter, and slather it on toast. This is a good way to ingest enough garlic to help you fight off a virus or bacterial infection—or maybe even nip it in the bud. If your digestion can tolerate it, do this two or three times a day. To help your garlic toast go down, keep a cup of hot ginger tea on hand. If you don't like to eat raw garlic, eat at least three cloves of cooked garlic in your meals, or take garlic in pill form, also known as "sociable garlic." (Take at least 5,000 mcg of allicin, the active compound in garlic, per day.)

Your Protective Shield: Final Thoughts

The principles of natural healing—from the contemporary Western approach to the ancient wisdom of Chinese medicine—can help you create a healthy immune system that will keep your entire body strong and vital. By using all the tools that we've discussed, and by choosing a lifestyle that continually nourishes and stimulates your immune system, you can have optimal health throughout your life.

The Essence of Chapter 2

- Protect your immune system and listen to its signals.
- Keep your Metal element balanced and maintain the strength of your immune system, especially if you are a Metal type.
- Use natural skin care products.
- Take a multivitamin every day and other supplements if needed.
- Nurture yourself, and manage your stress wisely.
- Bolster your immune system with Chinese herbal supertonics.
- Do hydrotherapy to stimulate your immune system and promote detoxification.
- If you get a cold or flu, treat it with natural medicine.

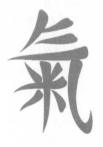

Chapter 3

Energy

Flowing Water: Protecting Your Kidneys, Your Source of Life

"We need the power of the Water Element's flow of water within our spirit to wash away the pollution which can affect the very core of our being."

—J. R. WORSLEY, *Classical Five Element Acupuncture*

KATRINA CAME to see me because at forty-five years of age she didn't think it was normal to have absolutely no libido. "I've always enjoyed a healthy intimate life with my husband," she said, "but now I'm simply too exhausted when we have time to make love, and I can't muster the energy it takes to enjoy sex." Katrina was under the impression that taking hormones would correct the problem, but she was concerned about their side effects. As it turned out, she didn't need to take hormones—she had regular menstrual cycles and her hormone levels were normal.

After discovering that Katrina had been under a great deal of stress, I recommended that we look at ways to build her kidney Qi, which can have a profound effect on a woman's libido and which can be depleted by chronic tension. After a few months on Chinese herbs, along with lifestyle changes to build her kidney Qi, Katrina said, "This approach took *time—it wasn't a quick fix—but not only has my libido increased, I feel totally revitalized on all levels!"*

❧❧

Your Kidney and Bladder Health

As Katrina was, you may be surprised to learn how the health of your kidneys can affect your overall vitality. Your kidneys serve you in countless ways. They are one of your primary organs of detoxification, they help maintain your body's fluid and mineral balance, and they clear waste products out of your system. If your kidneys didn't do their job of constantly cleaning your blood, you would either become excessively swollen from too many fluids or you would perish from dehydration.

Your kidneys work closely with your bladder to remove waste products from your body. Most women take their kidneys and bladder for granted until they become a source of irritation, which happens to a significant portion of the population. In the United States, urinary tract infections account for four million doctor visits each year.[1] Urinary incontinence, or involuntary release of urine, affects 14 to 16 million women in this country and some estimates are even higher.[2] Problems associated with the urinary system can have a major impact on the quality of women's lives.

In this chapter you will discover the many tools you need to maintain and enhance your kidney and bladder health from both a Western and a Chinese medicine perspective. You will find out how to evaluate the health of your kidneys and bladder, how to support them in ways that can improve your overall vitality and longevity, and how to strengthen your kidney Qi. And if you have a history of chronic urinary tract infections, interstitial cystitis, incontinence, or kidney stones, you will learn how to assist your body with these conditions using natural medicine.

The View from the West

Your two kidneys are located just beneath the lower ribs on either side of your lower back. They contain an amazing system of millions of tiny filtering units known as nephrons, which work around the clock to keep your blood clean. The kidneys dispose of the waste the nephrons filter out by making urine that flushes the toxins away. From the kidneys, the urine passes into small tubes called ureters that travel down to your bladder, until it is released when you feel the urge to go to the bathroom. You also rely on your kidneys to maintain a healthy pH level (the body's acid-alkaline balance), in addition to assisting in the synthesis of vitamin D—which is critical for your calcium absorption and your ability to maintain healthy bones. The kidneys also play a role in controlling your blood volume and blood pressure, and they secrete erythropoietin, a hormone that enables you to make red blood cells.

Protecting your kidneys and bladder from harm may not be something you've ever thought about, but dehydration and certain unhealthy lifestyle habits can create problems in these two organs. A lack of water or urine that is too acidic can trigger the formation of kidney stones. High-protein diets can eventually harm your kidneys, and a number of medications (such as nonsteroidal anti-inflammatory drugs) can damage their delicate filtration system. Bacteria from an untreated urinary tract infection could cause a kidney infection and lead to chronic urinary problems.

The View from the East

"The kidney abides within us like the bear in its cave, harboring the germ of being, the Essence, that feeds and renews our life force."

—HARRIET BEINFIELD AND EFREM KORNGOLD,
Between Heaven and Earth

In Chinese medicine, kidney Qi (remember, Qi is your essential energy) is thought of as the Source of Life because it is the very center of vitality. It is the well from which all creativity springs and the source of all yin and yang in the body. As in Western medicine, the kidneys and bladder are closely linked in the Chinese system; in fact, bladder Qi plays a very supportive role to kidney Qi, and the bladder and kidneys are classified as "paired organs" (a term used in Chinese medicine to refer to unique organ relationships that are useful when you need to take special care of a particular organ or system).

According to ancient Chinese texts, the kidneys are also the source of inherited wisdom. We each have a form of ancestral Qi, known as "Essence," that is passed down from one generation to another. Stored in your kidneys, it is often referred to as "kidney Essence," and it plays an important role in governing birth, growth, and reproduction. Your kidney Essence gave form to your brain, spinal cord, bones, teeth, and hair while you were still in the womb, and it supports these tissues throughout your life. If your kidney Essence is well nourished, you will have healthy mental and physical development, strong bones and teeth, and shiny, healthy hair. (Premature graying is a sign of deficient kidney Essence.)

Your kidney Essence, your spirit, and your overall Qi are called your Three Treasures. (In Chinese medicine, the word *spirit* is used much as it is in the West, often to connote an essential higher, transcendent, or nonphysical aspect of life; it has also been linked with the psyche, personality, and ego.) If you lead a life of excesses, squandering your Qi—that is, throwing it away unnecessarily with unhealthy lifestyle choices—you can deplete your Three Treasures. This can prematurely exhaust your vitality, increase your chances of developing kidney or urinary problems, and cause you to grow old before your time, leading to diseases associated with old age such as osteoporosis. For centuries, people in China have been taught the importance of pre-serving and strengthening their Three Treasures with practices such as Qi Gong and Tai Chi.

In Chinese medicine kidney Qi and Essence also direct physical and sexual de-velopment and keep the libido healthy. Decreased sex drive is a classic sign of depleted kidney Qi. Although the ancient text *The Art of the Bedchamber* makes it clear that ro-bust sexuality has long been considered a natural and healthy experience in China, tra-ditional Chinese medical philosophy cautions that too much sex, too often, can deplete your kidney Qi. If you have weak kidney Qi, you can also have reproductive problems such as an inability to conceive or maintain pregnancy. When your kidney Qi is strong, you will have greater vitality and will lead a more creative, abundant life.

The Water Element

Kelly, a successful career woman, came to see me with complaints of exhaustion, excess weight, and frequent illness. She had experienced chronic bladder infections and taken more antibiotics than she could count to treat them. When I asked Kelly about her emotional state, it became clear that she was a Water type and that she had ended up in a job that wasn't con-gruent with her true self. "My job demands that I am social all the time," she said. "I have to take clients to luncheons, give presentations, and manage about twenty people. Because I am most comfortable being my own boss, working alone and in a quiet atmosphere, the stress that I encounter at work is far greater for me than for someone who enjoys interacting with people all day."

Discovering that she was a Water type proved to be an enormous breakthrough for Kelly. It helped her rearrange her priorities and career so that she could make choices based on what she really wanted, rather than on other people's definition of success. Since then, her energy has returned and her life has been transformed. "Not only have I been much happier," she now says, "but my physical health has improved remarkably."

∽✕∽

Your kidney Qi, together with your bladder Qi, is responsible for controlling the wa-terways in your body, and it makes sense that in Chinese medicine the kidneys are represented by the Water element. If Water is your predominant element, you will find it particularly beneficial to pay close attention to the issues we will explore in this chapter. Even if you are not predominantly a Water type, this chapter will help you balance your Water element and strengthen your kidney Qi.

If you have a prevalence of the Water element, you are a seeker of wisdom. In your youth, you had the quality of being "wise beyond your years." As an adult you are a deep thinker, always searching for truth and meaning. You are a philosopher, comfortable in the world of your mind, and you often prefer your own thoughts to a superficial dialogue with others. You may enjoy elucidating your ideas in writing, and you are inclined to seek refuge among great books to do the work you are passionate about. Like water, you naturally gravitate to quiet places where you become tranquil and reflective. The old saying "Still waters run deep" perfectly embodies your spirit.

In Chinese medicine, kidney Qi has a unique connection with the sense of hearing; it is said that the kidneys "open to the ears." If you are a Water type, music has a special power to nourish and console you. You are apt to be a music lover and are likely musically talented, because music allows you to express yourself without having to articulate your feelings verbally. Music is a fluent medium, much like water; it has the capacity to move around objects and fill spaces, yet slip through your fingers and beyond your grasp.

When your Water element is balanced, you have a great deal of confidence and ambition. Your mind is sharp, you have a keen perception of life, and your spirit is strong and independent. You also have deep, well-developed values that you never compromise, no matter what the occasion, and you adapt yourself incredibly well to new obstacles in your path. Physically, you are healthy and vigorous. The Water element is strongly associated with salty tastes; when you are out of balance, you tend to either crave or abhor salty foods. You thrive on a low-salt diet with a minimum of spicy foods and lots of pure water, and exercises that stimulate your circulation, especially swimming. As long as you don't squander or dissipate your kidney Qi with a stressful lifestyle and a low-nutrient diet, you remain consistently healthy.

Your Water element is governed by the season of winter, the time of hibernation when the earth is still, cold, and silent and everything quietly waits for spring to burst forth. On a daily basis, your Water element rules the hours of darkness until the sun rises in the morning. As a Water type, you are a survivor, with enormous willpower and inner strength; you have all the stamina, endurance, and tenacity necessary to tough it out through the challenges of the long cold season or the "dark night of the soul." In *Wood Becomes Water: Chinese Medicine in Everyday Life,* Gail Reichstein points out that "water's power is not about action, or even preparation for action, but the power of potential action that we hold within."[3] Your Water element represents the period of time in which you are pregnant with possibilities but haven't yet begun to manifest them. This state of nonaction is full of promise, raw potential energy, and power.

But if you are predominantly a Water type, you may also have a tendency to spend too much time in solitude and waste your vital energy, either mentally or physically, by living too long in "survival mode." When this happens, your Water element can become imbalanced and disrupt your health on many levels. You are particularly prone to urinary tract infections and kidney stones, bladder problems, edema (swelling with water retention in your tissues), dehydration, stiff and painful joints, bone problems such as osteoporosis, and sexual difficulties such as diminished libido or an inability to achieve orgasm. On an emotional level, if your Water element is weak, your normally deep reservoir of inner strength can spill over into fear, especially when you are faced with the unknown. A Water type who is imbalanced and remains too long in isolation from others can become fearful, paranoid, despondent, or anxious. Instead of the usual mental and emotional clarity, there is forgetfulness and apathy.

If you are a Water type, the most important way to keep your kidney Qi in peak condition is to honor who you are rather than strive to become something you are not. Your challenge is to create a life that allows you to fully manifest your true nature. Our culture tends to be most supportive of ambitious Wood types or charismatic Fire types. Many Water types, like Kelly, try to be high-powered career women—and often succeed because they are strong-willed and resolute—but in the end find themselves deeply unhappy. Often, a breakdown in their health is what wakes them up to what they really want from life and to what they are best suited.

Are You a Water Type?

- Are you a seeker of truth and wisdom?
- Do you prefer being alone to being with company?
- Are you independent-minded?
- Do you have philosophical leanings?
- Do you consistently live according to deep religious or spiritual beliefs?
- Do you tend to be strong willed, even stubborn?
- Are you happiest when you are involved with a solitary project that you are passionate about?
- Do you prefer tranquil, secluded, secret places?
- Do you have a great deal of confidence and the ability to cope with challenges?
- Do you persevere long after others have given up?
- When you are not in good health, do you tend to become fearful, suspicious, or even paranoid of others?
- Do you enjoy exercises that stimulate your circulation?
- Do you have a particularly strong affinity for music?
- Do you tend to get kidney stones or have frequent urinary tract infections?

If you answered yes to most of the above questions, you are most likely a Water type. It is especially important for you to take the following steps to keep your body healthy, maintain strong kidney Qi, and balance your Water element:

Find tranquil, quiet places where you can be reflective.

Give yourself time to nurture your intellectual and spiritual pursuits.

Maintain a regular exercise routine in order to enhance your circulation; swimming is especially conducive to your Water element.

Choose a profession that you are passionate about and that supports your need to work in a quiet environment.

Play music to nourish your Water element.

Maintain a balanced lifestyle that doesn't squander your kidney Qi and Essence.

Avoid excessive salt and spicy foods in your diet.

Drink plenty of fresh, clean water.

Create time to socialize so that you don't become too isolated and emotionally inaccessible to others.

Is Your Kidney and Bladder Health Compromised?

In the following pages, you will discover how to evaluate your kidney and bladder health from the perspective of both West and East, and how to prevent or treat the most common kidney and urinary tract problems that women face. (Often the methods are the same, and prevention is always the best cure.) It's especially important to monitor the health of your kidneys and bladder if you are a Water type, because you are particularly prone to kidney and bladder problems. But kidney and bladder conditions—including urinary tract infections, interstitial cystitis, urinary incontinence, and kidney stones—affect a great number of women. Some kidney and bladder problems can be serious, so if you have kidney or bladder symptoms, it's best to see your physician.

In conventional Western medicine, your kidneys and bladder can be evaluated by your physician through laboratory tests, including a standard blood test, a urinalysis, a urine culture, and a pH test. These tests can tell you if your kidneys are functioning properly, if you have bacteria in your urine, or if the pH of your urine indicates an alkaline-acid imbalance in your body. They can help you determine whether you might have any of the urinary tract conditions that we will explore later in this chapter.

In Chinese medicine, the health of your kidneys and bladder is strongly influenced by the strength of your kidney Qi. You can assess your kidney Qi by examining your physical and emotional symptoms and by observing your tongue and pulse. There are many different types of kidney Qi imbalances; three of the most common are outlined in the "Kidney Imbalances from a Chinese Medicine Perspective" chart. Determining if you have any of these imbalances, and knowing your Chinese diagnosis, can help you choose the treatments and lifestyle changes that will best balance your kidney Qi.

Kidney Imbalances from a Chinese Medicine Perspective

SYMPTOMS	MOST LIKELY CAUSES	QUALITY OF THE TONGUE	QUALITY OF THE PULSE	CHINESE DIAGNOSIS
You have anxiety, tension, feelings of being tired yet agitated at the same time, scanty and dark urination, dizziness, poor memory, night sweating, afternoon fevers, insomnia, prematurely gray hair, constipation, thirst, a dry mouth at night, a sore back, achy bones, or feelings of heat in your palms and in the soles of your feet.	You have too much mental strain and stress, excessive sexual activity, chronic loss of blood, chronic illness, a lack of body fluids due to fever, or have taken too many yang-stimulating herbs.	Your tongue is red with crack lines and no coating.	Rapid and thin	Kidney yin deficiency
You have apathy, a lack of willpower and drive, frequent urination, an aversion to cold, infertility, poor appetite, weakness or water retention in your legs, a sore back, loose stools, or a feeling that you are "cold in your bones."	You have an excess of physically demanding work, too much sexual activity, spleen Qi deficiency leading to an excess of "dampness," or chronic illness; aging can also cause a deficiency of kidney yang.	Your tongue is pale, swollen, and unusually wet.	Weak and not easily felt on the surface of your skin	Kidney yang deficiency
You have decreased sexual drive and ability, hair loss, prematurely gray hair, loose and fragile teeth, poor memory, or problems with reproduction.	You have a stressful lifestyle, a high-protein, high-sugar diet, and exposure to toxins from your environment, food, and water; aging can also cause a deficiency of kidney Essence.	Your tongue is red, and its coating has a "peeled" appearance (the coating is absent in places).	"Floating and empty," which means you can feel it on the surface of your skin, but it isn't a full, strong pulse	Kidney Essence deficiency

Nourishing Your Kidneys

The Naturally Healthy Diet (outlined in Chapter 1) will keep your entire body healthy, preserving your kidney Qi and kidney Essence. In addition, certain foods can provide extra support for your kidneys. Eating a more alkaline diet (as discussed later in this chapter), choosing the highest-quality salt, and drinking plenty of clean water can all make your kidneys' job much easier and improve your overall health. And Chinese medicine has some very helpful suggestions for choosing foods to build your kidney Qi and nourish your Source of Life. In addition to your diet, you will discover that your kidney Qi and kidney Essence are nourished with Chinese herbal aphrodisiacs, Tai Chi, Qi Gong, meditation, aromatherapy, and flower essences.

In Chinese medicine, diet not only supplies the body with the nutrients it needs to function, but it also provides the foundation for Qi. Kidney Qi, which plays a critical role in the body's overall Qi, is particularly susceptible to imbalances in diet. Certain foods can help kidney Qi regain its equilibrium and also build kidney Essence.

For imbalances that are due to a kidney yin deficiency, it is recommended that you eat foods and herbs that are "cooling" in nature to build your kidney yin. They include tofu, squash, mushrooms, beans, sprouts, eggplant, watermelon, berries, grapes, blue corn, wild rice, seaweeds, spirulina, eggs, barley, black sesame seeds, and purple potatoes. For imbalances that are due to a kidney yang deficiency, it is best to eat "warming" foods and herbs, which have been used in China for centuries to build kidney yang. These include chicken, salmon, lamb, onion, garlic, walnuts, ginger, cloves, anise, pepper, and fennel. For imbalances that are due to kidney Essence deficiency, practice the Naturally Healthy Lifestyle. If your vitality is low from excessive stress, toxins, or a poor-quality diet, your kidney Essence is probably depleted. To rebuild it, increase your consumption of proteins such as low-mercury fish and soups made with the meat and bones of organically grown beef, chicken, or turkey. If you are a vegetarian, foods for rebuilding your kidney Essence include wheatgrass, barley greens, spirulina, royal jelly, and bee pollen.

Your pH Balance

Your pH level measures the balance of how alkaline or acidic your body is. You are healthiest when your pH is neutral or slightly on the alkaline side. The standard American diet, however, contains many low-mineral foods that make the body more acidic: foods high in protein, sugar, saturated fat, alcohol, processed grains, beans, and some nuts. Although it's healthy to eat protein, grains, beans, and nuts in moderation, consuming them in excess and at the exclusion of fruits and vegetables can create an excess of acid, putting undue stress on your kidneys and other organs and systems in your body.

Testing Your pH Balance

Your pH is measured on a scale of 1 to 14; a pH below 7.0 is acidic, and a pH greater than 7.0 is alkaline. Your body naturally keeps the pH of your blood at a constant 7.4, but the pH of your other tissues should be maintained at about 7.0. Keeping your pH in this range involves many factors, including diet, exercise, stress, and the actions of your kidneys, intestines, lungs, and skin. Your kidneys play an especially important role; if your diet and lifestyle create a chronically acidic pH in your tissues, your kidneys have to work harder to maintain equilibrium because they are unable to excrete urine with a pH lower than 5.0. To test the pH of your urine, you can use pH test papers found at your local health food store or pharmacy. It's best to test your urine pH in the morning, right after you wake up. The more acidic your urine is, the more acidic your body is. Your goal is to keep your urine pH at 6.5 or greater.

Stress can also make your body more acidic, as can many prescription medications. Another source of acid in your body is a by-product of excessive exercise, lactic acid (which is what makes your muscles sore after you exercise). The bottom line is that you don't feel well when your body is too acidic, and you can experience headaches, fatigue, greater susceptibility to infections, an increase in free radicals, and a decrease in your liver's ability to detoxify.[4] A chronically acidic pH could lead to yeast and bacterial overgrowth, autoimmune diseases, and degenerative conditions.

The good news is that your body has built-in mechanisms to remedy an acid-forming diet and lifestyle. It naturally buffers an acid state with alkaline minerals such as calcium and magnesium. If your body is too acidic as a result of eating the low-mineral standard American diet, however, you will make frequent withdrawals from your mineral "savings account"—your bones—to buffer the acids. For this reason, a diet and lifestyle that are chronically acid-forming can increase your risk of developing osteoporosis or osteoarthritis.

The foods that promote an acidic condition in your body are not necessarily the same ones that have an acidic taste in your mouth. Oranges, for instance, actually make your body more alkaline once they are metabolized. In general, foods containing the minerals calcium, magnesium, potassium, and sodium (such as fruits and vegetables) are alkaline-forming, whereas foods that contain high quantities of sulfur and phosphorus (such as meats and beans) are acid-forming. The following table indicates which types of foods make your body more acidic and which make it more alkaline.

Alkaline- and Acid-Forming Foods and Drinks

	ALKALINE-FORMING	LOW ACID-FORMING	ACID-FORMING
Vegetables	Most vegetables	Spinach, zucchini, and rhubarb	Carrots, chard, and tomatoes
Animal meats and eggs		Eggs, wild venison, and wild duck	Beef, veal, chicken, and pork
Seafood	Seaweeds	Fish and crab	Lobster, eel, shellfish, mollusks, and oysters
Dairy products	Ghee (clarified butter)	Sheep cheese, goat cheese, cream, butter, and yogurt from cow's milk	Cow's milk, goat milk, processed cheese, and aged cheese
Cow's milk substitutes			Soy milk
Grasses and sprouts	All grasses and sprouts		
Grains	Oats, quinoa, and wild rice	Brown rice, millet, kasha, amaranth, and triticale	Refined grains, wheat, corn, rye, oat bran, buckwheat, spelt, teff, farina, and white rice
Fats and oils	Flaxseed, cod liver, olive, and avocado oils	Grape seed, sunflower, and canola oils	Saturated animal fats, cottonseed oil, palm kernel seed oil, and lard
Fruits	Most fruits	Figs, dates, guavas, and pickled fruit	Plums, cranberries, pomegranates, and prunes
Nuts and seeds	Almonds, chestnuts, and most seeds	Pine nuts	Brazil nuts, walnuts, hazelnuts, pecans, peanuts, and pistachio nuts
Beans and legumes	Lentils	Kidney beans, fava beans, string beans, and wax beans	Pinto beans, white beans, navy beans, adzuki beans, lima beans, chickpeas, green peas, and snow peas
Sweeteners	Molasses, Sucanat, and rice syrup	Honey and maple syrup	Refined sugar, stevia, and saccharin
Beverages	Mineral water, green tea, and ginger tea	Kona coffee and sake	Coffee, soft drinks, black tea, beer, and alcohol
Spices	Sea salt, soy sauce, garlic, ginger, curry, and cinnamon		Table salt, nutmeg, cocoa, and vanilla
Vinegars	Apple cider and umeboshi vinegar	Rice vinegar	White acetic and balsamic vinegar

Source: Information derived from Dr. Russell Jaffe, *The Alkaline Way: Your Health Restoration* (brochure). These foods were analyzed based on total food composition and how the human body metabolizes them.

As the chart makes clear, the majority of the foods many people choose to eat are acid-forming. Popular high-protein, high-fat, low-carbohydrate diets, such as the one advocated by Dr. Atkins, create an acidic condition. The Atkins diet creates this acidity not only because it recommends foods that are acid-forming, but also because it produces ketones. Ketones are compounds that form when your body is digesting fat from your own tissues for energy—a state known as ketosis. This may seem like a favorable state for weight loss, but the presence of ketones in urine is not a sign of good health. (You form ketones if you deprive your body of food for long periods of time.) Ketosis puts a great deal of stress on the kidneys and the entire body.

Eating some acid-forming foods occasionally shouldn't be a problem, but I recommend that you eat primarily alkaline-forming and low acid-forming foods. Such mineral-rich foods—which include most fruits and vegetables—make you feel good, give you abundant energy, and make you less prone to disease. In addition, you should keep tabs on your diet by testing your urine pH periodically to make sure that you aren't eating too many acid-forming foods. You may need to increase your consumption of alkaline-forming foods during times when you are under a lot of stress, or if you have certain health conditions such as arthritis or an autoimmune disorder.

WHAT'S IN YOUR SALT?

When it comes to health, we should rephrase the old saying "You're worth your salt" to ask, "Is your salt worthy of you?" You probably haven't given much thought to what's in your salt shaker, but the commercial salt you purchase goes through a metamorphosis before it reaches your dinner table. It is heated, bleached, stripped of its trace minerals, and most likely treated with anticaking agents that contain aluminum. Some salts even have sugar added to them!

Salt, also known as sodium, is an essential mineral for every cell in the body. It helps regulate the heartbeat, blood pressure, nerve transmission, muscle contraction, stomach acid, and pH balance. The kidneys play an important role in balancing the body's salt level. If you have too much salt, your kidneys excrete it into your urine; if you have too little, your kidneys recycle it back to your bloodstream.

How much sodium do you need? The National Research Council recommends a daily intake of 1,100 to 3,300 mg of sodium each day for adults.[5] (One teaspoon of salt gives you 2,300 mg of sodium.) The average American consumes between 4,000 and 5,000 mg of sodium every day, and some sources estimate twice that amount. Anyone who consistently eats the standard American diet has no problem getting enough salt; processed foods are riddled with it. Rather, the problem usually lies in getting too much salt—and especially the wrong kind. From both a Western and a Chinese medicine perspective, high amounts of salt in the diet can cause calcium loss. Over time a chronically high consumption of salt can weaken your bones and increase your risk of developing osteoporosis.

High blood pressure has also been associated with ingesting too much salt. But researchers have found that simply removing salt from the diet is not enough. The key factor is the ratio of sodium to potassium—two components that work together in a unique way to regulate your water balance, which affects your blood pressure. Studies show that when sodium is decreased and potassium is increased, blood pressure can drop.[6] (And when you maintain the right ratio of sodium to potassium, your body is more alkaline.) The healthiest ratio is five times as much potassium as sodium. Yet most people on the standard American diet ingest twice as much sodium as potassium. The Naturally Healthy Diet, which includes plenty of fresh fruits and vegetables, will give you lots of potassium but very little sodium.

Table salt contains the minerals sodium and chloride, both of which are critical to health. But the refined salt in most salt shakers lacks important minerals and trace minerals found in unprocessed salt, including calcium, magnesium, sulfur, silicon, iodine, bromine, phosphorus, and vanadium. As a result, table salt is acid-forming. (Even the "sea salt" that is sold in health food stores has often been highly processed.) By contrast, unrefined salt that comes from the sea or is mined from ancient salt beds in the earth is alkaline-forming. For resources on how to obtain healthy, alkaline-forming salt, see Appendix B.

According to Chinese medicine, as we've seen, the Water element is associated with salty tastes. (When your element is out of balance, your desire for salt can be either exceptionally strong or weak.) Some salt is beneficial to kidney Qi, but too much can adversely affect it. As a mineral whose energetic qualities are contractive and moistening, salt can help you feel emotionally grounded and secure, but in excess it can induce emotional insecurity and fear. As Paul Pitchford, author of *Healing with Whole Foods: Oriental Traditions and Modern Nutrition,* points out, "Our desire for salt may reflect an internal wish for a more emotionally safe foundation . . . However, too much of an extreme substance such as salt causes its properties to reverse—kidney damage, fear, rigid legs and pelvis are all symptoms of a poor emotional and physical foundation resulting from excess salt."[7]

FLOWING WATER

"Water symbolizes both life and death: it is the womb from which all life emerges and the abyss to which it returns."

—GAIL REICHSTEIN, *Wood Becomes Water: Chinese Medicine in Everyday Life*

From both a Chinese and a Western medicine perspective, optimizing kidney function and maximizing the health of the whole body means drinking plenty of pure, clean water. But most people drink far too little water, and to make matters worse, they consume an excess of fluids like coffee and alcohol, which actually dehydrate them. A deficiency of water can lead to headaches, dry skin, constipation, poor detoxification, impaired immunity, urinary tract infections, and kidney stones. You should drink at least 48 ounces of water a day. And considering that your body weight is 50 to 60 percent water,[8] it makes a lot of sense to consume water of the highest possible quality.

The Environmental Working Group (EWG) has published numerous articles on water quality and contaminants in tap water. According to one article, "Weed Killers by the Glass," millions of Americans living in the Midwest have been exposed to high levels of pesticides by consuming tap water. "During peak runoff periods," the article reports, "pesticide contamination levels repeatedly exceed federal health standards and pose significant health risks."[9] But contamination of tap water is not limited to the Midwest. Chemicals that are used on farmland, or around your own property, can penetrate artesian wells and pollute groundwater after a heavy rainfall.

Chlorine in tap water is also a problem. It is added to public water supplies to kill bacteria, but it poses a significant health risk when it reacts with organic matter such as soil, fertilizers, sewage, or plant materials, because then it forms toxic by-products. The EWG points out that "a compelling body of scientific evidence—nearly 30 peer-reviewed epidemiologic studies—links chlorinated by-products to increased risks of cancer."[10] Research also shows that elevated levels of chlorine by-products in tap water—which have apparently risen as our rivers and reservoirs have become more polluted, resulting in ever more chlorine being added to kill bacteria—increase the risk of miscarriage and birth defects. Dumping more chlorine into the water supply to "clean" it is clearly not the answer; cleaning up our environment, the source of our tap water, is.

Recently, a number of water treatment facilities in the United States have been switching to a different chlorine compound, chloramine, to meet new standards requiring lower levels of chlorine by-products in tap water. But according to the EWG, the long-term effects of consuming chloramine by-products are essentially unknown; fish cannot survive in water treated with this compound, and kidney patients on dialysis are advised not to drink it.

Excess fluoride is another potential health hazard that may be in your tap water. Although it was originally added to public water supplies with the best of intentions—to help prevent tooth decay—its long-term effects are very controversial. The type of fluoride added to the water supply in most major American cities is hydrofluosilicic acid, a highly toxic by-product derived from the manufacture of phosphate fertilizer.[11] According to the head of preventive dentistry at the University of Toronto, Hardy Limeback, Ph.D., D.D.S., this form of fluoride, even when diluted to one part per million, "adds unwanted arsenic, beryllium, cadmium, lead, silicon, and even radioactive nuclides to the water."[12] He also expresses concerns about the potential effects of long-term accumulation of fluoride in bodily tissues, pointing out that "it likely affects thyroid function, may have neurological effects, may induce reproductive problems and may affect the pineal gland." Other studies indicate that chronic fluoride exposure could increase the incidence of osteoporosis.

Most countries in Western Europe, including Austria, Norway, Northern Ireland, Sweden, Denmark, Holland, France, Finland, Germany, and Belgium, do not fluoridate their public drinking water. Data from the World Health Organization has shown that people in these countries do not have higher amounts of tooth decay than people in countries where the water is fluoridated.[13] Clearly, the risks of being exposed to toxic compounds in water are not worth whatever potential benefits fluoride may provide; you can effectively prevent tooth decay with good dental care, regular brushing and flossing, and eating the Naturally Healthy Diet.

Whether your water is "soft" or "hard" also affects your health. Soft water contains a lot of sodium, and hard water has a higher amount of calcium and magnesium. Soft water is often considered desirable because it won't turn your clothes gray in the wash or leave a ring on your tub as hard water does. But soft water can elevate your daily sodium consumption and may increase your risk of hypertension. Another problem associated with soft water is that it can cause toxic heavy metals, including lead and cadmium, to be dissolved into the water supply from pipes in plumbing systems.

To a great extent, you can choose what kind of water you drink by using a water filter. I recommend that you use filtered water for all of your drinking and cooking. (Bottled water may taste good, but it can still contain undesirable chemicals.) Carbon filters, which you can attach right to your faucet, remove many substances—but not fluoride. To remove fluoride from your water, the best and most economical water filter is a reverse osmosis filter, which usually includes two or three different filtering methods and is connected to the water pipes under your sink. It protects you from chlorine, fluoride, bacteria, parasites, excessive sodium, heavy metals, and a host of other unwanted chemicals that may be in your tap water. This method has the added benefits of giving the water higher oxygen content and better taste. The drawbacks are that it wastes water (not all incoming water circulates through the filter) and removes minerals from the water, so make sure you are getting adequate minerals in your diet or in your supplements. If feasible, purchase a water filter for your entire house, so that you use filtered water when you bathe; your skin can absorb contaminants in unfiltered water. You can also purchase a small water filter that fits onto your showerhead.

CHINESE HERBAL APHRODISIACS

For centuries the Chinese have associated vibrant health and longevity with both abundant kidney Qi and strong libido. In Chinese medicine, kidney Qi and Essence direct sexual development and keep the libido healthy; improving the health of the kidneys often means increasing the health of the libido. Some of the most expensive and sought-after kidney-supportive Chinese herbal formulas (mixtures of herbs that have specific effects when combined together) have become known as aphrodisiacs; they enhance sex drive and performance because they build kidney yin, kidney yang, and kidney Essence. Many also enhance immunity, energy, and stamina, giving them a profound impact on overall health and longevity. According to Anne Marie Colbin, author of *Food and Healing,* "An aphrodisiac is a substance that will expand and relax someone who is sexually too tight, or contract and strengthen someone who is too spacey and scattered."[14] A number of Chinese herbal aphrodisiacs have both of these properties; they contain compounds that can stimulate as well as sedate your nervous system. This may sound surprising, but because of their dual actions Chinese herbal aphrodisiacs are legendary.

The Chinese have invested a few thousand years of research in perfecting herbal formulas for preserving sexual vitality. But it is sometimes difficult for Westerners to understand that these formulas are meant to be used within the context of boosting every aspect of your health. In the age of Viagra, it cannot be emphasized enough that taking a single drug or herbal formula does not make you sexually potent. Great health and vitality are what give you sexual vigor.

The health of your libido is measured not just by how much and how often you want to engage in sexual activity; it is much more than that. A woman's libido requires having energy and vitality, but also feeling relaxed and loving. Men tend to take herbal aphrodisiacs to build kidney yang energy for short bursts of sexual satisfaction, but women need to take them over a long period of time to build both kidney yin and kidney yang energy. Building only your kidney yang energy will ultimately exhaust your kidney yin and kidney Essence. By strengthening your kidney yin, kidney yang, *and* kidney Essence, herbal aphrodisiacs can fortify your sexual vitality by gently strengthening the health of your entire body.

The following are some of the best Chinese herbs with aphrodisiac properties. You can find them in many Chinese herbal formulas traditionally given to enhance libido and sexual performance, and in those prescribed for women who are infertile or menopausal. Here, these herbs are recommended primarily for their ability to enhance your kidney Qi and kidney Essence. Taking increased amounts of these herbs is not always beneficial; too much may have the opposite effect. For instance, taking an excessive amount of an herb that strengthens your kidney yang when you are lacking kidney yin can create an imbalance in your Qi and result in a lack of libido. For best results, consult with your Chinese medicine practitioner.

Chinese Ginseng. This powerful herb can strengthen Qi and help the body adapt to stress. It is used as a sexual tonic because of its modulating effects on the nervous system. If you are lethargic, it can give you sexual energy, and if you are tense, it can help you relax. Chinese ginseng contains compounds that may have effects on the body resembling those of certain sex and adrenal hormones. It does not act as an immediate sexual stimulant, but when taken long term it can enhance sexual vitality. It is usually used in combination with other herbal aphrodisiacs to increase sexual potency, kidney yang, and kidney Essence. In postmenopausal women ginseng can prevent atrophy of the vulvar and vaginal tissues. As a single herb, the recommended dose of ginseng is 200 mg taken two to three times a day. Chinese ginseng should not be taken by women with a deficiency of kidney yin because it can be too warming.

Rehmannia. Superb for nourishing kidney yin and kidney Essence, this herb is said to be "food for the kidneys," very rejuvenating, and with the potential to increase longevity. Rehmannia is usually used in combination with other herbs to build Blood and to strengthen yin and Qi. As a woman's herb, it can enhance sexuality and draw Qi and energy into the reproductive organs. You will benefit most from the prepared form of rehmannia that has been soaked in wine, steamed, and sun-dried. (This form should not be used if you have diarrhea.) Rehmannia is seldom prescribed as a single herb. One of the most popular Chinese herbal formulas containing rehmannia, along with other herbs for building kidney yin and kidney Essence, is Six Flavor Rehmannia Pills; the usual dose is eight pellets three times a day, depending on the type of product purchased.

Epimedium. This herb is considered to be the most powerful vegetarian sexual tonic in Chinese medicine, although surprisingly little is known of it in the West. For women, it is best used in combination with herbs like rehmannia, which strengthen or tonify yin, because epimedium has strong kidney yang-building effects. It may possess male hormone–like actions and is believed to work by stimulating the nervous system, especially the nerves in the genitalia. This herb has also been found to decrease high blood pressure, but it will not affect blood pressure that is too low. In addition, epimedium has powerful immunity-boosting and immunity-regulating effects. In Chinese medicine, it is also used for promoting health and longevity. Epimedium should not be used regularly by women who have an overactive sex drive, a high fever, or symptoms of kidney yin deficiency such as hot flashes, insomnia, or anxiety. It is best used in a Chinese herbal formula.

Cordyceps. This shining star among Chinese herbal aphrodisiacs builds sexual energy over time by enhancing kidney yang and replenishing kidney yin. Because of its dual nature, expansive yet contractive, cordyceps is a perfect sexual tonic for women. It also has immunity-enhancing properties. In China, cordyceps is highly valued. Fortunately, it has become more readily available as a result of modern cultivation techniques. The recommended dose of cordyceps as a single herb is 500 mg two to three times a day. Refrain from using it if you have a fever.

MOTION AND MEDITATION

As we have seen, Chinese medicine teaches the value of preserving and strengthening the Three Treasures—kidney Essence, spirit, and Qi—with practices such as Tai Chi and Qi Gong. These exercises were developed many centuries ago to build and regenerate Qi, and they have survived largely because of their ability to do so. Tai Chi and Qi Gong build strength and endurance with slow, deliberate movements; they emphasize nourishing kidney Qi and the Source of Life and help keep the Water element in balance. These exercises can also quiet your mind, tone your muscles, and help you get in touch with your inner power.

Tai Chi looks like a graceful dance—think of it as meditation in motion. Research has found that it can help prevent bone loss in postmenopausal women, and that seniors who regularly practice it have more muscle strength, better balance, and a decreased risk of falling. Other health benefits of Tai Chi include greater flexibility, increased immunity, and improved cardiorespiratory function.[15] Qi Gong, which as we saw in Chapter 2 can help support immunity, is the practice of working with your own Qi in specific exercises to increase health and vitality. The exercises are easy to learn and include breathing techniques, movements, and visualizations. You can explore Tai Chi and Qi Gong by taking classes from a skilled teacher or through videos and books.

Another great way to nourish your Source of Life and balance your Water element is meditation. It will give you clarity, an inner sense of serenity, and that precious quiet time that women often feel is lost in their lives. Many women find that early morning, before everyone else is up, is the best time of day to do their meditation.

AROMATHERAPY AND FLOWER ESSENCES

Aromatherapy can be a wonderful way to support your kidney Qi and keep your Water element balanced. According to Gabriel Mojay, author of *Aromatherapy for Healing the Spirit,* the following essential oils can have a significant impact on strengthening and balancing the Water element. You can add them to your favorite body lotion or your bath, or use them in an atomizer.

Cedarwood. This powerful remedy for kidney Qi can help with fluid retention by acting as a mild diuretic. The essential oil can be applied to your lower abdomen, above your pubic bone, to help with the cramping pain associated with bladder infections. On an emotional level, cedarwood can strengthen willpower; as Gabriel Mojay points out, it can help you to "hold firm, even against persistent external forces," and at the same time "restore a sense of spiritual certainty."[16]

Ginger. Ginger strengthens the yang energy of the kidneys and acts as a sexual tonic. Therapeutically, it is often used for poor circulation and lower back pain. On an emotional level, it can act as a catalyst if you feel that you are procrastinating and lack the drive to take action.

Juniper Berry. This herb works on both the urinary and the lymphatic systems. Through its stimulating and invigorating properties, it can help with fatigue and relieve cold hands and feet. On an emotional level, you can use the essential oil of juniper berry for rekindling your determination when you feel depressed or afraid of failure; Gabriel Mojay recommends it for consolidating willpower.

Water types may be especially responsive to certain emotional triggers that can throw you off balance. When you are exhausted, you tend to lack confidence and feel apathetic about things that are important to you. At these times, the following flower essences can create subtle shifts in your feelings to help you balance your Water element and reconnect with your wise, determined, and stoic side. The usual dose is a few drops or pellets under your tongue four times a day; you can also take flower essences once every two hours until your symptoms are alleviated. If a remedy hasn't helped your symptoms within twelve hours, you probably need to try a different one.

Mimulus. Mimulus is recommended if you lack confidence and are fearful and anxious about life's challenges. It is best used during times that you need to have a strong belief in yourself and build your courage—when you feel like the Lion in *The Wizard of Oz*.

Star Thistle. Star Thistle is recommended if you feel unfulfilled, either physically or spiritually, or if you tend to hoard your material possessions because you fear there won't be enough to go around. This flower essence may be especially appropriate if you live a reclusive life and don't trust others easily. It is used to help increase your feelings of abundance, your desire to share, and your need be connected to others.

Wild Rose. Wild Rose is recommended if you are dominated by feelings of apathy and a lack of hope. It is often used when a person has been ill for a long time, to help restore the vital force, bring back the will to live, and rejuvenate joy in life.

Gorse. Gorse is recommended if you are caught up in emotions of hopelessness, depression, and despair. It is used for supporting your Water element if you've been stuck for too long in the darkness of winter, literally or metaphorically, and you feel a need to restore joy and a positive outlook in your life.

What to Do When Your Kidney and Bladder Health Is Compromised

In the following pages, we will explore four of the most common problems that can affect a woman's kidneys, bladder, and urinary tract: urinary tract infections, interstitial cystitis, urinary incontinence, and kidney stones. As you will discover, there are many natural methods that you can use not only to help prevent these conditions but to treat them as well.

URINARY TRACT INFECTIONS

Clarissa told me she had gotten her first bladder infection about two years ago. She was treated with antibiotics and the symptoms went away, but as she told me, "it still seemed like every time I had sex I got another infection, and I was prescribed antibiotics again and again." Unfortunately, the antibiotics often gave her vaginal yeast infections that required treatment with more drugs. As she put it, "I was on a merry-go-round of medications." Frustrated with her situation, Clarissa said she didn't feel like she even wanted to have sex anymore. After a careful analysis of why she was prone to urinary tract infections, we were able to get her vaginal and bladder health back to normal.

Clarissa is not alone. In conventional Western medicine, women are often given antibiotics for a urinary tract infection. While this may work in the short term—antibiotics are able to kill off the bacteria that cause the infection—it doesn't completely address the underlying reasons for the infection. As a result, many women experience recurrent infections and the same merry-go-round of ineffectual treatment that Clarissa received.

Urinary tract infections are one of the most common reasons women seek out medical care. Statistics from the National Institutes of Health show that nearly 20 percent of women who get a urinary tract infection will get another one, and 30 percent of those women will be prone to yet another infection.[17] I've actually had patients who were told by their medical doctors that they would continue to have urinary tract infections unless they took antibiotics *after each act of intercourse*! If you have urinary tract infections, it's much smarter, and much better for your health, to look at why you are getting them in the first place and to prevent a recurrence.

Urinary tract infections can occur when bacteria take up residence in the urethra or bladder. Symptoms include pain, burning, pressure in the urethra or bladder, increased frequency of urination, and a strong sensation of having to urinate even though only a small of amount of urine is released. You can also develop pain in your lower back if bacteria travel up your ureters and infect your kidneys. In addition, you may have blood in your urine, or a fever.

Urinary tract infections are a clear illustration of how the state of your immune system can be critical in determining whether you will manifest good health. Most urinary tract infections are caused by bacteria that we are exposed to every day, yet you can have normal bladder health one day and a bladder infection the next. Why? Most likely because your immune system allowed bacteria to thrive where they normally wouldn't; an environment was created in your urethra and bladder that made you more susceptible to invasion by bacteria. This susceptibility can be caused by stress, diet, fluid intake, antibiotics, tissue irritation at the opening of your urethra or vagina, a bladder that doesn't fully empty when you urinate, or hormonal or anatomical changes during pregnancy and menopause. Being aware of these factors can help prevent urinary tract infections.

Stress contributes to the development of urinary tract infections because it profoundly depresses your immune system, creates a more acid pH, and can cause decreased urination. When you are under chronic stress, you release a lot of adrenaline, which inhibits urination. If you are under stress day after day, you tend to urinate less frequently—which can make you more susceptible to urinary tract infections. (This is because whenever you urinate, you naturally cleanse your bladder and urethra of undesirable bacteria. If you become dehydrated, bacteria can more easily gain an advantage, because you urinate less often.) Diet can also make you more vulnerable to urinary tract infections. If your diet is high in sugar, alcohol, and acid-forming foods, your tissues are less able to defend themselves from slight bacterial imbalances that naturally occur in the vulva, vagina, and urethra. A high-sugar diet also contributes to vaginal yeast infections, which create inflammation and irritation at your urethra that can open the door to a bacterial invasion. Your fluid intake affects how much, and how often, you urinate as well. Again, keeping yourself well hydrated is important; drinking at least 48 ounces of filtered water a day can help prevent urinary tract infections.

Antibiotics, although necessary in certain situations, can destroy the resident community of friendly bacteria that help prevent urinary tract infections. These friendly bacteria reside in your vagina, your urethra, and the mucous membranes of your vulva. Anything that harms your friendly bacteria promotes the growth of unfriendly bacteria and makes you more susceptible to urinary tract or bladder infections. When you consider that antibiotics can contribute to urinary tract infections, it seems ironic that some women are repeatedly given antibiotics to "treat" them. My patient Clarissa was able to get off her merry-go-round of infections and antibiotics only after she reintroduced friendly flora, which had routinely been killed off by her treatments.

You may also be prone to urinary tract infections if you have irritation or tissue trauma in your urethra or vaginal opening. One of the most common causes is sexual activity. Urinary tract infections are often referred to as "honeymoon cystitis" because many women get them after repeated intercourse. Considering that a woman's urethra is only millimeters away from her vaginal opening, it's a wonder that women don't have urinary tract infections more often. Many infections are naturally prevented by having adequate vaginal lubrication and urinating after sex.

Other causes of tissue trauma include vaginal infections, prolonged bike riding, wearing tight thongs, and using irritating vaginal douches or soaps. A number of my patients have had urethral irritation caused by perfumes in the soap they used in cleansing their vaginal area. Soaps can be irritating to your vulva, change the pH of your tissues, and allow bacteria to thrive. I recommend that you simply rinse your vulva with water and never apply soap directly to it.

An inability to eliminate all the urine in your bladder when you urinate can make you more susceptible to urinary tract infections. This is often seen in women with neurological or physical conditions (disorders of the nervous system or structural problems) and should be evaluated by a urologist.

It's common for pregnant women to be diagnosed with urinary tract infections. If untreated, they can lead to premature labor. According to Larrian Gillespie, M.D., author of *You Don't Have to Live with Cystitis,* pregnant women often have what she calls the "Shelf Syndrome."[18] When pregnant women sit on the toilet to urinate, they tend to lean back to accommodate their large bellies, resting with hands clasped above the belly (their "shelf"). This posture can cause urine to leak into the vagina, which can then become contaminated with bacteria; it also leads to chronically wet underpants, which further increases the chances of a urinary tract infection. To prevent urinary tract infections, pregnant women are advised to urinate leaning forward with their legs apart. This allows the urine to naturally cleanse bacteria from the vulva, perineum, and rectum.

Menopausal women who don't take estrogen may also experience recurrent urinary tract infections. This is because a low estrogen level can cause thinning and drying of the vaginal, vulvar, and urethral tissues, resulting in greater vulnerability to bacterial infections. If you are menopausal, you can use a low-dose natural estrogen cream directly on these areas of your body to enhance the integrity of the tissues. (For more information, see Chapter 10.)

For many women, a few simple techniques can reduce or eliminate many of these problems. Treating the underlying causes of a urinary tract infection is just as important as treating the infection itself. Here are some of the best natural therapies.

TREATING URINARY TRACT INFECTIONS

It's important to treat a urinary tract infection aggressively, as soon as it starts, because bacteria can move from your urethra and bladder up your ureters and cause an infection in your kidneys. I've found that natural medicines can be extremely effective for treating acute urinary tract infections early. If an infection has been present for over three days, however, the number of bacteria is usually high enough to warrant the use of antibiotics.

The most important thing you can do, if you start having symptoms of a urinary tract infection, is to immediately drink copious amounts of filtered water. This will promote your body's natural ability to flush bacteria out of your bladder and urethra. Natural medicines can also relieve symptoms, help prevent the infection from progressing, and in some cases cure it. Some boost your immune system, while others kill bacteria or prevent them from adhering to your cells' walls, where they take hold and cause an infection. You won't need to take all of the following remedies together, but for best results I recommend that you take at least two or three of them as soon as you begin to experience symptoms.

NATURAL REMEDIES

Vitamin A. This vitamin is useful for maintaining the health of your mucous membranes and boosting your immune system to fight infections. I recommend that you take 50,000 i.u. of vitamin A each day for up to a week; do not, however, take this high a dose for a prolonged period of time. This is a safe dose of vitamin A if you are not pregnant. If you are pregnant or think you might be pregnant, limit your intake of vitamin A to 10,000 i.u. a day.

D-Mannose. This remedy deserves the gold star when it comes to treating urinary tract infections, because it is very effective and has no side effects. It is a natural sugar found in pineapples and cranberries that interferes with the ability of bacteria to adhere to your bladder and urethral cell walls. D-mannose does not kill bacteria, as an antibiotic does; instead, it helps your body flush bacteria out when you urinate. It can be used long term, even by pregnant women. At the onset of a urinary tract infection, I recommend that you take half a teaspoon of D-mannose (the equivalent of approximately 1 g of D-mannose) every three to four hours. If your symptoms do not resolve within three days, see your health care provider and have a urine culture done. If you are prone to getting urinary tract infections after sex, take half a teaspoon of

D-mannose before and after intercourse to help wash undesirable bacteria out of your urethra. Remember to drink plenty of water.

Baking Soda. You can use baking soda to decrease painful urination during a urinary tract infection. Here's a simple home remedy: mix one teaspoon of baking soda in a cup of water, and drink this amount once or twice a day. This will decrease the acidity of your urine and make it less painful to your inflamed tissues.

Cranberries and Blueberries. These fruits can help treat urinary tract infections because they contain compounds that prevent the adherence of unfriendly bacteria to the cell walls of your bladder and urethra. When no other means are available, cranberries and blueberries can make the difference in whether you manifest a full-blown urinary tract infection. Cranberry juice and blueberries are usually available at your local grocery store. You can make blueberry juice by blending the fruit.

There are some drawbacks to using cranberries for treating urinary tract infections, however. They promote acidic urine, which can be irritating to tissues that are already inflamed due to an infection. In addition, the cranberry juice at most grocery stores is laden with corn syrup and other sugars that promote bacterial growth and are detrimental to your immune system. Buy pure, unsweetened cranberry juice (at your health food store), which tastes sour but is more effective. If you tend to have recurrent urinary tract infections, you can use cranberry extracts in pill form to help prevent them. If you have a chronic burning sensation in your bladder or the condition known as interstitial cystitis, do not use cranberry in any form because it could make the burning worse; use marshmallow tea (see below) to ease your symptoms. I recommend cranberries and blueberries only as a way to buy time until you can get a more effective and concentrated herbal or nutritional therapy. Be sure to follow up with your health care provider as soon as possible to evaluate your symptoms and have urine tests done. Remember, it is critical to treat a urinary tract infection soon after it starts, to prevent a kidney infection. (Note: Cranberry juice should not be taken in conjunction with the herb uva ursi.)

HERBS

Uva Ursi. This herb is excellent for the treatment of a urinary tract infection. It contains arbutin, a compound that does not kill bacteria directly but helps prevent their adherence to the cell walls of your bladder and urethra. Uva ursi also has a slight diuretic action, so you will urinate more often when you take it. It works best when your urine is more alkaline. Taking baking soda (as mentioned above) and eating a diet high in fruits (except cranberries, plums, and prunes, because they make urine more acidic) and vegetables will help you achieve this alkalinity. To relieve your symptoms, I recommend that you take uva ursi as a pill containing at least 10 percent arbutin; take 250 to 500 mg a day. Do not take uva ursi long term at high doses. If you have a tendency to develop recurrent urinary tract infections, I recommend that you use D-mannose instead. (Note: Uva ursi should not be taken in conjunction with cranberry juice.)

Marshmallow Root. This is one of the most important herbs for treating any kind of inflammatory condition in the urinary system. It soothes the mucous membranes of the bladder and urethra, decreases the pain associated with urinary tract infections, and helps restore the lining of your urinary tract so that you are less prone to repeat infections. It can also help to heal your bladder if you have interstitial cystitis. To make marshmallow tea, boil four cups of water and add two tablespoons of the root. Simmer on low heat for fifteen to twenty minutes, strain, and drink either hot or cold. During an infection, and for at least seven days afterward, drink a minimum of four cups a day. If making the tea is not convenient, I recommend you take marshmallow root in capsule form: take 900 mg two to three times a day.

HOMEOPATHIC REMEDIES

There are many homeopathic remedies for treating urinary tract infections. The three most commonly prescribed are Cantharis, Sarsaparilla, and Staphysagria. If you have the symptoms described below, I recommend that you self-administer low doses (of 30c or less) of the remedy that best matches your symptoms. (See Appendix A for information on how to use homeopathic medicine.)

Cantharis. This remedy is best used if you have an intolerable and constant urge to urinate with severe burning pain in your urethra, and if your symptoms improve when you keep moving. Cantharis is also recommended if your symptoms include blood in your urine.

Sarsaparilla. This remedy is recommended if you have pain at the end of urination, or if you have the urge to urinate but nothing comes out, or if just a small amount dribbles out. It is also recommended if you have bladder or urethral pain that tends to diminish if you are standing up.

Staphysagria. This remedy is specifically used for a urinary tract infection that comes on after sexual activity. It is recommended if you experience the sensation of needing to urinate but are unable to, and if you feel as if your bladder is never fully emptied. It can also be used if you have a burning sensation in your urethra and you feel irritable and chilly. On an emotional level, staphysagria is recommended if the onset of your symptoms coincided with feelings of anger and a sense of being taken advantage of.

DIET

In Chinese medicine, the most common cause of urinary tract infection is an accumulation of "damp-heat" in the bladder. This can develop if you've been overeating or ingesting too many foods (such as those containing dairy and sugar) that create a damp-heat condition. Eating "cold" and "cooling" foods can help you treat a urinary tract infection. (See pages 34–36 for a list of these foods.) It is recommended that you avoid sugar, foods that in Western medicine are found to have a high glycemic index, fruit juices, spicy foods, and dairy products.

SITZ BATHS

A type of bath known as a sitz bath is commonly prescribed by naturopathic physicians to relieve suffering from urinary tract infections. Although it may be cumbersome to perform, it is a very effective way to augment your body's ability to heal itself. The goal of the treatment is to increase the blood flow to your pelvic area.

To take a sitz bath, you need two basins wide enough to sit in and deep enough that water will reach the top of your pubic hair. Fill one basin with hot water and the other with cold. Place your bottom in the hot water first and remain there for one minute; then get out and sit in the cold water basin for thirty seconds. Alternate three times and end with the cold water. While you may be able to perform this feat in two large side-by-side kitchen sinks, you may find it more convenient to use two large basins placed on the floor. I recommend that you take a sitz bath twice a day while you are fighting a urinary tract infection.

INTERSTITIAL CYSTITIS

Interstitial cystitis is a chronic inflammation that occurs between the lining of a woman's bladder and the bladder muscle. It causes many symptoms similar to those of a urinary tract infection, such as increased urinary frequency and urgency and a painful, burning sensation in the bladder and urethra; the pain can be constant or intermittent, intense or mild. But in contrast to a urinary tract infection, with interstitial cystitis the urine culture is normal. (You don't have any abnormal bacteria.)

There is no definite known cause of interstitial cystitis, although chronic urinary tract infections may be an underlying cause. Larrian Gillespie, M.D., author of *You Don't Have to Live with Cystitis,* points out that interstitial cystitis may be caused by recurrent urinary tract infections resulting in a significant disruption to the mucous membranes of the bladder and urethra. The altered mucous membranes expose the blood vessels, nerves, and bladder wall to the caustic irritation of urine. Other possible causes of interstitial cystitis include immune disorders, environmental toxins, spinal misalignments, and endometriosis.

Dr. Tori Hudson, a naturopathic physician and leader in the field of women's health, calls interstitial cystitis "leaky bladder syndrome" because it results in chronic irritation of the bladder wall. Women with interstitial cystitis often have multiple food sensitivities that aggravate their condition. Interstitial cystitis is a complex condition, and treating it requires a multifaceted approach. The following is a step-by-step treatment plan.

Treating Interstitial Cystitis

Coat and Soothe the Lining of Your Bladder and Urethra. Marshmallow root tea is excellent for this purpose. To make it, see page 100.

Rebuild the Lining of Your Bladder. The bladder protects itself from irritants in the urine by maintaining a layer of protective cells. When this protective layer is disrupted by a urinary tract infection or some other factor, bladder pain and increased urinary frequency can result. Glucosamine sulfate, an inexpensive, readily available supplement that is known for its ability to relieve osteoarthritis, will help rebuild the lining of your bladder. Take 500 mg three times a day.

Eliminate All Foods That Aggravate Your Condition. Dr. Larrian Gillespie has compiled a useful list of foods and beverages to avoid in order to prevent flare-ups of interstitial cystitis and give your bladder wall and urethra a chance to heal. The list includes apples, apple juice, all citrus fruits, coffee, cranberries, grapes, ginger, spicy foods, apricots, cantaloupe, guava, peaches, pineapple, plums, rhubarb, strawberries, black tea, tomatoes, vinegar, and watermelon.

Keep Your Urine Alkaline. Alkaline urine will help diminish the bladder pain associated with interstitial cystitis. Eat an alkaline-forming diet (see page 86) and take a quarter teaspoon of baking soda twice a day, or 500 mg of calcium carbonate three times a day. You can test the pH of your urine to be sure that it stays at 6.5 or greater.

Drink a Lot of Filtered Water. Keep your urine as diluted as possible to avoid irritating your bladder wall with concentrated urine.

Prevent a Urinary Tract Infection. If you have interstitial cystitis, you may be prone to a urinary tract infection because the tissues of your bladder and urethra are chronically irritated. Use D-mannose to help prevent the adherence of bacteria to the cells in your urinary tract, but avoid using cranberry juice or cranberry pills, because they will aggravate interstitial cystitis.

Over time, by following these six simple steps, you can heal from interstitial cystitis. But if you are menopausal and have low estrogen levels, your vulvar, vaginal, and urethral tissues may have begun to thin, and you may need to take an additional step: use a low-dose estriol vaginal cream to rehydrate and strengthen your tissues. If you are opposed to using any estrogen, your naturopathic physician can provide you with black cohosh vaginal suppositories to help rebuild your tissues. (See Chapter 10 for more information on the use of vaginal creams.)

Some of the other potential causes of interstitial cystitis, such as immune disorders and environmental toxins, are addressed in Chapters 1, 2, and 4. If your interstitial cystitis doesn't resolve, I recommend that you consult your naturopathic physician to work out a comprehensive protocol that is specific to your needs.

URINARY INCONTINENCE

Urinary incontinence, or the involuntary release of urine, affects more than sixteen million women in the United States; some estimates are as high as thirty million. Women are five times more likely to develop urinary incontinence than men. The condition commonly occurs as a result of childbirth, but it has other causes as well. Urinary incontinence is characterized by an inability to hold back urine when coughing, sneezing, or laughing. It can lead to stressful and embarrassing situations that require major lifestyle changes. Urinary incontinence can range in degree and severity. Stress incontinence, which is the most common type seen in women, can be treated naturally. It is usually due to a weakness in the muscles that support the bottom of the pelvis, often referred to as the *pelvic floor.* (Other types of incontinence, which are beyond the scope of this book and should be managed by your physician, include urge incontinence, overflow incontinence, transient incontinence, and functional incontinence.)

Women who develop urinary incontinence after childbirth usually have stress incontinence. They can experience a leakage of urine whenever pressure is increased in their abdomen—for instance, when they sneeze, cough, laugh hard, lift a heavy object, or jump up and down. Many women with this kind of incontinence experience dramatic benefits from doing Kegel exercises, which strengthen the muscles of the pelvic floor.

Exercises to strengthen pelvic muscles are as old as Chinese medicine. For centuries, the ancient Chinese manual *The Art of the Bedchamber* has instructed women to exercise their vagina and pelvic floor muscles to enhance their sex lives. One exercise instructs women to do a "pelvic squeeze" during intercourse to increase vaginal sensations. In the 1940s, when medical doctor Arnold Kegel promoted Kegel exercises in the West for the treatment of urinary incontinence, some women who did the exercises faithfully were later surprised to experience orgasms for the first time in their lives. From both a Western and a Chinese point of view, Kegel exercises can increase blood flow to the pelvis, strengthen and tone the pelvic muscles, and enhance awareness of the pelvic area. From the Chinese perspective, Kegel exercises also increase the flow of Qi through the pelvis.

Your pelvic floor muscles are like a hammock that supports the organs in your pelvis. During childbirth, your hammock is flexible enough that it can stretch, allowing for the passage of your baby. Ideally, after childbirth these muscles return to their former positions. In reality, however, they often remain overly stretched and can become weak, resulting in stress incontinence. By doing Kegel exercises regularly, you can tone and strengthen the muscles that support your urethra and bladder. Many women have prevented, reduced, or entirely eliminated stress incontinence with Kegel exercises.

How to Do Kegel Exercises

To do Kegel exercises, you first have to become aware of the muscles that support your pelvic floor. One way to find them is to stop the flow of urine while you are urinating; the muscles you use are the muscles you will strengthen and tone with Kegel exercises.

You don't want to make a practice of stopping your flow of urine, but once you've become familiar with the sensation of tightening these muscles a few times, try contracting them when you are standing, sitting, or lying down. Keep your buttocks, abdominal muscles, and thigh muscles relaxed, and breathe normally. To be sure that you are contracting the right muscles, put your finger in your vagina; you should feel a tightening of your pelvic floor muscles around your finger.

There are two types of Kegel contractions: fast and slow. When you do fast Kegel contractions, you strengthen the fast-twitch fibers in your pelvic floor muscles, which are important for preventing leakage of urine when you cough or sneeze. When you do slow contractions, you build the slow-twitch fibers, which promote both strength and endurance and are responsible for muscle tone when your pelvic floor muscles are at rest. It's best to do a combination of fast and slow contractions, with an emphasis on the slow.

To do Kegel exercises, sit or lie down in a comfortable position and focus on your pelvic floor muscles. Begin with fast contractions by tightening the muscles of your pelvic floor, contracting your vagina and your anus at the same time. Hold each contraction for two seconds, then completely relax for two seconds, and repeat five times. Next do slow contractions, holding each contraction for ten seconds, then relaxing for ten seconds, and repeat five times. End your Kegel session with another series of fast contractions. As your muscles become stronger, increase the number of both fast and slow contractions to ten, and do the exercises three times a day.

To enhance the effectiveness of your Kegels, you can insert small weighted cones into your vagina. Your health care provider can prescribe these devices and give you instructions on how to use them in the privacy of your home. Cones of varying weights are used because as your pelvic floor muscles become stronger, you will be able to hold heavier cones in place for longer periods of time. Typically, a woman keeps a cone in her vagina for about ten to fifteen minutes once or twice a day.

KIDNEY STONES

Many women have described passing a kidney stone as the most excruciating pain they've ever experienced, worse than childbirth. In the United States more than a million people are hospitalized for the treatment of kidney stones each year. Certain medical conditions and genetic factors can increase your risk of forming stones, but many people form them because of their lifestyle and diet. Conditions that put you at higher risk for developing kidney stones can include dehydration, rapid weight loss, high protein diets, acidic urine, and excess salt in your diet.

There are different kinds of kidney stones, which form for different reasons. The most common are calcium oxalate stones. If you're concerned about the possibility of having this type of stone, either because you've formed one in the past or because of your family history, I recommend you take the following preventive measures:

- Eat alkaline-forming foods. (For a list of alkaline-forming foods, see page 86.)
- Avoid foods high in oxalates. These include leafy greens, rhubarb, chocolate, black tea, okra, nuts, beans, beets, wheat bran, and strawberries. Chinese cuisine can contribute to the formation of calcium oxalate stones because it often contains high-oxalate foods, such as peanut oil, bok choy, and soy protein. The MSG (monosodium glutamate) frequently found in Chinese dishes, as well as in many prepared Western foods, can also contribute to the formation of calcium oxalate stones. Limit your intake of vitamin C, because an excess of vitamin C can be converted to oxalates.
- Drink at least 48 ounces of filtered water a day to prevent dehydration and keep your urine diluted. This will enable you to wash out waste products more efficiently. Increased sweating, chronic diarrhea, and consuming drinks that dehydrate you (such as alcohol and coffee) will increase your need for fluids.
- Avoid rapid weight loss and high-protein diets. With rapid weight loss you begin burning fat for energy, which forms ketones that make your urine more acidic. Your urine can also become more acidic if you eat a high-protein diet like the one promoted by Dr. Atkins.

- Keep your urine alkaline by testing its pH every morning and evening to be sure that it remains at 6.5 or above. (Note: If you form a rare type of kidney stone comprised of calcium phosphate, you will need to keep your urine acidic to prevent forming another stone of this type.)
- Go easy on your salt shaker. The more salt you ingest, the more calcium you will have in your urine—which could increase your risk of forming a calcium oxalate stone.

If you already have a small stone that doesn't cause extreme pain, you can use herbs to help pass it and relieve the pain. Herbs that relax smooth muscle, soothe mucous membranes, and promote urination can be especially helpful. These include gravel root, hydrangea, marshmallow root, and horsetail. Gravel root and hydrangea root are effective antispasmodics, and both can decrease pain and inflammation in the urinary tract. Marshmallow root is an extremely effective herb for soothing the mucous membranes of the urinary tract, and horsetail is an excellent diuretic that provides support to the urinary tract tissues. I always recommend that marshmallow root be taken as a tea. (For a description of how to make tea from the root, see page 100.) You can take the other herbs as tinctures (extracts of the herbs in glycerin or alcohol; see Appendix B): mix gravel root tincture, hydrangea root tincture, and horsetail tincture together in equal parts and take one-fourth to one-half a teaspoon two to four times a day. These herbs should be taken for at least two months to relieve mild aches associated with small kidney stones.

Flowing Water: Final Thoughts

As we've seen in this chapter, the Naturally Healthy Lifestyle is essential to protecting the vitality of your kidneys. By nourishing your kidneys with alkaline-forming foods, natural salts, and clean water, you can significantly affect the health of your kidneys and your entire body. We've also explored many ways that you can support the energetic functions of your kidneys. Keeping your Water element in balance can help prevent many kidney and bladder problems, especially if you are a Water type. Preserving your Three Treasures with Chinese herbal medicines, meditation, and ancient Chinese exercises can also help you create a healthier, longer life. And natural medicine can help you prevent or treat a number of kidney and bladder disorders, such as urinary tract infections, interstitial cystitis, urinary incontinence, and kidney stones. Remember what Chinese medicine has to teach us about the importance of kidney health: taking care of your kidney Qi is integral to your well-being, because it is your Source of Life, at the very center of your vitality, and the wellspring from which all your creativity flows.

The Essence of Chapter 3

- Preserve your Three Treasures: your kidney Essence, your spirit, and your Qi.
- Keep your Water element in balance, especially if you are a Water type.
- Support your kidneys by increasing alkaline-forming foods in your diet.
- Use natural salt, and drink plenty of clean water.
- Increase the vitality of your kidneys and enhance your sexual energy with Chinese herbs.
- Support your kidney Qi with Tai Chi, Qi Gong, and meditation.
- Take simple steps to prevent urinary tract infections; if you have a urinary tract infection, treat it immediately with natural medicine.
- Treat interstitial cystitis with natural medicine.
- Do Kegel exercises to prevent and treat urinary incontinence.
- Prevent kidney stones with your lifestyle and diet.

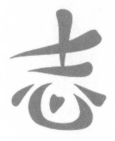

A m b i t i o n

New Shoots:
Restoring Your Liver and
Your Essential Vitality

"Growth itself contains the germ of happiness."
—PEARL S. BUCK, *To My Daughters, with Love*

WHEN JULIE came to see me, she'd been having debilitating migraine headaches. To treat them, her physician had prescribed an antidepressant and an unlimited supply of drugs to kill the pain. As Julie told me, "The antidepressant caused weight gain and the painkillers only partially masked the pain. Even though I was miserable, I lived like this for years.

"Then I entered perimenopause. The migraines got worse, my digestion went haywire, and I had hot flashes that made me feel like I would spontaneously combust. I was so uncomfortable in my body that I had to quit my job and spend several days a month in bed. The headaches hit two to three times per week and would take at least twenty-four hours to go away.

"Desperate for help," she went on, "I saw a neurologist who prescribed a cocktail of drugs—another antidepressant, sleeping pills, and an anticonvulsant for my migraines. I had to take blood tests regularly to see if the drugs were damaging my liver. I tried hormone replacement therapy in hopes of alleviating my symptoms, but to no avail."

Although Julie had been taking a barrage of medications to help with her symptoms, they failed to treat the underlying cause of her problem—her liver. And in fact, the medications were causing congestion in her liver and further compromising her liver health. I prescribed a liver cleanse, and within a month her health had turned around. "There was improvement in all areas of my body," she said. "By six weeks, the difference was dramatic: the migraine cycle was broken, the hot flashes were gone, and my digestion was normal! I feel healthier than I have in years; in fact, I feel great! My mind is clearer and I am migraine-free. I have my energy back, along with a new sense of well-being. I now have hope that my future will be healthy and productive."

✿

Your Liver Health

Your liver is your organ of regeneration. It is your master cleanser, filtering your blood and neutralizing toxins so that your health is continually renewed. Your liver helps you create and maintain vitality in every cell in your body. In both Western and Chinese medicine, keeping the liver functioning optimally is essential to keeping the body, mind, and spirit healthy.

When your liver is working well, you have energy in the morning when you wake up, you can think clearly, you are easily able to maintain your blood sugar levels, and you have a sense of well-being. You also have a healthy digestive system and strong immune defenses. If your liver isn't working well, you can experience many physical and emotional symptoms. These include fatigue, headaches, migraines, foggy thinking, premenstrual syndrome, abdominal bloating, high blood pressure, fluid retention, allergies, mood swings, depression, constipation, poor digestion, nausea, and poor immune function. An unhealthy liver can be the precursor to many diseases, including cancer and autoimmune disorders.

What would prevent your liver from functioning at its best? The most likely answer can be summed up in one word: toxins. In our industrialized society, toxic chemicals are ubiquitous. You are exposed to them everywhere in your daily life. They may be in the products you buy, the food you eat, the water you drink, and the air you breathe. Every person and every ecosystem on the planet has been affected. The statistics are alarming. According to the Environmental Working Group, thirty billion pounds of pesticides, which can have especially toxic effects, have been released into the environment since the 1940s. Today two billion pounds are used annually, of which 850 million pounds are used on food.[1]

Toxic chemicals, including heavy metals such as mercury, are found in exceptionally high concentrations in both animals and humans; they are stored in our fatty tissues, our nervous system, and our bones. Mercury gets all the bad press these days, but the presence of other heavy metals (including arsenic, lead, and tin) in your body is not to be taken lightly, either. Heavy metals can take a heavy toll on your health.

Many toxins interfere with your liver's ability to detoxify, which can result in even more toxic compounds creating havoc in your body. Some toxins, such as dioxin, can mimic estrogen and activate estrogen-sensitive cells, and may cause other hormone-related disorders, or initiate cancer. Increased exposure to environmental chemicals may also contribute to infertility, learning disabilities, neurological symptoms, and autoimmune diseases.

The good news is that there are many ways you can limit your exposure to toxins and help your liver break them down, and there's a wealth of information available to help you do it. This chapter will give you the tools you need to support your liver through diet, supplements, herbal medicines, and cleansing. It also includes a detailed plan to safely and effectively detoxify your liver. Starting today, there is a lot that you can do to enhance the quality of your life by nurturing your liver health.

The View from the West

"To a very large extent, our health and vitality are determined by the health and vitality of our liver."
—Joseph Pizzorno, N.D., *Total Wellness*

Your liver, the grand filter and detoxifier for your entire body, is your largest internal organ. It resides under your rib cage, in the upper right side of your abdomen, and consists of many different kinds of cells that work together to keep you healthy. When you eat a meal, all the food particles that are absorbed in your small intestine are carried through your portal vein to your liver. Your liver is responsible for keeping your blood clear of toxins that are in your food or that result from your own body's metabolism. It also filters toxins that entered your bloodstream after being absorbed through your lungs and your skin. In addition to neutralizing toxins, it breaks down hormones, maintains your blood sugar level, produces cholesterol, stores vitamins, makes bile, prevents chronic disease by destroying invading bacteria and viruses in your blood, and more.

If you had lived before the industrial revolution, your liver's greatest challenge would probably have been dealing with toxins naturally found in the foods you ate and those produced by your body. In today's world, so much more is being demanded of your liver. The enormous increase in synthetic environmental toxins during the past century has added a new, unnatural burden to liver health. In addition, your liver's ability to function optimally can be impaired by hormone replacement therapy, birth control pills, bacterial toxins from abnormal intestinal flora, alcohol, and a number of pharmaceutical drugs.

Why is it that some people can tolerate relatively little exposure to environmental toxins while others can smoke, drink alcohol, and work in toxic environments and seem to suffer no ill effects? Nobody knows for sure, but I suspect that in many cases it boils down to liver health and how efficiently a person's liver can break down toxins. Let's look at how the liver goes about this essential process.

The liver has two detoxification systems, referred to as Phase I and Phase II, which are especially important to health. Phase I breaks down most toxins and neutralizes them, but some toxins actually become *more* toxic after Phase I, and the Phase II detoxification system is called into action to make sure the toxins are fully broken down so that the body can dispose of them. These two detoxification systems have been described as a two-phase wash cycle. Sometimes the first wash cycle isn't powerful enough to get everything clean, and the second wash cycle is necessary to finish the job. The second wash cycle may also be critical to neutralizing the damaging effects of toxins produced by the first cycle. If the two-phase wash cycle isn't working as it should (for example, because of interference from environmental chemicals), toxins can accumulate in the liver and in the rest of the body and cause cell damage, immune disorders, and even damage to your DNA, potentially resulting in cancer and other diseases.

After toxins have been through the wash cycles in your liver, they are mixed with bile and deposited into your gallbladder, a small pouch that lies under your liver. The toxins, now bound up with bile acids, are escorted out of your body through your stools. If the bile flow out of your gallbladder is impaired, in a condition called cholestasis, toxins remain in your liver for longer periods of time. Many women who have cholestasis suffer from premenstrual syndrome, gallstones, fatigue, headaches, constipation, allergies, multiple chemical sensitivities, and poor digestion. As we will see, a liver cleanse can relieve many of these symptoms; it can also enhance all the actions of your liver and gallbladder and promote detoxification.

I often ask my patients to view the importance of liver cleansing in this way: if your organ of detoxification, the master detoxifier for your entire body, becomes overburdened with toxic chemicals to the point where *it* isn't working properly, then it can no longer effectively detoxify your system. It is crucial that you purify your purifier.

In addition to cleansing your liver, there's a lot you can do to change your external and internal environments to maximize your liver health. As you read on, you will discover, for example, that your liver needs sufficient amounts of amino acids, vitamins, minerals, and antioxidants to function properly and to effectively neutralize toxins. Certain amino acids and antioxidants, such as alpha lipoic acid, are especially important for maintaining and restoring the essential vitality of your liver.

The View from the East

From a Chinese perspective, the liver is extremely important to health; it is responsible for new growth and transformation, and it orchestrates the flow of Qi throughout the body. When your liver is healthy, your Qi flows freely, generating health in your body, mind, emotions, and spirit. You feel happy, creative, and "on top of the world," and you have an abundance of energy. You also have balanced hormones, good digestion, strong muscles, and high vitality.

If the liver is unhealthy, Qi does not flow freely and the rest of the body suffers. This is most commonly caused by stress, including emotional distress, but it can also be brought on by drugs, toxins, or overeating. If your liver Qi becomes stagnant, your creativity is blocked and you can easily become frustrated, irritated, overwhelmed with strong emotions, and beset by outbursts of rage. You may also be subject to a number of other symptoms, including headaches, migraines, insomnia, fatigue, depression, abdominal swelling, muscle twitches, stiff tendons, fevers, dizziness, tremors, and constipation.

The internal rhythms of your body depend on your liver's ability to coordinate the flow of your Qi. Your breathing patterns, your appetite for food, and many of your other daily routines are the end result of careful and deliberate "planning" by your liver Qi. In addition, your liver Qi governs your hormonal cycles, determining which hormones are released and in what amounts. When your liver Qi is imbalanced, you are more likely to suffer from premenstrual syndrome, menstrual cramps, irregular menstrual cycles, thyroid and adrenal problems, and other hormonal imbalances.

In Chinese medicine, the uterus and ovaries are considered to be extensions of the liver. If you have fibroids, heavy menstrual bleeding, or ovarian cysts, your liver is usually treated as well. Your liver Qi stores your Blood and regulates menstruation; the seven-day period before ovulation is described as being dominated by the liver, when the uterus is preparing for a fertilized egg and sexual desire is building.

In Chinese medicine it is said that liver Qi "opens to your eyes." This means that your eyes are a reflection of the health of your liver. When your liver is healthy, your eyes are clear and bright. If your eyes are continually dry, or if the whites are red, your liver Qi may be out of balance. Your liver influences your vision in a metaphorical sense as well, by shaping the way you perceive your future.

Your liver Qi also plays a role in controlling your body's immune response, by helping you identify what is foreign to your body and establish boundaries to protect yourself. When your liver is not working optimally, these boundaries can become blurred and allergies or autoimmune diseases can develop.

Just as the liver and gallbladder are closely linked in the Western system, in the Chinese system they are considered "paired organs," working together to balance health on many levels. The gallbladder, which is known as the "honorable minister," fosters good judgment and helps you make decisions. If your liver and gallbladder are out of harmony, you can become indecisive, display poor judgment, and experience frequent headaches.

The Wood Element

Linda sought out natural medicine because she felt sick and tired too often to be able to enjoy life. As she put it, she "needed a new body." A few years earlier she had been diagnosed with a thyroid condition and undergone surgery. "The surgery alone was enough to put my body into shock," she told me, "but my lifestyle at that time didn't help. For years I've worked as a defense attorney. I'm good at this job, it suits my personality, and it gives me a decent paycheck. Unfortunately, the job pushed me so hard all the time that my body never had time to recover."

When Linda realized that she was a classic Wood type, she began actively exploring new ways to get her health back on track by balancing her Wood element. "Discovering that I was a Wood type helped me to see my life in perspective," she said. "I knew that I couldn't leave my high-paying job, but I could try to balance my Wood element with creative activities that nourished my other elements and different parts of myself. I started singing and language classes. I also started exercising on a regular basis, and putting me first instead of my job. Over the past few years, I've regained a true sense of health in my body. I no longer get sick frequently, and I don't have to sleep all the time. I feel so much more in control of my destiny now that my Wood traits are no longer consuming me."

The liver is represented by the Wood element in Chinese medicine. The Wood element, which promotes regeneration and growth, flourishes in the springtime, when new shoots are sprouting from the earth with determined energy, reaching upward and outward, and competing for nutrition, sunlight, and space.

If you have a dominance of the Wood element, enhancing your liver function is of the utmost importance because the liver is where this element has its greatest influence. Even if you are not predominantly a Wood type, you will benefit from boosting your liver health and balancing your Wood element, since you have each of the Five Elements within you.

If you are a Wood type you have an ambitious, strong type A personality and high vitality. Like a new shoot in springtime, you are vigorous and aggressive, you love life, and you are eager to succeed. You thrive on action, exercise, and movement. Naturally setting high goals for yourself, you enjoy creating structure in your life, making plans, and following through with them. Through hard work and sheer determination you attain your goals. The process is not as important to you as the goal or finished product, and you take great pride in your achievements.

As a Wood type, you are very productive and capable of accomplishing a lot in your life. With your assertiveness and confidence, you can really make things happen. You are apt to be a "winner" in your chosen field and hold a high-power position. Extroverted and driven, you have what it takes to be the CEO of a big company or run for public office. You can attain just about anything you set your mind to because you are doggedly determined. Many famous athletes, adventurers, risk-takers, and world leaders are Wood types. As a physician, I've noticed that once Wood types are convinced that their health is critical to obtaining their ultimate goals, they become totally committed to taking care of themselves. When they discover that a healthy diet, regular exercise, and maintaining a balanced lifestyle are critical components to their success, nothing will stop them.

On a spiritual level, if you are a Wood type, you have a strong sense of hope, vision, and purpose, and you see great potential for the future. You have the spirit of a seedling pushing out of the earth, gathering energy to accomplish your dreams. You know that your mission is to become a sapling, and then a tree, and you will get there even if it is against all odds. It is said in Chinese medicine that a healthy liver allows the creative spirit to thrive; it also enables you to be flexible and yielding, both physically and emotionally, like a tree in the wind.

If you have a dominance of Wood, you can be more prone to certain emotional and physical imbalances. You are particularly affected by stress because your liver is responsible for managing stress in your entire body. As a Wood type, you characteristically find it hard to relax—you tend to be so goal-oriented that you forget to smell the roses along the way—so it's important for you to learn to pay attention to the signs that your body gives you if you are under excessive stress. When your Wood element is balanced, your liver Qi is abundant and thriving, but when you work too hard for too long in pursuit of your goals, you can squander your precious vital energy and exhaust your liver Qi.

When stress finally catches up with you, it is most likely to take the form of premenstrual syndrome, hormone imbalances, breast and ovarian cysts, high blood pressure, headaches (including migraines), painfully tight muscles, eye problems, digestive imbalances, heart disease, and cancer. On an emotional level, it may thwart your usual sense of purpose in life; all of your ambition, creative energy, and decisiveness can seem to disappear, and you become depressed. If this happens, you have a tendency to seek out new projects to immerse yourself in, but this is counterproductive. You will benefit most during these times by focusing your energy inward to heal yourself rather than outward on some new external project. Quiet, introverted activities such as yoga, Tai Chi, Qi Gong, meditation, counseling, and psychotherapy can be especially helpful in balancing your Wood element and replenishing your vital energy.

If you are a Wood type, it is important to create time for play in your life. Playtime revitalizes your liver Qi, which you need in order to continue pursuing your goals. All work and no play can make you dull and might even make you ill. Your diet is also critical, because you tend to believe you can eat and drink anything, at any time, and still be able to keep on pushing yourself to work harder. In fact, a diet without coffee, sugar, alcohol, and fatty foods will nourish your Wood element and keep you strong and healthy, and you will accomplish much more in the long run.

In Chinese medicine it is thought that sour-tasting foods can stimulate liver Qi and help balance the Wood element. If you are a Wood type, you probably have a predilection for sour flavors, unsweetened yogurt, pickles, or vinegar. Wood types often crave lemons and may even enjoy sucking on them. (In an interesting parallel with Western medicine, naturopathic physicians have used lemons for more than a century to help detoxify the liver.)

The voice quality of the Wood type is normally loud and confident; when your Wood element is balanced, you speak with a tone of calculating certainty. You can demand attention simply with the power of your voice. But if your Wood element is imbalanced, your voice will seem monotone and lacking in vigor, or else you will resort to raising your voice and shouting. Anger is the primary emotion expressed by the Wood type (which means that anger is more apt to be expressed by a Wood type than by the other element types), and frustration is common when the Wood element is out of balance. If you rant and rave, it is because you want to be in charge, but by acting out you appear to be out of control, and you usually get the opposite response than the one you intended. When your Wood element is imbalanced, others may perceive you as having a domineering personality.

Keeping your Wood element in harmony with your other elements is essential to your health. If your Wood element is out of balance, your other elements will also be imbalanced. Linda's story, which you read above, is a good example of issues that often affect Wood types. While her dominant Wood element enabled her to achieve her professional goals, in excess it exhausted her Qi and resulted in illness. Linda was able to restore her health by making conscious choices to nourish her body and the other aspects of herself.

Whether or not you are a Wood type, liver cleansing is a good idea, not only because it revitalizes your liver Qi but also because the liver has such a strong influence on all the Five Elements. Cleansing your liver can help release physical toxins and heavy metals that you are exposed to, and it can also discharge "emotional toxins." Both can cause stagnation in liver Qi and lead to imbalances in the Wood element. Many people have described experiencing a kind of emotional catharsis during a liver cleanse.

Are You a Wood Type?

- Are you ambitious?
- Do you enjoy reaching the goal more than the process?
- Are you a workaholic?
- Do you have a clear sense of purpose in your life?
- Are you highly active and productive?
- Do you create a lot of structure in your life?
- Do you enjoy planning your projects?
- Do you tend to organize and lead others?
- Do you have a strong vision of your future?
- Are you an adventurer or a risk-taker?
- Do you tend to push yourself to the breaking point?
- Do you tend to get angry and irritable when overstressed?
- Do you thrive on competition?
- Do you get migraines?
- Do you crave sour foods?
- When tense, do you have tight, painful muscles, headaches, and digestive problems?
- Do you tend to avoid taking care of yourself until you simply collapse?
- Do you thrive on exercise and movement?
- Is it hard for you to just relax?
- Do you tend to have a domineering personality?
- Do you become argumentative if you don't get to do things your way?
- Do you ever become depressed when you are exhausted?

If you answered yes to most of these questions, you most likely have a dominance of the Wood element. The following guidelines will help you balance your Wood element and maintain health in your body, mind, and spirit:

> Exercise regularly to keep your Qi moving.
> Create time to take care of yourself, and playtime to balance your work time.
> Do a liver cleanse.
> Avoid overextending yourself and squandering your Qi.
> Seek out counseling if you tend to get angry easily or have controlling behavior.
> Become conscious of how your aggressive behavior can work for you or against you.
> Practice yoga, Tai Chi, or meditation to quiet your mind and balance your extroverted nature.
> Learn to enjoy the process of moving toward your goals as much as you enjoy achieving them.
> Avoid alcohol, coffee, sugar, and fatty foods.
> Remember that attaining great health will allow you more success in reaching your life goals.

How Toxic Are You?

As we've seen, in both Western and Chinese medicine the health of the entire body is intimately connected to the health of the liver. By answering the following question-naire, you can get a good idea of how well your liver is functioning and how toxic you are. Circle the number in each row that best applies to you.

0 = You *never* experience the symptom.
1 = You *occasionally* experience the symptom.
2 = You *regularly* experience the symptom.

Do you have dark circles under your eyes?	0	1	2
Do you have breast tenderness before your period?	0	1	2
Do you have mood swings before your period?	0	1	2
Do you frequently have low blood sugar or hypoglycemia?	0	1	2
Do you have allergies?	0	1	2
Are you sensitive to perfumes or chemicals?	0	1	2
Do you get frequent headaches?	0	1	2
Do you have insomnia?	0	1	2
Do you wake up exhausted and feel sluggish throughout the day, despite getting a good night's sleep?	0	1	2
Do you frequently feel nauseated for no apparent reason?	0	1	2
Are you ultrasensitive to medications?	0	1	2
Do you frequently experience muscle aches and pains?	0	1	2
Do you get diarrhea or a lot of gas when you eat fatty foods?	0	1	2
Do you have migraines?	0	1	2
Do you have poor concentration?	0	1	2
Do you often feel sleepy or fatigued after eating?	0	1	2
Do you have bad breath?	0	1	2
Do you have a strong body odor?	0	1	2
Are the whites of your eyes yellow or chronically bloodshot?	0	1	2
Do you have hemorrhoids?	0	1	2

Add up your score for each column:

Tally your total score by combining your scores from all three columns:

- If your total score from all three columns combined is 10 or less:
  Your liver's ability to detoxify is most likely not impaired.
- If your total score from all three columns combined is between 10 and 25:
  Your liver's ability to detoxify is probably somewhat compromised.

• If your total score from all three columns combined is 25 or greater:
  Your liver's ability to detoxify is most likely impaired.

Even if your score indicates that your liver's ability to detoxify is not significantly impaired, it is important to become aware of the ways you may be unwittingly exposed to toxins and to limit your exposure to them. (See "Removing Toxins from Your Environment" on page 121.)

If your liver's ability to detoxify is somewhat compromised or most likely impaired, I recommend that you look into why. Consider whether toxins may be responsible for throwing your health out of balance: examine your lifestyle, dietary habits, prescription drug use, and recreational drug use (including alcohol). Take a look at your work and home environments. For instance, you may have been regularly exposed to toxins if you've worked in a hair salon or if you've lived for an extended period of time near an industrialized area, a location where agricultural insecticides and pesticides are used, or a golf course. You can't change your past exposure to toxins, but you can make healthier choices for the future. And you can help your liver process many of the toxins you have already been exposed to with the liver cleanse that begins on page 126.

TESTS TO EVALUATE LIVER HEALTH

Most Western doctors evaluate liver function by looking at a standard blood test that includes a measurement of the liver enzymes. If the test shows the liver enzymes are high, it means the liver cells are dying off at a rate faster than normal. This is common if you are suffering from hepatitis or inflammation of the liver. But even if the level of your liver enzymes is normal, the test doesn't tell you how well your liver is able to detoxify.

In the event that you want more information to evaluate how effectively your liver is functioning, your naturopathic physician can order special tests. The following are the tests most commonly used when more information is required to get the liver back on track.

NAME OF TEST	HOW THIS TEST WORKS/WHAT IT TELLS YOU
Liver detoxification profile*	This comprehensive test evaluates both Phase I and Phase II (the two-phase wash cycle) of the liver's detoxification system. It measures urine, saliva, and blood to assess how well these phases are working.
Antioxidant test	You can do this test at your naturopathic physician's office. It is a urine test that can tell you if you have adequate antioxidants in your system at the time of collection. If you have an abundance of antioxidants, your liver is better able to protect your tissues from the ravaging effects of toxins.

NAME OF TEST	HOW THIS TEST WORKS/WHAT IT TELLS YOU
Tests for environmental chemicals*	Blood and urine tests may give you some indication of the levels of environmental chemicals (such as DDT, PCBs, chlordane, or malathione) in your body. But these tests don't always provide you with a definitive assessment of your body's burden of these kinds of chemicals, because they are stored in your body fat; in some cases, a fat biopsy will give you more accurate results.
Heavy metal tests*	Your naturopathic physician can order a urine, stool, or hair test to evaluate you for heavy metals. To remove heavy metals from your body, work closely with your naturopath to devise a detoxification plan. (The supplements taken to remove heavy metals are by prescription only.) While you are taking these supplements, I recommend you do the liver cleanse outlined in this chapter. This will help your body remove heavy metals from your system more effectively.

*Laboratories that perform these tests are found in Appendix C.

EVALUATING YOUR LIVER HEALTH WITH CHINESE MEDICINE

From a Chinese perspective, evaluating the health of the liver means looking at physical and emotional symptoms, observing the quality of the tongue, and assessing the pulse. The conditions listed below are all considered excessive Wood, or liver, conditions. If you see yourself in one of these categories, you will benefit enormously from a liver cleanse, both physically and "energetically." The goal of a liver cleanse is to move Qi and Blood, clear heat and dampness, and ultimately to bring the entire body back into balance.

Liver Imbalances from a Chinese Medicine Perspective

SYMPTOMS	QUALITY OF THE TONGUE	QUALITY OF THE PULSE	CHINESE DIAGNOSIS/ CONDITION
Moodiness, depression, frustration, irritability; irregular and painful periods, pain before periods, breast swelling, breast cysts, PMS, poor appetite, and abdominal distension.	Normal or slightly purplish	Tense, tight, or wiry	Liver Qi stagnation
Irregular and painful periods, dark menstrual blood, clots in menstrual blood, uterine fibroids, abdominal pain, ovarian cysts, and endometriosis.	Purple, sometimes with dark purplish spots	Tense, tight, or wiry	Liver Blood stagnation
Irritability with outbursts of anger, headaches (especially at the temples), dizziness, a red face and eyes, a bitter taste in the mouth, constipation, dry stools, and ringing in the ears.	Red and dry, with a slightly yellow coating	Tense, tight, or wiry; full and fast	Liver fire blazing upward

SYMPTOMS	QUALITY OF THE TONGUE	QUALITY OF THE PULSE	CHINESE DIAGNOSIS/ CONDITION
A sense of fullness or pressure in the chest and upper abdominal area; jaundice; a bitter taste in the mouth, nausea, vomiting, a vaginal discharge that causes itching, loss of appetite, and abdominal swelling.	Red, with a thick yellow coating	Tense, tight, or wiry; "slippery" and fast	Damp-heat in the liver and gallbladder

How to Support Your Liver

The Naturally Healthy Lifestyle and Diet will help keep your liver in good health. But there are certain key lifestyle issues that were not addressed in Chapter 1 that specifically pertain to your liver. For example, you can use aromatherapy and flower essences to support your liver by nurturing your Wood element. When your liver is running smoothly from an energetic point of view, the health of your entire body benefits. Of course, your liver needs to be cared for physically as well. By removing toxins from your environment and doing everything you can to minimize your exposure to them, you can profoundly enhance your liver health.

AROMATHERAPY AND FLOWER ESSENCES TO BALANCE YOUR WOOD ELEMENT

According to Gabriel Mojay, author of *Aromatherapy for Healing the Spirit,* the essential oils bergamot, everlasting, and sweet orange will relieve stress and tension associated with stagnant liver Qi. Using these essential oils can help keep you on an even emotional keel and balance your Wood element. Add them to your favorite body lotion or your bath, or use them in an atomizer. If you carry a small vial of oil in your purse, you can dab a few drops on your wrist and deeply inhale the aroma when you feel agitated or stressed.

Bergamot. Recommended for depression due to chronic unrelenting stress and repressed emotions, bergamot is a musky-smelling oil that harmonizes your liver Qi and allows you to relax.

Everlasting. This essential oil can help resolve headaches and migraines resulting from stress and tension. It moves your Qi as well as your Blood, so it is used for muscle aches and pains. Gabriel Mojay points out that everlasting is helpful if you are "blocked" on an emotional level and are experiencing deep resentment, anger, and bitterness.

Sweet Orange. Sweet orange is recommended if you tend to strive for perfection but in the process become tense and irritable. It is also used for digestive problems that arise from stress.

Flower essences can also help you create subtle shifts in your emotions and balance your Wood element. They may be especially useful if you are a Wood type and tend to become angry and frustrated when you push yourself too hard for too long. If you find yourself in this uncomfortable state, use one of the following flower essences to engender a sense of inner peace and calm. The usual dose is a few drops or pellets placed under the tongue four times a day, but you can take flower essences once every two hours until the symptoms are alleviated. If the flower essence hasn't helped you within twelve hours, consider changing the remedy to one that better fits your particular symptoms.

Impatiens. This essence will help you cope with your emotions when you are excessively busy, impatient, and irritable. It is recommended if you feel rushed and agitated, unable to slow down and be in the moment, cut off from experiencing your true feelings, or burned out from exhaustion.

Dandelion. This essence is recommended if you experience tension from trying to achieve too much. It can help you feel more at ease if you find yourself overwhelmed with responsibilities and not paying attention to your body's needs.

Cayenne. This essence can be used when you feel emotionally "stuck" and resistant to change. It can help you create new growth and transformation in your life and get past whatever is blocking you from moving forward.

REMOVING TOXINS FROM YOUR ENVIRONMENT

Naturopathic physicians Stephen Barrie and Peter Bennett, authors of *7-Day Detox Miracle,* compare exposure to toxic chemicals in modern society to a leaky faucet that continually drips toxins into the body, which acts like a bucket. The liver keeps trying to empty the bucket, but when toxins overwhelm it, or it lacks the nutrients it needs to do its job, the bucket fills up and overflows. That overflow can be the beginning of many diseases and disorders. Though ancient Chinese texts of course do not mention environmental toxins, a traditional Chinese medical perspective would unquestionably view toxins as having a detrimental effect on liver Qi, increasing susceptibility to the condition known as stagnant liver Qi.

Although you can't escape being exposed to certain toxins, you can reduce your rate of contact with them—how fast the faucet leaks into your bucket—and make an enormous difference in your liver's ability to process and eliminate them from your body. And by regularly cleansing your liver—or emptying the bucket—you can further improve your overall health.

The best place to start decreasing your exposure to toxins is right in your home, the place where you have the most control over what you are exposed to. Without realizing it, you may be bringing a steady stream of toxic substances into your home and into your body. I recommend that you decrease your exposure on an ongoing basis, because although you can do a lot of good by immediately minimizing your exposure, the health benefits of removing toxins from your environment are cumulative, and some may come only after many years of making healthy choices.

In one study the Environmental Protection Agency analyzed six hundred homes over a five-year period and found that they contained more than twenty toxic compounds, some of which are linked to cancer and birth defects.[2] Many of the compounds you are exposed to in your home are likely to come from aerosol sprays, new furniture and rugs, paints, and cleaning solvents; these products often release gases that, when concentrated in your living space, can adversely affect your health. Other sources of household toxins include dry-cleaned clothing, tap water, yard and garden products, and personal items such as cosmetics, hair dyes, and nail polish.

Manufacturers claim that the amounts of toxic chemicals used in foods, cosmetics, furniture, and cleaning products are within ranges considered safe for humans, but an overwhelming amount of data shows links between these chemicals, hormone imbalances, and cancer. In small amounts your body can process toxins, but in large amounts—or perhaps in combination with other chemicals or your own hormones—they can lead to numerous health problems.

Increasing evidence shows that exposure to environmental toxins is only part of the picture. It appears that the *timing* of the exposure can also be critical. Children and unborn fetuses, because of their immature and developing immune and nervous systems, are much more susceptible than adults to the damaging effects of environmental chemicals. Research suggests that girls exposed to high levels of estrogen-mimicking chemicals during puberty can be at higher risk for breast cancer later in life.[3] Other studies, such as those cited by the authors of *Our Stolen Future* (a far-ranging look at the impact of man-made chemicals on health), suggest that environmental toxins that mimic estrogen may be responsible for the increased incidence of endometriosis in young women and estrogen-responsive breast cancer in postmenopausal women.[4] According to a study published in the *Archives of Environmental Health,* fatty tissue derived from women who had breast cancer showed higher levels of environmental chemicals than that of women who didn't have breast cancer.[5]

The following list will help you decrease your exposure to toxins in your everyday environment. Although this list doesn't address every situation in which you may be exposed, following its recommendations can make a big difference in your total exposure.

Use a Water Filter. Depending on where you live, your tap water may be a soup of toxic chemicals including heavy metals, agricultural products, fluoride, and chlorine. (See Chapter 3.)

Use an Air Filter. HEPA filters are good for removing dust mites and sequestering airborne chemicals from furniture, new clothes, and bedding and can also help clear the air of secondhand cigarette smoke. They are freestanding, low-maintenance machines that plug into any wall outlet. If you need to eliminate molds, use an ozone air filter (but not while you are in the room).

Bring Plants into Your Home That Help Detoxify the Air. These include aloe vera, spider plants, bamboo palms, Boston ferns, arrowhead plants, banana plants, Chinese evergreens, devil's ivy, English ivy, mums, peace lilies, philodendrons, and umbrella plants. These plants can remove both benzene and formaldehyde from a living space.[6]

Choose All-natural Biodegradable Cleaning Products. Many household cleaning products contain toxic chemicals such as phenols, formaldehyde, toluene, butane, and xylene, which can damage the immune system and overwhelm the liver's detoxification systems. You can find Seventh Generation and other liver-friendly cleaning products at your health food store.

Be Aware of the Potential Toxic Chemical Release from New Products in Your Home. If you've ever hung a new vinyl shower curtain in your bath, you've probably noticed the smell lingering in your bathroom as it gives off gases; air out a new shower curtain for several days before using it. New furniture can also emit toxins used in the manufacturing process. (Before you use new furniture, let it off-gas by leaving it for a few days in a room that you don't regularly use, with your air filter on.) Many new clothes, sheets, and comforters retain some amount of synthetic chemicals from the manufacturing process and should be washed before you use them.

Avoid Using Outdoor Lumber Products That Contain Arsenic. You can order a test kit to measure if there is arsenic in your picnic table, deck, or your child's play set. See Appendix B for information on how to order.

Use All-natural Pesticides in Your Yard. Some synthetic pesticides can mimic estrogen and act as hormone-disruptors in both women's and men's bodies, potentially inducing hormone-related disorders and cancers. Alternative pest-control products include Safer Garden Fungicide, Safer Tree and Shrub Insect Attack, and Safer Yard and Garden Insect Attack.

If You Have Pets, Avoid Using Flea and Tick Collars. You may be exposed to toxins in the collars when you touch your pets. If you use another method of flea or tick control, such as Frontline, on your pets, be sure not to touch them where you've applied the chemical.

Avoid Using Toxic Chemicals and Poisons to Exterminate Pests in Your Home. There are many natural nontoxic pest control products. One company, Fleabusters, uses a nontoxic product to dehydrate and kill bugs. Other alternative household pest-control products include Perma Proof Diatomaceous Earth, Perma Proof Drax Ant Gel, and Black Flag Roach Ender Roach Control System. Be aware that many rat poisons contain arsenic, a toxic heavy metal. Old-fashioned snap-traps are much better for your health!

Use All-natural Cosmetics and Personal Care Products. Many cosmetics contain toxic chemicals that you can absorb through your skin or inhale. A 2002 *New York Times* article cited a study showing that synthetic chemicals known as phthalates may cause birth defects. Phthalates, which were found to interfere with the reproductive development of male fetuses, are an ingredient in numerous deodorants, fragrances, hair gels, mousses, hair sprays, nail polishes, and body lotions. Of seventy-two products containing phthalates that were studied, only fifty-two listed the chemical on their ingredient labels. The Centers for Disease Control and Prevention measured levels of phthalates in humans and found that virtually all the 289 people tested had been exposed to them. They also found that the levels of phthalates were highest among women of reproductive age, presumably because of exposure from their personal care items. There are many other ingredients in cosmetic and personal care products that you should avoid; the list is too lengthy to include here. The easiest way to steer clear of them is to purchase all-natural products.[7]

Avoid Dry-cleaning Your Clothes. Approximately 90 percent of dry cleaning involves the use of a solvent called perchloroethylene, also known as Perc. Long-term exposure to Perc has been linked to increased risk of cancer in animals, and Perc is a potential carcinogen in humans. If you must have your clothes dry cleaned, request Perc-free dry cleaning or air out your clothes in a well-ventilated area (preferably outside your home) for a few days before you wear them.

Use Stainless Steel, Cast Iron, or Glass Cookware. I don't recommend using aluminum cookware because it can add a significant amount of aluminum, which is a toxic heavy metal, to your diet. If you use nonstick (Teflon) cookware, be sure that it isn't scratched or chipped, and avoid using it at extremely high temperatures. You can safely use copper cookware if it is lined with stainless steel.

Limit Your Exposure to Plastics. Many plastics are constantly off-gassing, and some chemicals in plastics, such as biphenyl-A or nonylphenol, can mimic estrogen. Avoid drinking water that has been kept in plastic containers and exposed to heat for extended periods of time. Heat can increase the levels of these chemicals in water stored in plastic, and the longer the water has been stored, the higher their concentration. Although bottled water may taste better and have fewer contaminants in it than most unfiltered tap water, it is a good idea to abstain from drinking any water that has been stored in plastic and left in the sun. Also avoid eating food that has been heated with any type of plastic wrapping in a microwave oven.

Avoid Getting Toxic Chemicals on Your Skin or Inhaling Their Fumes. These can include glues, paints, turpentine, car grease, and many other substances that may be commonly used in and around your home.

Be Aware of How You Pump Your Gasoline. Benzene, a known carcinogen, has been found on the clothing and skin of people after pumping gas. When you pump your gas, face away from the pump, try not to breathe the fumes, thoroughly wash your hands afterward, and change your clothes as soon as you get a chance.

Replace Silver Dental Fillings with Porcelain or Gold Fillings. Silver fillings (mercury amalgams) are a source of mercury and other heavy metals. Ask your dentist to use a dental dam in the process of removing them, so that you don't swallow debris from the old fillings. Some dentists have special equipment that can decrease your exposure to mercury as it is being removed from your teeth. If you replace your fillings with gold, be sure your dentist uses pure gold and not gold combined with the metal palladium. Take at least 1,000 mg of vitamin C before and after your fillings are removed. Dentists sometimes give their patients intravenous vitamin C to protect them from the deleterious effects of heavy metals they may be exposed to during the procedure.

Avoid Vaccines Containing Thimerosal. Thimerosal is a mercury-containing preservative. If it's necessary for you to be vaccinated, ask your health care provider to order a vaccine for you that is thimerosal-free. (The Merck pharmaceutical company makes thimerosal-free vaccines.)

Avoid Alcohol and Other Toxic Drugs. (See Chapters 5 and 8 for information on the deleterious effects alcohol can have on your health.)

For more information on how to find products that are environmentally friendly and don't compromise your liver health, see *The Safe Shopper's Bible* by David Steinman and Samuel Epstein, M.D.

The Liver Cleanse: Restoring Your Essential Vitality

Now that you've started helping your liver by decreasing your exposure to toxic chemicals in your environment, it's time to enhance your liver's ability to detoxify. I've designed the following liver cleanse to maximize your liver health from the standpoint of both Western and Chinese medicine; it will alleviate the physical burdens on your liver and can vastly improve your health—at the same time that it is balancing your liver Qi.

This cleanse includes the use of diet, supplements, herbs, and other ways of promoting the removal of toxins from your body. Although the liver is the central organizer of detoxification, it is one of many organs that remove toxins from the system; the skin, lungs, intestines, and kidneys all play important roles. This is why skin brushing, spa therapy, and regular exercise are important aspects of a liver cleanse; by helping eliminate toxins, they help your body detoxify and make your liver's job easier.

Cleansing your liver is easy and fun—and you will most likely feel fantastic while doing it. The goal is to help your liver do a better job by moving toxins out of your body, and ultimately to recharge your energy. Even if you are already healthy and feel great, this cleanse can give your liver an extra boost and make you healthier in the long run. I recommend that you do a liver cleanse at least once a year, continuing with your cleanse for a minimum of two weeks and a maximum of two months. How long you continue depends on how toxic your liver is and how well you respond to the treatment.

Most people feel great while they are doing a liver cleanse, but not everyone feels great during every phase of a cleanse. Some people experience side effects such as fatigue, headaches, insomnia, skin rashes, or other symptoms. These side effects can happen when you begin moving toxins out of deep storage in your body, where they may have been entrenched for a long time. If you experience side effects, you have a choice: you can either continue with your cleanse and work through the symptoms, or you can decrease the intensity of your cleanse until the symptoms dissipate. In this case, extend your cleanse for a longer period of time, to ensure that you adequately decrease your body's burden of toxins.

Consult your naturopathic physician if you have symptoms that don't go away when you decrease the intensity of your cleanse, or if you are on prescription drugs. Your liver may metabolize drugs more quickly while you are on a liver cleanse. For example, anticonvulsant drugs require steady levels in your bloodstream in order to maintain a nonseizure state; a liver cleanse could decrease the levels of the drugs and potentially result in seizures.

From a Chinese perspective, it's best to do a liver cleanse in the springtime. Spring is the primary season of the Wood element, when liver Qi is the strongest, and the time for rebirth and renewal. During the winter most people eat a heavier, higher-fat diet and lead a less active lifestyle, which can cause liver Qi imbalances. Symptoms of these imbalances include premenstrual syndrome, menstrual irregularities, painful periods, abdominal swelling, constipation, nausea, headaches, moodiness, depression, irritability, and anger. Your liver cleanse can alleviate all of these symptoms, help balance your liver Qi, and restore your essential vitality.

Every aspect of the liver cleanse is important. When combined, their cumulative effects can powerfully revitalize your liver. Let's look at each one in turn.

- **Eat a healthy vegetarian diet, choose organic foods, and avoid alcohol, caffeine, and processed foods.**

The diet I recommend for your liver cleanse is a modification of the Naturally Healthy Diet (outlined in Chapter 1), with special emphasis on maximizing liver health and empowering the body's natural ability to detoxify. From the standpoint of both Western and Chinese medicine, a diet that enhances overall health will increase the effectiveness of the liver cleanse in many ways.

It's best to eat a vegetarian diet while on your liver cleanse because most animal products contain environmental toxins, especially in their fat. From a Chinese perspective, some "warming" foods and spices may help with the cleanse, but many "neutral," "cooling," and "cold" foods can be especially beneficial in promoting detoxification. You help your liver enormously by eating organic foods, because they are free of pesticides. And as we saw in Chapter 1, organic foods may also be higher in antioxidants than nonorganic foods. Antioxidants are important for both wash cycles of your liver (Phase I and Phase II of your detoxification system) to function optimally.

It is important to avoid alcohol during your liver cleanse, because alcohol is toxic to the liver in any amount. The whole point of the liver cleanse is to detoxify; the last thing you want to do is add toxic substances to your body. Also steer clear of caffeine during the cleanse; you need to take as much stress off your liver and adrenal glands as possible. Processed foods should be avoided as well; they are full of synthetic preservatives and colorings. It is important to avoid ingesting unnatural chemicals while you are on your liver cleanse.

- **Eat adequate protein and take specific amino acids to enhance your liver detoxification.**

You can significantly enhance your liver's ability to detoxify by providing it with the proteins it needs to function. People who are on a chronically low-protein diet do not detoxify as well as those who ingest adequate amounts of protein.

While you are on your liver cleanse, eat plenty of beans and legumes. Other vegetarian protein sources include wheat seitan, eggs, and nonfat yogurt. If you are unable to eat a vegetarian diet for any reason, choose to eat small amounts of low-mercury fish and organic poultry. Be sure to eat frequent meals to avoid experiencing low blood sugar or hypoglycemic symptoms such as light-headedness, irritability, weakness, and foggy thinking.

The amino acids glycine and glutamine can raise the level of the most important antioxidant working in your liver. This antioxidant, glutathione, is critical for your liver's second wash cycle to operate. To promote your liver function during your cleanse, take 500 mg of glycine three times a day, and 500 mg of glutamine three times a day.

- **Drink lemon water every day.**

Lemons are a sour food and therefore have a strong action on the liver. In Chinese medicine, it is said that lemons draw impurities out of the liver because they are an astringent. Lemons contain a compound in their peel, D-limonene, which can assist with liver detoxification because it is a potent stimulator of the first and second wash cycles. To make lemon water, squeeze a whole organic lemon into 48 ounces of filtered water and grate in some of the peel; drink this amount over the course of each day during your cleanse.

- **Drink dandelion root tea.**

Dandelion root tea can increase bile flow, which enhances your body's ability to eliminate toxins through your gallbladder. It can also decrease lymph congestion and decongest your liver. In Chinese medicine, dandelion is an effective herb for promoting detoxification because it clears toxic heat and dampness.

To prepare dandelion root tea, simmer two tablespoons of the root in four cups of filtered water on low heat for ten to fifteen minutes. Strain, and drink one cup twice a day. (Note: Dandelion root is a diuretic, so you may have to urinate more often while taking it.)

- **Increase your dietary intake of liver-supportive foods.**

Liver-supportive foods include such vegetables as Jerusalem artichokes, globe artichokes, burdock root, beets, garlic, and beans. They also include cruciferous vegetables, such as broccoli, cabbage, brussels sprouts, bok choi, kale, kohlrabi, turnips, and cauliflower. Broccoli sprouts (the tiny shoots from broccoli seeds) are especially supportive of the liver. Jerusalem artichokes and burdock root contain an immune-enhancing, liver-friendly compound called inulin. Globe artichokes help the liver produce bile.

Naturopathic physicians have included beets in liver detoxification programs for decades because they contain betaine. Betaine can induce the liver's second wash cycle to kick into gear.[8] (It can also enhance the breakdown of homocysteine, a compound found to increase the risk of heart disease.) In Chinese medicine, beets are known to nourish Blood and clear the liver; they are also excellent for women who have menstrual disorders and constipation, which can both be caused by poor liver function.

Garlic and beans are loaded with sulfur compounds that help the liver's second wash cycle work more efficiently. Although garlic is considered energetically "hot" in Chinese medicine, small amounts can stimulate the liver Qi to help remove toxins. Avoid eating garlic in excess; too much will stagnate your liver Qi, which can impair your ability to detoxify. I recommend adding one clove of chopped garlic to your food each day as part of your liver cleanse.

Cruciferous vegetables contain indole-3-carbinol, a cancer-fighting compound that also stimulates detoxification in the intestines and in both wash cycles of the liver.[9] Indole-3-carbinol also assists the liver with estrogen metabolism, promoting the formation of friendly estrogen compounds rather than unfriendly, potentially cancer-causing estrogen compounds.

Eat broccoli sprouts often during your cleanse; I recommend at least one cup each day. They are full of antioxidants that increase the rate of liver detoxification. In Chinese medicine, broccoli has the energetic function of clearing heat, which is beneficial to your liver cleanse.

- **Avoid grapefruits and grapefruit juice.**

Grapefruit contains naringenin, a compound that can significantly impair the liver's ability to break down toxins. Research has shown that many pharmaceutical drugs remain in circulation in your body longer than expected if they are taken with grapefruit juice.[10] Grapefruit juice could cause increased toxic side effects from these drugs or other toxic substances.

I recommend that you always limit your intake of grapefruit and grapefruit juice, even after your cleanse.

- **Eat oranges and tangerines.**

Oranges and tangerines contain compounds that help your liver break down toxins in both your first and second wash cycles.[11] You can also make your own fresh orange or tangerine juice.

- **Use the herbs turmeric and dill weed in your diet, and avoid cayenne.**

I recommend you increase your consumption of curries containing turmeric during your liver cleanse. Turmeric contains curcumin, which can increase the breakdown of cancer-causing agents by its direct action on the liver.[12] In Chinese medicine, turmeric is also considered to be excellent for liver Qi stagnation.[13] Increasing your consumption of dill weed will also help with your liver cleanse. The oils in dill weed can activate your liver's ability to break down toxins. In Chinese medicine, dill weed is beneficial if you have liver Qi stagnation because it can move Qi, which helps with liver detoxification.

It's a good idea to limit your consumption of cayenne pepper while you are cleansing your liver. Cayenne contains capsaicin, a compound that can inhibit the liver's first wash cycle. In Chinese medicine, cayenne pepper is considered a "hot" herb, and although a small amount can benefit you by moving your liver Qi, too much can cause your liver Qi to become stagnant. It is best to have your liver Qi flowing freely during your cleanse to assist with detoxification.

- **Drink vegetable-fruit smoothies or juices twice a day.**

From a Western medicine viewpoint, vegetable-fruit smoothies can assist with your liver cleanse because they are full of fiber, which helps remove toxins from the body. They also are full of antioxidants and other compounds that assist the liver with detoxification. According to Chinese medicine, most vegetables and fruits are energetically "neutral," "cooling," or "cold" foods and can help remove toxins (which tend to be energetically "hot").

If you use a superblender to make your smoothies, you get the added benefits of all the fiber in your vegetables and fruits. (A regular blender is not powerful enough to liquefy some ingredients, such as carrots; see Appendix B for information on superblenders.) If you are using a juicer rather than a superblender, it's best to increase your fiber intake by adding a tablespoon of psyllium husk to each smoothie. (With a juicer, you discard the fiber.)

Make a fresh vegetable-fruit smoothie or juice twice a day during your cleanse, and make only what you can drink at the time; if you store your smoothie or juice in the refrigerator for future use, it can lose much of its antioxidant content. The following is a simple recipe that you can alter depending on the vegetables and fruits available.

Basic Vegetable-Fruit Smoothie/Juice

1 carrot
½ cup fresh parsley or spinach
½ apple
1 to 2 cups filtered water
1 tablespoon psyllium husk (if you use a juicer)

For variety, and to increase your consumption of raw fruits and vegetables, add any of the following: a few slices of cucumber or raw beet, a tomato, a banana, a stalk of celery, or ½ cup beet greens.

Some people choose to do a juice fast as part of their liver cleanse. Juice fasting can accelerate the detoxification process. During a juice fast, it's important to continue to take the supplements outlined for the liver cleanse. To do a juice fast, stop eating all solid food and ingest only vegetable-fruit juices or smoothies. (You can use either a juicer or your superblender to do a juice fast.) You can do a juice fast for up to three days, but I recommend that you begin juice fasting after you've been on your liver cleanse for at least a week and that you continue your liver cleanse for at least a week after your juice fast has ended. You can do a juice fast once or twice a year, but juice fasting should not be done if you're pregnant or lactating, or if you have diabetes or hypoglycemia.

- **Take a daily multivitamin to assist your liver with detoxification.**

Your multivitamin will provide you with many nutrients that help with liver detoxification; minerals and the B vitamins are especially important. When it comes to supporting liver health, minerals support the body's Qi, and B complex vitamins nourish, soothe, and rectify liver Qi. The amounts of each nutrient that should be found in your daily multivitamin are listed in Chapter 2.

- **Take antioxidants to enhance your liver function.**

Antioxidants are important for liver health. They assist in liver detoxification by supporting the two-phase wash cycle in many ways. As inner bodyguards, they take stress off the liver by putting themselves in the way of free radicals. Free radicals are generated by environmental stressors, chemicals, sunlight, and your own metabolism. The more antioxidant potential you have, the more able you are to effectively neutralize the damaging effects of toxins and free radicals.

Certain antioxidants, such as vitamin C, alpha lipoic acid, and selenium, are especially important because they keep the liver operating in top form by recycling glutathione, an essential compound necessary for the liver's second wash cycle. I recommend you take the following amounts of these antioxidants every day during your liver cleanse: 3,000 mg of vitamin C, 200 mcg of selenium, and 100 mg of alpha lipoic acid. (Check your daily multivitamin; it will probably not contain these amounts of vitamin C and alpha lipoic acid, so you will need to take additional supplements to make sure that you are getting a total of these amounts.) In Chinese medicine, vitamin C is especially beneficial to the liver because it helps eliminate toxins by clearing heat.[14]

- **Take a lipotropic complex.**

Lipotropic complexes, which are nutritional supplements consisting of vitamins, amino acids, and herbs, are designed to enhance the liver's ability to function. You can find lipotropic complexes at your local health food store. They usually contain vitamin B6, magnesium oxide, choline, inositol, methionine, and the following herbs: milk thistle, dandelion root, Oregon grape root, and celandine. Take one pill three times a day with meals while you are on your liver cleanse.

The nutrients in a lipotropic formula are aimed at helping your liver's detoxification systems (your two-phase wash cycle) function optimally. One of the most beneficial herbs for this purpose is milk thistle; it not only protects the liver from the damaging effects of toxins, it also increases your liver's ability to break toxins down. In addition, milk thistle helps damaged liver tissue regenerate, acts as a potent antioxidant, and prevents the depletion of glutathione.[15] In Chinese medicine, milk thistle is used to treat liver Qi stagnation and revitalize the Blood.

- **Do a liver flush to help your liver release toxins.**

A liver flush is sometimes referred to as a gallbladder flush, because it can induce your gallbladder to release the bile (and toxins bound up with bile) stored there. You should refrain from doing a liver flush if you've been diagnosed with gallstones because the flush could release stones from your gallbladder into your bile duct; if they are of a certain size, they could become lodged in your bile duct, resulting in a medical emergency.

If you don't have gallstones, begin your liver flush one week after you've started your liver cleanse. To do your liver flush, take the following on an empty stomach first thing in the morning: one tablespoon of lemon or lime juice mixed in two tablespoons of organic extra-virgin olive oil. Do this every morning for three to six days.

- **Release toxins through spa therapy.**

Perspiration can enhance the body's ability to eliminate toxins that have been stored in the fatty tissues. One of the best ways you can shed toxins through sweating is with a sauna. Researcher and clinical nutritionist Russell Jaffe, M.D., Ph.D., a leading expert on low-heat dry sauna use, recommends using a sauna at a temperature of

105 to 110 degrees Fahrenheit for forty-five to ninety minutes, three to five times a week.

According to Dr. Jaffe, "Low-temperature 'spa therapy' can release fat-soluble toxins such as PCBs, pesticides, solvents, and phthalates that are stored in your fatty tissues." It is important to be in a low-heat dry sauna for a prolonged period of time in order to get the full benefits of spa therapy. He advises staying in the sauna until an oily film forms on your skin. If temperatures are too high or the duration of time too short, you will eliminate mainly water and electrolytes. When you have been in a low-heat dry sauna for at least forty-five minutes, you begin to release toxins that wouldn't otherwise be mobilized out of your body.

After spa therapy, vigorously wash your skin to remove any toxins that have been released, which could otherwise be reabsorbed; Dr. Jaffe suggests that you use a loofah sponge and glycerin soap. For people who have a high burden of toxins in their fatty tissues due to frequent exposure or occupational hazards, he recommends a low-heat sauna five to seven days a week, for three to six months; he also advises taking adequate protective antioxidants to reduce the risk of these chemicals harming the body while they are being released.

If spa therapy is not an option for you, another way to detoxify by sweating is to enroll in Bikram yoga classes. The classes are conducted in an environment heated to 105 degrees, and they last up to ninety minutes. This form of yoga is great exercise: you will most definitely sweat. (Be sure to shower as soon as possible after each class to remove the newly eliminated toxins from your skin.) Drink plenty of fluids before and after any therapy or activity that involves a lot of sweating. Refrain from doing spa therapy or Bikram yoga if you have high blood pressure or advanced heart disease or are pregnant.

If you have imbalances in your liver—such as the conditions known in Chinese medicine as Liver Fire Blazing Upward or Damp-Heat in Your Liver and Gallbladder (see the "Liver Imbalances" chart on pages 119–120)—you should refrain from saunas or hot yoga classes until your fire has cooled down. You will know that your fire has cooled down when you no longer experience the symptoms of Liver Fire Blazing Upward (such as irritability, anger, and constipation) or of Damp-Heat in Your Liver and Gallbladder (such as a feeling of fullness in your chest and upper abdomen, nausea, and loss of appetite). Adding more heat to these conditions could make your symptoms worse. Wait until you've been on your liver cleanse for at least a week and some of your symptoms have dissipated before you begin heat therapy of any kind.

- **Do skin brushing once a day.**

By stimulating your circulation of blood and lymph, skin brushing can help your body detoxify. It also removes dead skin cells from the surface of your body. I suggest you use a soft shower brush once a day, before your bath or shower, to gently brush your skin. Always brush toward your heart, because this is the direction in which your venous blood flows. Cover every area of your skin from your neck down, and use a washcloth on your face.

- **Do aerobic exercise at least four times a week.**
  Aerobic exercise is an important part of your liver cleanse because it increases the blood flow through your liver, releases toxins through sweating, and helps with detoxification by bringing more oxygen to all your tissues. At the same time, it improves the circulation of your lymphatic fluids, which assists in the removal of toxins from your tissues. Aerobic exercise is also recommended during a liver cleanse from a Chinese medicine perspective, because it releases heat and moves liver Qi and Blood. You may find that while you are on your liver cleanse, exercising gives you a greater-than-usual sense of energy and power in your body.

Your Master Cleanser: Final Thoughts

After you've completed your liver cleanse, you can incorporate many of the tools you discovered during the cleanse into your daily routine. For example, it's a good idea to keep drinking lemon water on a regular basis, ingesting vegetable-fruit smoothies a few times a week, and choosing organic, high-fiber foods that best support your liver; I also recommend that you continue with regular aerobic exercise and other methods we've explored for increasing sweating.

When your liver is working optimally, you feel great because your body efficiently processes toxins and removes them from your system. Your liver is also your organ of regeneration, continuously renewing your health and orchestrating the flow of Qi. As long as you keep your liver healthy, you are regenerating the essential vitality of your entire body, your mind, and your spirit. By following the plan I've outlined in this chapter, you can keep your liver healthy from both a Western and a Chinese medicine viewpoint. Remember to nurture your Wood element, especially if you are a Wood type. All your life goals, all your future successes and achievements, may ultimately depend on your ability to keep your liver healthy and your Wood element balanced.

The Essence of Chapter 4

- Be mindful that your liver is the master cleanser for your entire body.
- Keep your Wood element balanced: it strongly influences your liver, which maintains the flow of Qi throughout your body.
- Assess your liver function and your ability to detoxify.
- Use aromatherapy and flower essences to keep your Wood element in balance.
- Remove toxins from your environment, or limit your exposure to them.
- Do a thorough liver cleanse to help your master detoxifier do its job.
- Incorporate into your daily life some of the tools you discovered doing your liver cleanse.
- Remember, especially if you are a Wood type, that great health is critical to achieving your life goals.

Chapter 5

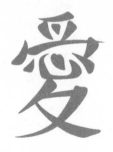

Love

A Fire Within:
Creating Health in Your Heart
and Spirit

*"The heart is the sovereign of all organs and represents the
consciousness of one's being. It is responsible for intelligence, wisdom,
and spiritual transformation."*

—The Yellow Emperor's Classic (THIRD CENTURY B.C.)

W HEN *I first saw Jennifer, she was concerned about her heart health because her blood
tests showed that her cholesterol and triglyceride levels were higher than normal. She
also had borderline high blood pressure. She was tired and frustrated and said that she felt
"worked to the bone." But she wanted to take charge of her health and do everything she could
to avoid taking various drugs to prevent heart disease as other family members did.*

*I learned that Jennifer was forty years old and living a busy life as a full-time teacher
and mother of two. With the birth of her second child three years earlier, her exercise routine
disappeared, and she had gained weight. It became clear that she needed time to take care of
her heart, including her spiritual and emotional heart. After supporting her heart for a few
months with diet, exercise, herbal and nutritional supplements, and lifestyle changes,
Jennifer was happy to inform me that, to her medical doctor's surprise, not only did her blood
tests show marked improvement, but her blood pressure did, too. "I discovered that by taking*

care of my heart both physically and emotionally," Jennifer said, "I was also taking care of the part of me that could bring joy into my life, my work, and my family."

A Healthy Heart

The heart plays a central role in virtually every function in the body. The heart and its blood vessels are like branches springing from a tree, giving life. They are ceaseless in their efforts to provide nourishment and deliver the most precious substance, oxygen, to every cell in the body.

But a woman's heart is so much more. Many women come to see me because they are concerned about the health of their hearts; what I help them understand is that by nurturing their emotional hearts, they can profoundly affect their physical health. My goal is to help them see that by shifting toward themselves some of the nurturing energy they give so freely to others, they can not only feel more emotionally balanced but create positive physical changes as well.

Nowhere is the mind-body connection more evident than with your heart. From ancient Chinese texts to a modern-day perception, the heart represents emotions, particularly love. The Chinese say the spirit is stored in the heart and a healthy heart can experience abundant joy. Recent scientific studies have confirmed that laughter can enhance heart health.[1] I recommend that my patients laugh often and "heartily."

Your heart deserves special care. Diseases of the heart are the leading cause of death for women in the United States. In fact, heart disease affects more women than the disease women seem to fear most—breast cancer. According to the National Heart, Lung, and Blood Institute, one in ten American women forty-five to sixty-four years of age has some form of heart disease, and this increases to one in four women over age sixty-five.[2] In addition, millions of women have suffered from strokes, and 93,000 women die of stroke each year.

The good news is that heart disease is largely a preventable condition. With a healthy diet and lifestyle, you can create excellent heart health and avoid heart disease. It's important to begin taking care of your heart at an early age because many heart diseases, especially hardening of the arteries, start many years before symptoms appear.[3] But it's never too late. When it comes to matters of your heart, you have a lot of power to control your destiny.

According to Chinese medicine, the heart is represented by the Fire element and requires balanced Qi for optimal health. Among the qualities the Fire element represents are laughter, joy, heat, and love. Creative visions and your ability to bring them to fruition come from your heart; when your Fire element is in balance and your heart

Qi is strong, you're capable of manifesting love, including self-love, in its highest form as unconditional love and acceptance.

The Naturally Healthy Lifestyle—which consists of excellent nutrition, regular exercise, balanced Qi, and adequate detoxification—can strengthen your heart, keep levels of harmful cholesterol within an optimal range, and protect your blood vessels from injury. Making such heart-healthy choices will enable your cardiovascular system to function optimally throughout your life.

The View from the West

Your heart muscle keeps pumping, without conscious thought or effort, every day of your life. One side of the pump sends blood to your lungs to be refreshed with oxygen; the other sends the blood saturated with oxygen out to every cell in your body. Your arteries, which carry the oxygen-rich blood from your heart, are powerful conduits that end in minuscule capillaries. Oxygen is dropped off at your capillaries, and then your blood begins its journey back to your heart and lungs through your veins. Each breath saturates your blood with oxygen essential for life. Your heart beats 100,000 times every day, and the cycle repeats itself a staggering number of times over the course of your life. Your heart and its blood vessels (the arteries, capillaries, and veins) make up what is called your cardiovascular system.

Your heart is a muscle not unlike your biceps but far more specialized. It's made up of three different types of muscle and is encased in a protective tissue layer called the pericardium. Another layer of tissue, the delicate endothelium, lines the insides of your arteries. Protecting your endothelium from damage is critical to preventing the onset of atherosclerosis, or clogging and narrowing of the arteries, the most common heart disease.

The View from the East

We can find no wealth above a healthy body and a happy heart.
—Chinese proverb

In Chinese medicine, the heart is the king, the part that loves, and the place where the spirit resides. The heart also houses the mind. A healthy heart allows for clarity of mind and peaceful sleep and enables laughter and feelings of joy and happiness.

Western medicine is confirming what has been known for centuries in the

East—that a healthy heart is a joyful one. Research has shown that laughter and a good sense of humor may protect you from heart disease and that emotions can have a profound effect on stress levels, the heart, and the immune system.[4] A study published by Duke University in 1999 demonstrated that maintenance of emotional well-being is critical to cardiovascular health.[5] In the 1970s author Norman Cousins sparked the interest of researchers when he outlined his recovery from a chronic degenerative disease in his book *Anatomy of an Illness;* he watched funny movies and laughed his way back to health. Many others have advocated laughter as the best medicine, from Patch Adams, M.D., founder of the Gesundheit! Institute, to Bernie Siegel, M.D., author of *Humor and Healing.*

In the West, many health care practitioners use visualization and positive thinking to tap into the power of the mind for healing. Visualizations can be as simple as envisioning yourself as "the little engine that could," imagining yourself enjoying optimal health free of pains or worries, or seeing yourself winning an athletic competition or a victory over disease. Many Westerners assume that the heart has no part in this process, but Chinese medicine—because it holds that the heart has such an intimate relationship to the mind—sees a healthy heart as playing an important role in empowering the mind to help people achieve their full potential.

According to Chinese medicine, the heart has important connections to many other organs and systems in the body. Since your heart Qi manifests on your face, your complexion glows when you have a healthy heart. As the great Taoist sage Chuang-tzu wrote in the third century B.C., "Those whose hearts are in a state of repose give forth a divine radiance, by the light of which they see themselves as they are."[6]

The Fire Element

Kula, a thin and exuberant young woman, came to see me because she was experiencing anxiety and insomnia. Her anxiety had started after a prolonged period of stress; she had been preparing diligently for her acting finals. She couldn't sleep at night because her mind was racing, so she was drinking coffee in the morning to keep herself awake. Kula expressed a number of Fire personality traits; she loved working with people and being the center of attention. She disliked being alone. She told me that whenever she pushed herself too hard, she would get insomnia. Kula was very talkative and expressive, and she laughed a lot during our visit.

A perfect example of the Fire type, Kula was passionate about acting, driven by her excitement and enthusiasm, and fueled by an intense desire to be in the limelight. I told Kula that when she was under increased stress, she'd probably always have some imbalance in her Fire element. Knowing her own tendencies, Kula could be aware of the emotional imbalances that can result from stress and make choices to nurture her Fire element when she knew she'd be going through a stressful time. I recommended that she stop drinking coffee, begin gentle yin exercises, and eat cooling foods that would have a yin effect on her body.

The heart is represented by the Fire element in Chinese medicine. The Fire element symbolizes love and rules summer, the months of intense growth and heat, when the year is reaching its fullest potential. It governs the south, where temperatures are warm and summerlike, and it is associated with heat and the color red.

As you have seen, we all have all of the Five Elements—Wood, Fire, Earth, Metal, and Water—within us, but one element can dominate. If you are a Fire type, you have exuberant energy and enthusiasm and an abundance of joy and creativity. You are full of love and passion, you like drama, and you thrive on travel. When your energy is balanced, you are emotionally stable and easily able to separate what's important in your life from what's trivial. You have harmony in your body, and protection for your physical and emotional heart. You can stay focused, think logically, and at the same time be passionate about your friends, family, and personal interests. When it comes to relationships, you have an enormous amount of what I call "social Qi," a seemingly boundless energy for social interaction. You absolutely love to be with people.

In Chinese medicine, the heart connects directly with the tongue and governs speech; if you are a Fire type, you especially enjoy expressing yourself verbally and speaking rapidly. In fact, you do just about everything quickly, and you thrive on sports involving constant motion. You can get so excited about what you're doing that your breathing becomes hurried and shallow. Your most productive time of day is between eleven A.M. and three P.M. When you are healthy, you soar; when you are unhealthy, you crash hard to the ground.

Since your heart is your king, when your Fire element is in balance, your other elements (Earth, Metal, Water, and Wood) will also be in better balance. The more balance created among your elements, the better your health will be. Because the Fire element represents love, a balanced Fire element enables you to create self-love, the place from which much healing comes. And because your mind and spirit are housed in your heart, a healthy heart means a healthy mind and spirit—which also means a healthy body.

As a Fire type, you experience imbalances—excess fire flaming upward or a fire that has gone out—when you push too hard for too long, thriving on excitement but ultimately burning out. Too much or too little fire can lead to a number of physical and emotional symptoms. For example, when your fire is too low, you can have difficulty staying focused and separating your thoughts from your feelings, or you may lack your usual spontaneity and creativity, feel tongue-tied, or become depressed. When your fire is too high, you are agitated, easily irritated, and boisterous and can experience insomnia and hypertension. Your Fire can also become imbalanced when there's too little water, or yin, to offset it, which often occurs with prolonged stress, as in Kula's case.

Since your heart controls your blood, you can experience menstrual irregularities if your Fire element is imbalanced. Your heart also controls your body temperature and your perspiration; when your Fire element is out of balance, you may have a pale complexion or perspire excessively.

According to Chinese medicine, the Fire element includes the heart's three ministers: the "triple burner," the pericardium, and the small intestine. These three ministers act as imperial bodyguards to the king—the heart—who is critical to the operation of all of the other organs in the body.

The triple burner can be thought of as the Qi in the chest, abdomen, and pelvis. With a "burner" in each of these areas, it performs energetic functions related to the heart, digestive system, and kidneys. In your heart, your triple burner works to create harmony and emotional well-being. For instance, it helps you maintain sincere, long-lasting commitments. If you have an imbalance in your triple burner, you may have an abundance of ideas for exciting new projects, but once the excitement wears off you tend to shelve them and your commitments to them dissolve. You may have a history of finding the "love of your life" one week, only to move on to a new relationship the next. For a Fire type, this is reflected in the quality of fire flaring up suddenly and then dying out just as quickly.

In Chinese medicine, the pericardium, the layer of tissue surrounding the heart, plays a significant role in defending the heart from disturbance and insult. The heart is seen as being so important to the spirit that it requires the special bodyguard of the pericardium to protect it against any physical or psychological trauma. Your pericardium is responsible for safeguarding your intimate relationships and for protecting the very center of your being from the shocks of the world.

The small intestine is intimately connected to the heart, separating the pure from the impure. It sorts through food and assimilates the nutrients. The heart can even alleviate some of its excess fire by shifting it to the small intestine. When this happens, you can experience poor digestion and "heartburn," metaphorically a most fitting term. On a mental and spiritual level, the small intestine plays a vital role in sorting through information and emotions. Healthy small-intestine Qi allows you to figure out which aspects of your life are most important. When your small intestine Qi is weak, you have trouble sorting not only through the food you eat but also through your experiences to clarify which choices, feelings, ideas, values, and relationships are healthy and which ones aren't. You can keep your small-intestine Qi strong by eating healthy food and maintaining optimal digestion. (See Chapter 6.)

The three ministers—the triple burner, the pericardium, and the small intestine—all help protect the heart from disharmony. Your heart becomes imbalanced only after more subordinate organs are thrown off balance. For example, when your kidney becomes deficient in yin, or water, other organ systems become dry and stressed. Your heart is profoundly affected when this happens, and your body can manifest symptoms of insomnia, hot flashes, and anxiety. But it takes a lot of chaos to overthrow your king, and taking the steps outlined in this chapter can keep the heart on its throne.

Are You a Fire Type?

- Are you outgoing?
- Are you charismatic?
- When you have a new idea, are you full of excitement and enthusiasm?
- Are you loquacious?
- Do you seek out drama and sensation?
- Are you extremely emotional?
- Do you tend to share how you feel with others?
- Are you often excessively empathic to others' needs?
- Do you get overly sentimental?
- Do you prefer to be with company?
- Do you thrive on change?
- Do you love to travel?
- When you're nervous, do you tend to laugh?
- Is it easy for you to feel love for others?
- Do you thrive when you regularly create time to nurture yourself?
- Are you most productive from eleven A.M. to three P.M.?
- Do you love summer more than any other season?
- Are you genuinely friendly to strangers?

If you answered yes to most of these questions, your personality is most likely dominated by the Fire element, and it is especially important for you to nourish your heart. Your goal is to keep your fire burning steadily—not too high and not too low. You can take the following steps to keep your Fire element balanced:

Keep your energy focused on what's really important in your life.
Maintain healthy emotional boundaries with others.
Create a schedule that includes time to nurture yourself.
Follow your Naturally Healthy Diet to nourish your physical and "energetic" heart.
Eat regular meals; don't allow yourself to get too hungry.
Limit your intake of hot and spicy foods.
Practice deep breathing on a regular basis.
Engage in activities that bring you joy and nourish your heart Qi.
Quiet your mind through meditation, visualization, and peaceful thoughts.

Assessing Your Heart Health with Western Medicine

From a Western medical perspective, the cardiovascular system is considered healthy when the blood vessels are clear of debris—free of plaque in the vessel walls—and the heart can perform its pumping action without distress. Although most people think of a heart attack as the most common result of heart disease, the heart will often give many signals before serious heart problems result. What are the signals for heart disease that you should learn to watch out for? One of them, high blood pressure, or *hypertension,* is exactly what it sounds like. When the heart and blood vessels are performing under a lot of pressure, your cardiovascular system is under an increased amount of stress. Over time this stress can damage your blood vessels, increase your risk of both arteriosclerosis and atherosclerosis, and lead to a heart attack or stroke.

Arteriosclerosis is also known as "hardening of the arteries" because it can cause the arteries to lose their elasticity and become inflexible. This condition usually develops when a person has chronic high blood pressure, consistently high cholesterol, diabetes, or other risk factors. Atherosclerosis, the most common form of arteriosclerosis, is a condition in which the blood vessels become narrowed and clogged with cholesterol deposits, or plaque. This condition develops in the endothelium, the delicate layer of tissue lining the arteries, and can eventually impede blood flow and the amount of oxygen that gets to your tissues. Coronary artery disease is a condition that develops when your coronary arteries, which directly supply your heart, fill with plaque. This can ultimately result in a heart attack, a condition in which heart muscle actually dies. Other heart conditions include angina, arrhythmia, congestive heart failure, stroke, and palpitations.

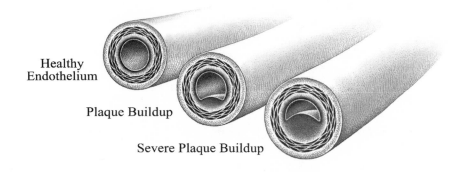

Healthy
Endothelium

Plaque Buildup

Severe Plaque Buildup

Many women first come to me with concerns about their heart health when they begin to see signs like increased cholesterol levels, increased triglycerides, and high blood pressure. Let's look at each of these factors and what they mean for your heart and your whole body—and how evaluating your own risk for heart disease is important for assessing the health of your cardiovascular system.

CHOLESTEROL AND TRIGLYCERIDE LEVELS

As you've seen, cholesterol, a waxy substance produced by your liver and found in the foods you eat, can play a critical role in the development of problems in your heart and blood vessels. You need cholesterol because it's part of every cell membrane in your body. Your cholesterol level is linked to your hormones; too little cholesterol can lead to abnormally low hormone levels. But too much cholesterol, especially the wrong kind, can increase your risk of heart disease.

It's important to maintain a favorable ratio of good to bad cholesterol. The heart and blood vessels favor "good" HDL cholesterol and are not fond of "bad" LDL cholesterol that can clog their conduits with plaque. As the accompanying box illustrates, it's important to keep your total cholesterol level at less than 200 mg per deciliter of blood, your LDL level low, and your HDL level high. Research has hailed HDL cholesterol as the most accurate predictor of heart disease risk. Exercise and a balanced diet can increase HDL cholesterol.

Total Cholesterol Level
   Less than 200: desirable
   200 to 239: borderline high
   240 or higher: high

HDL (Favorable) Cholesterol
   Less than 40: low
   60 or higher: high

LDL (Unfavorable) Cholesterol
   Less than 100: optimal*
   100 to 129: near or above optimal
   130 to 159: borderline high
   160 to 189: high
   190 or higher: very high

Source: *Third Report of the Expert Panel on Detection, Evaluation, and Treatment of High Blood Pressure* (2001).[7]

Measurements are in mg/dl.

*The National Institutes of Health recommends that the goal for LDL cholesterol levels be less than 70 mg/dl for those who are at "very high risk" for a heart attack.

Triglycerides are fats that circulate in the blood. They come primarily from fats, alcohol, and simple carbohydrates in the diet. Chronically high triglyceride levels in women over fifty are a strong predictor for the development of coronary artery disease. You can reduce triglyceride levels by following the Naturally Healthy Diet, making lifestyle changes (such as decreasing stress), and exercising.

BLOOD PRESSURE AND PULSE

Blood pressure measures the work capacity of the heart as it circulates the blood through the cardiovascular system. When your blood pressure is taken, you are given a reading with an upper number and a lower number. The upper number (the *systolic* blood pressure) represents how hard your heart has to work to push blood out; the lower number (*diastolic* blood pressure) represents the pressure in your heart when it's resting between contractions. Your blood pressure can vary during the day—for instance, when you exercise or experience stress.

Annual measurements of your blood pressure are sufficient unless you're more than sixty years of age, are on medications that can increase blood pressure such as birth control pills, or have a history of abnormal readings. In a phenomenon called *white coat syndrome,* people may register transiently high readings when they have their blood pressure taken at the doctor's office; when the measurement is taken in the comfort of their own homes, it is within normal range. One high reading doesn't necessarily mean you have high blood pressure. If your blood pressure reading is higher than normal, it's a good idea to take readings at different times of the day to see if they are consistently high. A diagnosis of high blood pressure is given only after three different high blood pressure readings have been taken at separate doctor visits.

High blood pressure is a major risk factor for heart disease, heart attack, and stroke. Extra pressure on the vessels can damage the delicate endothelium and lead to increased deposition of plaque. Hypertension increases with smoking, obesity, atherosclerosis, stress, lack of exercise, caffeine ingestion, high alcohol consumption, and a standard American diet. Pregnancy, certain kidney diseases, and hormone replacement therapy—including birth control pills—can also cause high blood pressure.

Testing Your Blood Pressure

	SYSTOLIC		DIASTOLIC
Normal	<120	and	<80
Pre-hypertension	120–139	or	80–89
Hypertension:			
Stage 1	140–159	or	90–99
Stage 2	> or = 160	or	> or = 100

Source: *Seventh Report of the Joint National Committee on Prevention, Detection, Evaluation, and Treatment of High Blood Pressure, 2003*[8]

Your physician will also take your pulse when assessing your cardiovascular function. This measures the rate of blood flow through your arteries. A normal pulse rate is between 60 and 100 beats per minute, but it changes with various stressors. For example, when you're anxious, your pulse rate can increase well above normal range;

when you're in a state of shock, it decreases dramatically. Exercise naturally increases your pulse rate; when you stop exercising, it slowly returns to normal.

RISK FACTORS AND SPECIAL TESTS FOR THE HEART

Since heart disease is the leading cause of death for women in the United States, another important consideration in determining your heart health is evaluating your risk factors for heart disease. The major risk factors are well known; as we've seen, they include high cholesterol, high triglycerides, and high blood pressure. Other major risk factors are obesity, lack of exercise, genetics, increased age, cigarette smoking, and diabetes.

Your risk for a heart attack increases with the number of risk factors you have. If you have only one of the major risk factors, you are at 30 percent greater risk of getting a heart attack than someone who has none. But if you combine factors, your overall risk can multiply dramatically. For example, if you have both high cholesterol and high blood pressure, your risk for a heart attack increases 300 percent![9]

If you're particularly concerned about preventing heart disease because you have some of the major risk factors, you can ask your physician to order comprehensive laboratory tests that will give you a more complete assessment of your heart. These include an electrocardiogram (ECG), which measures your heart's electrical rhythm, and blood tests to measure your serum ferritin, homocysteine, fibrinogen, lipoprotein-a, insulin, C-reactive protein, and thyroid hormones.

Knowing your risk factors for heart disease and taking diagnostic tests if necessary enables you to make healthier choices and take measures to protect your heart. A healthy heart is one that not only looks perfect, according to typical Western diagnostic tests, but also is cared for by the Naturally Healthy Lifestyle, which includes balanced Qi. In the following pages, you will explore many ways that natural medicine can make dramatic changes in your heart health.

Assessing Your Heart Health with Chinese Medicine

My patients are often surprised to learn the difference between Western and Chinese diagnoses of the heart. For example, in Western medicine, if your blood pressure readings are high, you are diagnosed with hypertension and are typically treated with prescription drugs. In Chinese medicine, there is no exact correlating diagnosis; in fact, blood pressure isn't traditionally taken. Instead, the Chinese view what we in the West call hypertension as a manifestation of imbalanced heart Qi, which is the result of lifestyle, diet, and emotional stressors. If you have hypertension, you could have a number of Chinese diagnoses, but the classical symptoms are most clearly seen in deficiency of heart yin, too much heart yang, or stagnation of heart Qi and Blood. Later in this chapter we will explore ways that each of these conditions can be treated with different foods, herbs, aromatherapy, and flower essences.

Some conditions not commonly associated with the heart in Western medicine are intimately linked with heart Qi in Chinese medicine. As you can see in the "Common Heart Imbalances from a Chinese Medicine Perspective" chart, these conditions, which include insomnia, irritability, anxiety, dizziness, and poor memory, can be due to imbalances in the "energetic" heart. Knowing your condition from an Eastern perspective can help you to make better choices in creating balance in your body, mind, and spirit.

From a traditional Chinese medical perspective, your pulse is an important part of your diagnosis, and it's important to know the *quality* as well as the *rate* of your pulse. By taking your pulse, your Chinese medical practitioner can gather much critical information—not only about your heart, but about the strengths or weaknesses of the Qi flowing through your body.

Common Heart Imbalances from a Chinese Medicine Perspective

SYMPTOMS	QUALITY OF YOUR TONGUE	QUALITY OF YOUR PULSE	CHINESE DIAGNOSIS
Palpitations, fatigue, shortness of breath with exertion, a pale complexion, and you sweat easily.	Pale or normal in color	Not easily felt	Deficient heart Qi
Insomnia, night sweats, hot flashes, afternoon fevers, anxiety, heat sensations in the hands and feet, a dry mouth, and poor memory.	Red at the tip	Fine and rapid	Deficient heart yin
Palpitations, cold sensations (especially in the hands), weariness, shortness of breath, and a sense of congestion or stuffiness in the heart region.	Pale, wet, and swollen	Weak	Deficient heart yang
Dizziness, palpitations, insomnia, poor memory, anxiety, pale lips, and a dull, pale complexion.	Thin and slightly dry	Fine and difficult to feel	Deficient heart Blood
Insomnia, a reddish complexion, irritability, heartburn, and thirst; tongue and mouth may have canker sores; a bitter taste in the mouth.	Red; swollen at the tip	Rapid and strong	Excess heart fire
Emotional tension, dull chest pain, shortness of breath, restlessness, frequent sighing, and cold hands from stress.	Dark purplish	Like a knotted, taut string	Heart Qi and Blood stagnation

In some ways, the Chinese understanding of cholesterol mirrors the Western view. Cholesterol wasn't measured in traditional Chinese medicine, but it is generally perceived as a yin substance. If you tell a modern-day practitioner of Chinese medicine that your cholesterol is high, he or she will usually consider it a symptom of a stressful lifestyle. This is because the more yang, or stressful, your lifestyle is, the more your body will respond by releasing the yin substance cholesterol in an attempt to balance it.

Nourishing Your Heart

Nourishing your heart means making your heart a priority in your daily life. The good news is that many of the ways you can nourish your heart are also the ways you can best prevent heart problems. With heart disease, as with other key aspects of health, prevention is the best cure, and the distinction between prevention and treatment is often blurred. Garlic, for example, can be used to prevent heart disease by keeping cholesterol low and at the same time to treat high blood pressure.

Every day you have tremendous power to influence your heart's destiny through your dietary choices. The Naturally Healthy Diet is great for your heart; it supplies you with the right kind of fats, lean proteins, whole grains, and an abundance of fruits and vegetables. Because diet is so important to protecting and maintaining your heart health, the following pages present a number of foods that are particularly heart healthy. And regular exercise, detoxification, nutritional supplementation, herbs, aromatherapy, and flower essences can all help keep your heart healthy and treat heart imbalances from both the Western and the Eastern view.

FOODS, SPICES, AND TEAS AS HEART MEDICINE

Nature provides us with an abundance of opportunities to support the heart through diet, from both a Western and a Chinese perspective. For example, fruits and vegetables, the most heart friendly of foods, provide an abundance of antioxidants that protect the blood vessels from potential damage; berries in particular have heart-protective properties. In Chinese medicine, most fruits and vegetables are "cooling" or "neutral" in nature, so they are often recommended for heart conditions when there is too much "heat" or yang, such as in cases of deficient heart yin and excess heart fire. In addition, the Chinese view holds that bitter flavors found in dark green leafy vegetables like spinach, kale, and Swiss chard can nourish the heart.

There is a wonderful alignment between Western and Chinese medicine when it comes to fats in the diet. In the Western view, some fats are good for the heart, because they help prevent heart disease, but too much fat is bad for the heart because an overabundance of calories from fats increases the risk of heart disease. In the Chinese view, fat has yin qualities because it's moistening and nourishing; but if you consume too much fat it can have a yang action on your body. In excess, this can lead to the accumulation of phlegm and "dampness," which can result in what is known in the West as atherosclerosis.

The following foods, spices, and teas have been shown to be especially beneficial for the cardiovascular system.

Oats. Oats can be nourishing to an exhausted nervous system. You can obtain their relaxing effects by ingesting them as oat straw tea or as an oat groats cereal. The fiber from oats has been shown to help lower cholesterol levels by reducing the amount of cholesterol that is absorbed in the intestines. For depression, oat straw tea can be combined with skullcap. (See page 162.) In Chinese medicine, oats are particularly nourishing to the nervous system because they build Blood, Qi, and Essence; they also provide nourishment if you have a chronic heart disease. For tea, I recommend that you steep one or two teaspoons of oat straw in a cup of boiling water for ten minutes. As a cereal, cook one cup of oat groats in two cups of boiling water for approximately ten minutes.

Garlic. An effective agent for lowering cholesterol and triglyceride levels, garlic also reduces blood pressure, thins blood, and as a bonus, has strong antibacterial and antifungal properties. In Chinese medicine, garlic has long been used for fatigue, cold limbs, and a lack of vitality; it strengthens yang, increases circulation, and can be used for high blood pressure due to a stagnation of heart Qi. Garlic must be eaten raw or lightly sautéed to retain its potency. For your heart health I recommend a dosage of one or two cloves a day.

Avoid Coffee and Lower Your Risk of Heart Disease

Coffee can increase your blood levels of cholesterol and homocysteine, an amino acid that can increase your risk of heart disease. A study reported in the *American Journal of Clinical Nutrition* found that eliminating coffee from the diet can lower the risk of heart disease.[10] Many of my patients enjoy coffee substitutes found in health food stores— Caffix, Pero, Roma, Inka, and Postum.

Ginger. Ginger can help increase circulation, thin blood, and lower both blood pressure and cholesterol. In Chinese medicine, ginger is also beneficial to the heart because it increases circulation and yang. I recommend that you simmer one or two teaspoons of sliced ginger root per cup of water for at least ten to fifteen minutes, strain it, and drink as needed.

Cayenne. A strong stimulant for the cardiovascular system, cayenne can decrease blood clots, lower cholesterol levels, and stimulate the heart and circulation.[11] Cayenne may be helpful if you have heart palpitations. In Chinese medicine, cayenne has been used to treat ailing hearts for centuries; if you have a heart condition with symptoms of intolerance to cold, fatigue, and shortness of breath, cayenne can help increase your circulation and your heart's yang energy. Rather than taking cayenne as a supplement, I recommend you use it to spice up your favorite dishes.

Note: In Chinese medicine, ginger and cayenne are considered energetically "hot" and should be avoided if you have heat signs such as insomnia, anxiety, hot flashes, or a red tongue.

Turmeric. Turmeric, which contains the compound curcumin, is used in many curry recipes. Curcumin, a potent antioxidant, has been shown to reduce "bad" LDL cholesterol and also has anti-inflammatory properties.[12] Add turmeric to your favorite dishes to get the benefits of this heart-friendly spice.

Green tea and black tea. Tea contains flavonoids and other healthy compounds that can help lower your cholesterol, protect your LDL cholesterol from damage due to oxidation, and protect your blood vessel walls. Green and black teas have been used in China for thousands of years. I recommend a dosage of one or two cups of *decaffeinated* green or black tea daily. Because green tea has powerful anticancer properties, it's also available as a nutritional supplement; the recommended dosage for heart health is 150 to 300 mg a day in a form standardized to contain 70 percent polyphenols.

Is Chocolate Medicine for Your Heart?

To the delight of chocolate lovers everywhere, a study published in the *American Journal of Clinical Nutrition* in 2001 reported that chocolate may be good for heart health.[13] Chocolate contains flavonoids that act as antioxidants and decrease damage due to "bad" LDL cholesterol, thus preventing one of the major causes of heart disease. But the study didn't take into account all the heart-unfriendly sugar and fat mixed with the chocolate to make it taste so delightful! If you can't live without chocolate, try creating recipes using dried cocoa and the herbal sweetener stevia to satisfy your taste buds and protect your heart.

ALCOHOL AND YOUR HEART

In recent years the media has touted the purported benefits of drinking alcohol to help prevent heart disease. But drinking alcohol may not be the best choice when looking at the health of your heart or your whole body. Let's look at the pros and cons.

The Pros: Red wine has been shown to contain flavonoids that can be beneficial for heart health. Some studies have also shown that alcohol can have positive effects on blood fats and clotting factors, both of which can lower the risk for coronary artery disease.[14] It is important to know that this lowered risk was primarily found in middle-aged people—men over fifty years of age and women over sixty who limited their alcohol intake to one or two drinks a day.[15] Some of the research suggests that people who already had coronary artery disease benefited the most.[16]

The Cons: Alcohol is an addictive substance and is toxic to the body. It damages liver cells, diminishing their ability to metabolize fats, and interferes with immune function. One study indicated no evidence that moderate alcohol consumption in premenopausal women will prevent heart disease.[17] Consumption of alcohol among women is highest between the ages of twenty-six and thirty-four, and no data exist suggesting that alcohol intake in this age group can help prevent heart disease.[18] Alcohol can contribute to your risk for breast cancer (see Chapter 9), as well as cancers of the mouth, throat, esophagus, and liver.[19]

Since alcohol can increase excretion of minerals such as calcium and magnesium, excess alcohol consumption can increase your risk of osteoporosis. Furthermore, it is well known that excess alcohol consumption can lead to hypertension, cirrhosis of the liver, and death.

Traditional Chinese medicine believes that alcohol produces excessive "heat" and "dampness" in the body, which can result in hypertension and atherosclerosis.

At best, alcohol may help only a limited number of women prevent heart disease. Because it has numerous adverse effects on the entire body, I don't recommend drinking alcohol for heart health—especially when abundant evidence shows the positive effects that diet, lifestyle, and nutritional and herbal supplements can have without potential side effects.

NOURISHING YOUR HEART WITH EXERCISE

Designing Your Heart-Healthy Exercise Program: Getting the Best of East and West

Choose an activity that brings you joy.

Work out within your target heart rate.

Always warm up and cool down.

Be consistent: exercise a minimum of thirty minutes five to six times a week.

Your heart, like any muscle, works best when it's in good shape. Exercise strengthens it and enhances circulation so that every cell in the body receives more blood and oxygen. Western medicine dictates that the way to strengthen the heart is through consistent aerobic exercise. The principles of ancient Chinese medicine offer a different perspective when it comes to exercise and the heart.

From a Chinese medicine standpoint, the goal of exercise is to help balance your yin and yang; the heart can be strengthened not only through appropriate physical exercise but also through peaceful thoughts and meditation. When you are considering which form of exercise to do on a regular basis, remember that your heart is the organ of joy, and that creating joyful exercise in your life will nurture your heart in more ways than one. If you are a Fire type, you may need to choose sports that involve interacting with others, because you love company. But if in your daily activities you have constant interaction with people, you may wish to choose an exercise that's more solitary to keep your energy balanced.

In Chinese medicine, the heart is responsible for perspiration; if you sweat too much and too often, your heart Qi can become deficient. The exercises most commonly recommended in Western medicine for strengthening the heart and the entire cardiovascular system are what I call, from the perspective of Chinese medicine, "yang exercises." If your Qi is strong and you do these exercises in moderation, they are excellent for enhancing circulation and promoting health. But done in excess, they will consume your Qi and create heavy, tight muscles that can cause muscle and joint problems.

While too much yang exercise can consume your Qi, too much "yin exercise" may not provide you with sufficient cardiovascular benefits. You want to balance exercises that are yang and that cause excessive sweating (such as aerobic activity) with exercises that are yin and don't involve excess sweating (such as yoga and Tai Chi). To nourish your heart Qi, you may need to make your yang exercises more yin simply by slowing down the pace. (For a list of yin and yang exercises, see Chapter 1.)

According to both Western and Chinese medicine, you don't have to exercise to the point of exhaustion in order to strengthen your heart. Rather, exercise to your target heart rate (see the "Determining Your Target Heart Rate" chart). If your heart rate is slower than the low end of your target heart rate, you need to increase the intensity of your exercise to get the cardiovascular benefits. If your heart rate goes too high, you're pushing your body too hard. When you push too hard, you put yourself at higher risk for injury and, according to Chinese medicine, you sweat excessively. As your cardiovascular strength improves, you'll find that your target heart rate changes.

Determining Your Target Heart Rate

1. Take your resting heart rate by feeling your pulse at your wrist or your neck and counting the number of beats for 15 seconds while you are perfectly rested. Multiply the number of beats by 4 to get your resting heart rate. For example, if you count 15 beats during the 15 seconds, your resting heart rate is 15 times 4, or 60 beats per minute.

2. Subtract your age from 220 to calculate your estimated maximum heart rate. For example, if you are 40 years old, your estimated maximum heart rate is 220 minus 40, or 180 beats per minute.

3. Subtract your resting heart rate from your estimated maximum heart rate. For example, 180 minus 60 equals 120 beats per minute.

4. Multiply the number you arrived at in step three by 60 percent. For example, 120 times 60 percent equals 72.

5. To calculate the *low end of your target zone*, add the step you arrived at in step four to your resting heart rate. For example, 60 plus 72 equals 132 beats per minute, the low end of your target zone.

6. To calculate the *high end of your target zone*, multiply the step you arrived at in step three by 80 percent and add it to your resting heart rate. For example, 120 times 80 percent equals 96 and 96 plus 60 equals 156 beats per minute, the high end of your target zone.

To summarize, this means that when you exercise, your heart rate should stay between 132 and 156 beats per minute for optimal heart health.

Source: American College of Sports Medicine, *ACSM's Guidelines for Exercise Testing and Prescription*, sixth ed. (Philadelphia: Lippincott Williams & Wilkins, 2000), pp. 147–151.

You can even walk your way to a healthy heart. Walking is an easy, heart-healthy exercise you can do every day. It can be done as a yin exercise by walking slowly or as a yang exercise by walking briskly. The program known as 10,000 Steps a Day encourages walkers to count their steps using a pedometer. Most people take 3,000 to 5,000 steps in the normal course of a day, but you can be creative and increase that number by choosing the stairs instead of the elevator, and the parking spot that's farthest from your destination instead of the one you have to wait for. One patient told me that she was never able to stick to a regular fitness program, but by filling her quota of 10,000 steps daily, she consistently met her exercise and weight-loss goals. She couldn't find time to go to the gym, but somehow she could take a brisk walk at the end of the day if her pedometer read less than 10,000. By taking 10,000 steps, you will be walking approximately five miles and, at an energetic pace, burning 300 to 500 calories every day.

AN ANCIENT CHINESE EXERCISE

In Chinese medicine, exercising the heart can mean something very different from what it means from a Western perspective. Dr. Nan Lu, author of *A Woman's Guide to a Trouble-Free Menopause,* recommends what he calls "one of the most powerful ancient exercises you can do for your heart."[20] You can help heal your heart, he says, by doing the following: "Face the mirror and smile at yourself—really smile at yourself—from your heart." To "really smile," according to Dr. Lu, is to openly express your genuine innermost joy and happiness. "Smiling at yourself," he explains, "from your heart—not just a fake smile—actually has a physical effect. It can help make Blood and Qi flow throughout your whole body." Once you have mastered this exercise, he suggests that you try smiling at others from your heart. He believes this practice is "much more effective than physical exercise" for your heart Qi.

To further nourish your heart, Dr. Lu recommends clearing your mind with meditation. To fit meditation into your busy life, he has a simple solution: from time to time, take a few moments—perhaps even just thirty to sixty seconds—to be quiet and calm. Do this before starting daily activities such as turning on your computer or car, beginning a meal, falling asleep, or making an important decision. At the end of the day, you'll find that all of these borrowed moments have added up to a quieter mind, and a quieter mind means a more balanced Fire element and a healthier heart.

DETOXIFICATION

Although your heart and blood vessels don't specifically break waste products down, your bloodstream carries wastes for removal from your body, and your arteries and capillaries are susceptible to injury if they're carrying waste products that can damage your blood vessel walls. Toxic free radicals and other irritants can damage the delicate lining of your blood vessels (the endothelium) and set the stage for atherosclerosis.

Studies have indicated that high levels of mercury in the body may damage the lining of the blood vessels and increase the risk of heart disease. One study suggests that mercury promotes the formation of free radicals and reduces the antioxidant effects of selenium and other enzymes that are important in breaking these substances down.[21] As we have seen, it's clear that mercury can have many other damaging effects, and that heavy metal detoxification can help remove it from your body. If you've been exposed to high levels of mercury or other heavy metals through dental work, high consumption of contaminated fish, or your work, refer to Chapter 4, to see how you can test for heavy metals.

Another toxin that can potentially increase your risk of heart disease is chlorine, a chemical added to public drinking water to prevent bacterial growth. Jonathan Wright, M.D., a well-known author and researcher in the field of complementary medicine, points out, "There are few, if any, communities around the world with chlorinated drinking water that have a low incidence of atherosclerosis. Chlorine is a powerful oxidizing agent, which is capable of causing severe damage to blood vessels. In animal studies, chlorine has been found to promote the development of atherosclerosis."[22] Dr. Wright suggests removing chlorine from tap water by boiling it for five to ten minutes, or by adding a pinch of vitamin C. You can also purchase a water filter for your faucet and shower head. (See Chapter 3 for information on water filters).

Exercise helps you detoxify because it enhances your circulation, bringing more oxygen to each and every cell in your body. In addition, it helps your cells remove wastes more quickly. By causing you to sweat, exercise removes toxins from your body through your skin. Although excessive sweating can consume your heart Qi, you will be much less likely to have problems if you adequately replenish your fluids and electrolytes.

HYDROTHERAPY

In Chapter 2 we saw how you can do hydrotherapy to enhance your immune system by strengthening your Wei Qi or protective Qi. In Chapter 4 we saw that low-heat saunas can promote detoxification. Studies have also confirmed that regular sauna use may help prevent atherosclerosis by improving the function of the endothelium.[23] In fact, your entire cardiovascular system can benefit from hot and cold water therapy (also known as "contrast hydrotherapy"; see page 66); it invigorates your whole body and stimulates your heart. You can make contrast hydrotherapy a part of your daily routine. It can be an extremely relaxing therapy—alleviating stress, calming your spirit, and soothing your nervous system—at the same time that it is increasing your circulation and keeping your heart and blood vessels healthy. (Caution: Contrast hydrotherapy should not be used if you have uncontrolled high blood pressure or advanced heart disease.)

NUTRITIONAL SUPPLEMENTATION

By now, you can see that you can enhance your heart health through the daily choices you make in your diet and lifestyle. As you move toward a Naturally Healthy Lifestyle, you can also take a number of nutritional supplements to enhance your heart health and help prevent heart disease. The goals of taking nutritional supplements for your heart include:

- Protecting your blood vessel walls from damage
- Preventing the formation of atherosclerotic plaque
- Preventing the oxidation of LDL cholesterol
- Keeping your overall cholesterol within normal range
- Ensuring an abundance of HDL cholesterol
- Enhancing your overall cardiovascular function
- Keeping your heart Qi balanced

The following nutritional supplements can support your heart and cardiovascular system.

ANTIOXIDANTS

Antioxidants are the most important nutrients for protecting the heart and blood vessels from the damage that can lead to atherosclerosis. Antioxidants protect against the formation of free radicals that can damage cells and, ultimately, tissues. Numerous studies have elucidated the powerful role they can play in the prevention of many diseases, including cancer. Antioxidants are found in a wide variety of foods, but taken as supplements they can provide you with therapeutic doses that are nearly impossible to get through diet alone.

Vitamin C has many heart-protective properties and is one of the most beneficial antioxidants you can take for preventing heart disease. It can elevate good HDL cholesterol, prevent oxidation of "bad" LDL cholesterol, and protect and strengthen blood vessel walls.[24] Vitamin C can be found in abundance in oranges, peppers, watermelon, grapefruit, cantaloupe, papayas, and kiwis. In Chinese medicine, vitamin C is also beneficial to the heart because it is considered "cooling," which means it can clear heat and calm your spirit. The recommended dose for prevention of heart disease is 1,000 mg a day, which you can get in your daily multivitamin.

Vitamin E is another important antioxidant for preventing heart disease; by incorporating itself into "bad" LDL cholesterol, it can prevent some of the damaging effects that LDL cholesterol can have on your blood vessel walls. It also plays a role in protecting your blood vessel walls from free radical damage.[25] When buying vitamin E, always choose a brand containing mixed tocopherols; most vitamin E that you find on the shelves is made with only alpha tocopherol. Mixed tocopherols, which combine the alpha, gamma, delta, and beta forms of vitamin E, offer you much better antioxidant protection. From a Chinese medicine perspective, vitamin E can nourish Blood and yang energy and be especially helpful for some heart conditions. If you are at risk for developing heart disease, take 800 i.u. a day, which is twice the amount that you will find in your multivitamin.

Tocotrienols, which are associated with vitamin E, are powerful antioxidants—more powerful than vitamin E alone—and can also decrease your cholesterol levels.[26] For lowering cholesterol, take 80 mg of tocotrienols a day.

B VITAMINS

If you are concerned about your heart health, I recommend that you learn more about your risk by having a blood test that measures the amino acid homocysteine. If your results are high, make sure you are supplementing your diet with B vitamins (B_6, B_{12}, and folic acid). Homocysteine can increase your risk for heart disease, especially if you are genetically susceptible to it. Women who take birth control pills, or seniors with multiple nutritional deficiencies, can have elevated levels of homocysteine.[27] B vitamins can help prevent heart disease and strokes by working synergistically to lower your level of homocysteine. The daily dosages necessary for lowering homocysteine are 10 mg of B_6, 400 mcg of B_{12}, and 650 mcg of folic acid. Most daily multivitamins contain enough B vitamins to provide these amounts.

Should You Take Aspirin for Heart Health?

Many physicians recommend aspirin to help thin the blood and prevent blood clots and strokes. But according to Stephen T. Sinatra, M.D., author of *Heart Sense for Women*, "If you don't have a documented history of heart disease, I do not recommend aspirin therapy. In women over the age of seventy-five, aspirin can increase the risk of stroke. And there is strong data to show that aspirin is poorly tolerated by a lot of people, with gastrointestinal bleeding being a major adverse side effect."[28] The good news is that there are many natural compounds that can give you the same benefits, without the undesirable side effects of aspirin. Dr. Sinatra encourages women to drink ginger tea every day to thin their blood and decrease inflammation. To thin your blood and help prevent blood clots and strokes, I recommend ginger, ginkgo biloba, and the friendly omega 3 fats found in fish and flax oils. In addition, I recommend the antioxidants vitamin E and tocotrienols, which are also blood-thinning compounds.

MINERALS

Minerals are essential to many functions in your body. They can work together to keep your heart's electrical system running optimally and to regulate your blood pressure. The following two minerals are especially helpful—in my practice I have seen that they can markedly decrease heart palpitations due to stress and menopausal changes.

Potassium. Potassium is one of the most important minerals for a healthy heart. If you have hypertension, it's important to pay special attention to your potassium/sodium balance. A five-to-one potassium-to-sodium ratio is ideal for your heart. In the standard American diet, unfortunately, sodium usually dominates potassium, which contributes to high blood pressure. Your potassium/sodium balance can be further affected if you lose significant amounts of potassium from excessive sweating, diarrhea, or vomiting. Most fruits and vegetables contain potassium, and exceptionally high amounts are found in bananas, apples, oranges, carrots, avocados, apricots, and peaches. It's best to simply decrease your sodium intake and boost your intake of potassium-rich foods, but supplementation can be helpful when you can't get enough potassium in your diet. You can purchase potassium in 99-mg tablets. I recommend that you take three tablets twice a day for high blood pressure, and three tablets once a day for treating palpitations.

Magnesium. Magnesium is also an important heart-supporting mineral. In addition, it's essential for producing the energy that your heart cells need to function. If you have atherosclerosis, magnesium can dilate your blood vessels and prevent spasms. Wheat germ, tofu, nuts and seeds, whole grains, vegetables, and many other foods have a high magnesium content. In supplement form, the recommended dosage is 300 to 600 mg a day for high blood pressure or palpitations. (When you take magnesium, it's always a good idea to take about twice the amount of calcium with it.) Note: Taking an excessive amount of magnesium can cause diarrhea.

Treating Common Conditions Related to the Heart

A number of heart-related conditions, such as high cholesterol and high blood pressure, can be treated successfully with nutritional supplementation, herbal remedies, aromatherapy, flower essences, amino acids, and Chinese medicine. In the following pages, we will explore approaches you can use to treat common conditions related to your heart.

NUTRITIONAL SUPPLEMENTS TO TREAT
HIGH CHOLESTEROL

If you've made dietary and lifestyle changes to lower your cholesterol but you still remain in the moderate-to-high-risk categories for heart disease, you may want to consider taking a cholesterol-lowering supplement. You have many options for lowering your cholesterol effectively, naturally, and without resorting to the pharmaceutical medications known as statin drugs, which can have numerous side effects. Choose one of the following cholesterol-lowering supplements, and recheck your cholesterol three months after you start taking it. If your cholesterol is still high, see your naturopathic physician for further guidance.

Policosanol. One of the most important cholesterol-lowering agents, policosanol works by decreasing your liver's ability to produce cholesterol (much as the statin drugs do, but without their adverse effects). Policosanol decreases "bad" LDL cholesterol, and some studies have shown that it elevates "good" HDL cholesterol.[29] Because it also acts as a blood thinner, I recommend that you avoid other blood thinners, like aspirin, when using policosanol. I prescribe policosanol as a general cholesterol-lowering agent and because it has antioxidant properties and low toxicity. The recommended dosage is 5 to10 mg, two times a day.

Guggulipid. This supplement is made from guggul, a resin from the mukul myrrh tree, and is used in traditional Ayurvedic (Indian) medicine. It reduces unfavorable LDL cholesterol and triglyceride levels and increases favorable HDL cholesterol. Guggulipid works in the liver by inhibiting production of cholesterol and can assist in the elimination of cholesterol through the bile and stool.[30] I recommend guggulipid if you have high cholesterol and low thyroid function, because it can enhance your thyroid hormone function as well.[31] The recommended dosage is 500 mg (each 500-mg tablet containing 25 mg of standardized guggulsterone extract) three times a day.

Pantethine. The activated form of vitamin B_5 (pantothenic acid), pantethine is used to decrease cholesterol levels. It has been shown to lower "bad" LDL cholesterol and increase "good" HDL cholesterol. Pantethine is chosen over other cholesterol-lowering compounds when your blood tests show repeatedly high triglycerides, because it's particularly effective in lowering triglyceride levels.[32] The recommended dosage is 300 mg, three times per day.

Tocotrienols. These potent antioxidants, found in rice bran and barley oils, can lower your cholesterol level by inhibiting your liver's ability to manufacture cholesterol.[33]

Tocotrienols can also help prevent atherosclerosis by protecting your blood vessel walls, and strokes by thinning your blood and inhibiting the formation of blood clots. Like policosanol, tocotrienols are recommended as general cholesterol-lowering supplements and because they have antioxidant properties and low toxicity. The recommended dosage is 40 to 80 mg a day.

Garlic. When taken in supplement form, garlic can play an important role in lowering your cholesterol. You can take powdered garlic supplements that have been prepared so as to maintain its cholesterol-lowering properties. Garlic is preferred over other cholesterol-lowering agents if you tend to feel cold and have poor circulation—symptoms of yang deficiency in Chinese medicine—and if you have high blood pressure. Your garlic powder supplement should provide you with at least 5,000 mcg daily of allicin, which is the active component in garlic.

Niacin. Also known as vitamin B_3, niacin is the most extensively researched nutritional supplement recommended for lowering cholesterol. But niacin can cause numerous side effects, including reddening, itching, and burning sensations in the skin. It can also cause liver stress if taken at too high a dose for too long. Instead, I prescribe a derivative of niacin, inositol hexaniacinate, which offers many of the same cholesterol-lowering benefits without the undesirable side effects of niacin. (Even with inositol hexaniacinate, it's a good idea to have your doctor check your blood for any signs of liver stress.) Inositol hexaniacinate is recommended over other natural cholesterol-lowering supplements when you have high cholesterol and poor circulation. The recommended dosage of inositol hexaniacinate is 500 mg three times a day with food.

What About Chelation Therapy?

Many people who have been diagnosed with atherosclerosis choose chelation therapy to remove plaque buildup in their blood vessel walls. Chelation involves taking a drug called EDTA intravenously. Twenty to forty three-hour sessions are required, and the cost is $100 to $150 per session. Although the effectiveness of this therapy has been debated for many years and the established medical community doesn't generally endorse it, many medical doctors prescribe chelation for what I call "Roto-Rootering" the arteries. Both Alan Gaby and Jonathan Wright, nationally respected holistic medical doctors, use chelation therapy in their practices. Dr. Gaby writes that he and Dr. Wright have "seen chelation work medical wonders in patients with atherosclerotic disease."[34] In some cases I refer patients to doctors who specialize in chelation therapy. But "Roto-Rootering" your blood vessels won't take care of the problem unless you make significant diet and lifestyle changes as well. I recommend that my patients with atherosclerosis follow a program for reversing heart disease such as the one outlined by Dean Ornish, M.D. This program has proven that through significantly lowering intake of dietary fats and making heart-healthy lifestyle changes, heart disease can be reversed. It's quite holistic in its approach and draws from principles that have long been upheld by naturopathic medicine: a nontoxic, noninvasive way of working with your body's ability to heal itself. If you've been diagnosed with atherosclerosis, I suggest you read *Dr. Dean Ornish's Program for Reversing Heart Disease: The Only System Scientifically Proven to Reverse Heart Disease Without Drugs or Surgery* (New York: Ivy Books, 1995).

HERBS FOR YOUR HEART

Herbal remedies have been used for centuries in both Western and Chinese medicine to nourish and heal hearts. I prescribe herbs regularly in my practice to help my patients achieve optimal heart health. They not only have active constituents that you can use medicinally but they also have "energetic" properties that can help you balance your heart and spirit. Because the emotions and nervous system are so intimately linked to the heart, treatment of any heart condition will include treatment of the emotions and nervous system as well. Many herbs have an effect on the physical heart as well as on the emotional heart. For example, one of my favorite herbs, melissa, is very calming; it can lower blood pressure and relax an overanxious nervous system.

The following herbs can be used individually or in combination with other herbs, depending on the diagnosis. Note the striking similarities between the ways many herbs are used in Western medicine and in the Chinese tradition.

Motherwort. Its Latin name, *Leonurus cardiaca,* tells you right away that this wonderful herb is of special significance for the cardiac system. Motherwort strengthens the heart and is used to treat arrhythmia and heart palpitations caused by tension or anxiety. In Chinese medicine, it tonifies heart Qi, moves Qi and Blood, and is used for rapid heartbeat, heart palpitations, shortness of breath, or anxiety. Because of its calming effects on the cardiovascular system, motherwort can lower your blood pressure temporarily. It also affects the uterus, so it should not be used during pregnancy. The recommended dosage is one teaspoon of motherwort steeped in one cup of boiling water for ten minutes; strain and drink this amount three times a day.

Mistletoe. This herb has a relaxing and restoring effect on the nervous system and is used to treat mild cases of high blood pressure. In Chinese medicine, mistletoe is said to "move the Blood," which means it increases circulation; it is used to treat hypertension because of its ability to move Qi, decrease yang, and tonify yin. It's safe to use mistletoe for prolonged periods of time. The recommended dosage is two teaspoons of the herb steeped in one cup of boiling water for ten minutes; strain and drink this amount three times a day.

Skullcap. This herb is used for heart palpitations, to treat depression, for premenstrual tension, and to relax the nervous system. In Chinese medicine, skullcap is "cooling" and is used to calm the spirit, circulate heart Qi, and clear "heat." The recommended dosage is one teaspoon steeped in a cup of boiling water for fifteen minutes; strain and drink this amount two or three times a day, or as needed.

Hawthorn Berry. This herb contains flavonoids that can dilate blood vessels, decrease blood pressure, reduce atherosclerosis, and improve overall heart and cardiovascular health. In Chinese medicine, it's used to strengthen heart Qi, revitalize heart Blood, support heart yin, move stagnant heart Qi and Blood, and calm the spirit. Hawthorn berry is considered safe for long-term use but should not be used if you have diarrhea or chronically loose stools. The recommended dosage is 250 mg (containing 10 percent procyanidin) three times a day.

Ginkgo Biloba. This herb promotes blood flow throughout the body and strengthens blood vessel walls. It increases circulation to the brain and can help improve memory in the elderly (though it has not been shown to improve memory in young people with good circulation).[35] It's also an antioxidant and can thin your blood. In Chinese medicine, ginkgo biloba is used to move heart Qi and Blood. The recommended dosage is 40 mg (as a standardized extract of 24 percent ginkgo flavonglycosides) three times a day. Note: Side effects of ginkgo biloba are rare, but some people report mild stomach distress or headaches. You should avoid using ginkgo biloba if you are taking blood-thinning medications.

HERBS AS AROMATHERAPY FOR THE HEART

The sense of smell appears to have an immediate connection to the limbic system—the emotional center of the brain—through the olfactory nerve. This gives essential oils a unique potential to directly affect your moods and feelings and even to lower your blood pressure. Many herbs contain volatile oils; when concentrated, they can act as strong medicines on both the physical and emotional heart. The following are two of my favorite heart-nurturing essential oils; both are especially useful if you are a Fire type.

Lavender. This herb has a long and colorful history as both a medicine and a perfume. It acts as a stimulant, as well as a sedative, to the cardiovascular and nervous systems. If you suffer from nervous exhaustion, lavender can restore your vitality; if you're agitated and anxious, it can calm you. In Chinese medicine, lavender is used to circulate heart Qi and relieve tension.

A delightful way to enjoy the benefits of lavender as aromatherapy is to add dried lavender or its essential oil to your bath. You can also make tea from the dried herb. The recommended dosage is one teaspoon of the herb steeped in one cup of boiling water for ten minutes; strain and drink as needed.

Melissa. Also known as lemon balm, this herb contains a volatile oil that has a calming and restoring effect on your heart. It's used to treat heart palpitations resulting from depression or agitated nerves. Melissa is included in a number of herbal formulas for high blood pressure because of its soothing effects on the nervous and cardiovascular systems. It can help relieve both agitated manic states and depression. In Chinese medicine, melissa calms the spirit and is especially useful for circulating heart Qi.

You can apply the essential oil of melissa to your skin, add a few drops to your bath, or inhale it by using an atomizer. Melissa is a safe herb that you can use long term as a relaxant, with one exception: it shouldn't be used during pregnancy because it can mildly stimulate the uterus. To drink melissa as a tea, the recommended dosage is two or three teaspoons of the dried herb steeped in one cup of boiling water for fifteen minutes; drink this amount two or three times a day.

FLOWER ESSENCES FOR YOUR EMOTIONAL HEART

As you've seen throughout this chapter, the physical heart and the emotional heart are deeply connected; each intimately affects the other. In Chinese medicine, an imbalance in the heart or its ministers profoundly affects the nervous system and psyche. Flower essences can affect your heart through their ability to affect your emotions. They may help lift your spirit and calm your heart if it is agitated. The recommended dosage for flower essences is four drops or pellets under your tongue, four times a day. To strengthen the effects of a remedy, you should take it more frequently rather than increase the number of drops per dosage. Up to five different remedies can be added together, although usually only one or two in combination are used. You can choose which remedies to use based on your emotional symptoms. Flower essences can be added to drinking water, applied to your skin—either as they are or mixed into a lotion, cream, or oil—or added to your bath.

Rescue Remedy. This combination of five flower essences—Impatiens, Clematis, Rock Rose, Cherry Plum, and Star of Bethlehem—can be used for any situation that traumatizes the emotional heart. It calms you when you feel you need to be "rescued"; for example, if you're in shock or experiencing sudden panic. You can also use it to deal with the nervousness, fear, or anxiety surrounding an upcoming event such as a medical procedure or dental work. In Chinese medicine, it would be most appropriately used for moving heart Qi and strengthening heart yin.

Elm. This flower essence can be used by mothers and other caregivers who feel they have spent so much of themselves that they have nothing left to give; who feel empty, depressed, or despondent. It can help to reignite your passion for your work, especially if you feel burned out. In Chinese medicine, this flower essence would be best used for a lack of yang, or heart fire.

Impatiens. This flower essence is recommended if you are a type A personality, always impatient, wanting to get things done in a hurry, and irritated by others who work at a slower pace. Impatiens is used to induce a calming effect. In Chinese medicine, it would be appropriate for moving Qi and Blood and decreasing yang.

Yerba Santa. This flower essence can release constriction in your heart region due to profound sadness or grief. In Chinese medicine, it would be used for moving Qi and Blood because it restores joy in the heart by releasing the unresolved feelings and pain that can lead to emotional stagnation.

Aloe. Aloe may be useful if you exhaust yourself working too hard and forget to take care of yourself. It can help to rejuvenate you and balance your energy with your physical needs. In Chinese medicine, aloe would be used to strengthen yin and rekindle energy—particularly if you are a Fire type, and your fire flares up with bursts of creativity and enthusiasm, burns too high, and flames out.

Amino Acids to Help an Ailing Heart

Amino acids are the building blocks of protein. They're found in protein-rich foods such as meat, eggs, and beans. The following amino acids are used to treat conditions in which the heart is already stressed, such as high blood pressure, coronary artery disease, and irregular heartbeat.

L-taurine can have a profound impact on your heart. When taken as a supplement in therapeutic doses, it can positively influence the electrical activity of the heart and has also been shown to help lower high blood pressure.[36] The recommended dosage is 500 mg three times a day.

L-arginine dilates blood vessels, which is great news if you have hypertension or atherosclerosis.[37] In addition, L-arginine lowers cholesterol levels and thins blood. The recommended dosage is 1,000 mg three times a day.

LOWERING YOUR BLOOD PRESSURE

Nutritional supplements and herbal medicines can be effective for lowering blood pressure and relaxing an overanxious nervous system. At any stage of hypertension you can help lower your blood pressure by implementing the Naturally Healthy Lifestyle and Diet. It's always important to decrease your sodium intake and increase your potassium intake. In addition, I recommend the following for each stage.

If you have pre-hypertension (systolic pressure is 120 to 139 or diastolic is 80 to 89), use the Chinese dietary recommendations, herbs, and flower essences outlined in the "Special Methods for Treating Hypertension" chart (page 166) to nourish your heart.

If your blood pressure is in the Stage 1 hypertension range (systolic pressure is 140 to 159 or diastolic is 90 to 99), use the Chinese dietary recommendations, herbs, and flower essences outlined in the chart, and supplement your diet with L-arginine and potassium (available in 99-mg pills; the recommended dosage is three pills twice a day). I also recommend that you increase your intake of potassium-rich foods.

Depending on your Chinese diagnosis (see the "Special Methods for Treating Hypertension" chart), in Stage 1 hypertension you can use single herbs, or combine them, to help lower your blood pressure. For example, for high blood pressure due to *excess heart fire,* you can use herbs such as lavender, motherwort, melissa, and mistletoe. An excellent formula for those with high blood pressure due to *deficient heart yin* (often seen in menopause) or *heart Blood and Qi stagnation* (due to stress and nervous tension) can be prepared by combining equal parts of mistletoe, hawthorn, and melissa. The recommended dosage is two teaspoons of the herbal mixture steeped in one cup of boiling water for ten minutes; drink one cup of this preparation three times a day.

If your blood pressure is in the Stage 2 hypertension range (systolic pressure is 160 or over, or diastolic is 100 or over), take L-arginine and potassium (as described above for Stage 1 hypertension) and L-taurine. You can also incorporate the Chinese dietary recommendations, herbs, and flower essences outlined in the chart. It may be necessary for you to take pharmaceutical medications to lower your blood pressure while you are treating the underlying cause of your hypertension.

For Stage 1 and Stage 2 hypertension, it's best to see a licensed naturopathic physician for further advice. If you are taking prescription medicine to lower your blood pressure, you will especially need qualified guidance regarding nutritional supplements and herbs.

Special Methods for Treating Hypertension

WESTERN AND CHINESE DIAGNOSES	SYMPTOMS	RECOMMENDED CHINESE DIET	RECOMMENDED HERBS AND AROMATHERAPY	RECOMMENDED FLOWER ESSENCES
High blood pressure and excess heart fire	Insomnia, a reddish complexion, irritability, heartburn, and thirst	Eat "cold" foods to decrease heart fire; avoid greasy, "warming," and "hot" foods	Motherwort Mistletoe Lavender Melissa	Impatiens
High blood pressure and deficient heart yin	Insomnia, night sweats, hot flashes, afternoon fevers, anxiety, and heat sensations in hands and feet	Eat "cold" foods to nourish heart yin; avoid "hot" foods and alcohol	Mistletoe Skullcap Hawthorn Melissa	Rescue Remedy Aloe
High blood pressure and heart Qi and Blood stagnation	Emotional tension, shortness of breath, restlessness, frequent sighing, and cold hands from stress	Eat "hot" foods to disperse stagnant heart Qi and Blood; avoid "cold" foods	Motherwort Mistletoe Hawthorne Ginkgo biloba Melissa	Rescue Remedy Impatiens Yerba Santa

Your Dynamic Heart: Final Thoughts

"The love that we receive from the Fire element bathes every part of our lives. It fires our spirit . . . allowing us to share in the spirit that pervades everything in the universe. It flows through our relationships with our partners, our families and our friends, and it is the power by which we transform ourselves and one another."

—J. R. WORSLEY,
Classical Five Element Acupuncture

In my practice, I am constantly rewarded by seeing the profound transformations that can happen when people take the simple measures I've outlined in this chapter. After all, your heart is much more than merely a muscle that pumps blood throughout your body; it is the king and the home of your spirit. Your heart and its ministers provide you with the ability to nurture others and take care of yourself. You can prevent heart disease and create optimal heart health by taking care of your body, mind, and spirit, and by listening to your heart. Your heart is in your hands: you have a tremendous amount of power to influence its destiny.

The Essence of Chapter 5

- Create joy and laughter in your life, and keep your Fire element balanced.
- Keep your blood pressure and cholesterol within normal ranges.
- Follow the Naturally Healthy Diet to nourish your heart, and avoid coffee and alcohol.
- Exercise regularly.
- Decrease your exposure to heavy metals, and avoid drinking chlorinated water.
- Practice contrast hydrotherapy.
- Protect your heart health with vitamins and minerals.
- Take herbs and supplements if you need to lower your cholesterol and blood pressure.
- Use Chinese and herbal medicine to balance your heart Qi.
- Smile!

Chapter 6

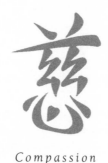

Compassion

Gifts of the Earth:
Nourishing Your Digestive Health

"The Element Earth is our connection with mother Earth herself."
—J. R. WORSLEY, *Classical Five Element Acupuncture*

WHEN I first saw Suzanne, she had been suffering from digestive problems for many years. She'd been in a downward spiral and wanted a way to make her body healthy again. "Since I was a teen," she said, "I'd been prescribed antibiotics off and on to treat acne. The medicine didn't clear it up, and instead caused some major side effects in my digestion. I became constipated and bloated all the time. I was so uncomfortable that I wasn't able to participate with my dance troupe. To cope with the stress, I would head for the sweets, which just made me gain weight, exacerbated my digestive symptoms, and triggered depression."

Suzanne had the classic symptoms of imbalanced bacteria in her intestines. She also had food allergies, which were aggravating her symptoms. After changing her diet and doing an intestinal cleanse, her digestive problems disappeared. In addition, Suzanne later said, "I was happy to discover that my acne dramatically cleared up—for the first time since I was an adolescent."

A Healthy Digestive Tract

As we've seen in previous chapters, choosing the right foods is the first step in creating optimal health. But great health also depends on your body being able to process the food you eat and thus provide nutrition to every cell in your body. It is through your digestion that the external world meets your internal environment. If you eat an apple at breakfast, it becomes part of who you are by dinner.

When your digestive system is working well, this process happens smoothly; you have a strong foundation for your vitality, and it is easy to maintain your normal weight and to continue to make healthy food choices. If your digestion is not working well, you may experience stomach or intestinal pain after you eat certain foods, or develop symptoms in other parts of your body—such as skin rashes, joint pains, or migraines—which you might be surprised to discover are the result of poor digestive health.

On their first visit to my office, I always ask my patients in detail about their digestion because so much depends on it, and it can be the underlying cause of so many health problems. Digestive imbalances have become an epidemic as people continue to eat the standard American diet—which includes many low-nutrient, high-calorie foods—and take commonly prescribed pharmaceutical drugs such as steroids, birth control pills, and antibiotics. Correcting digestive imbalances caused by these activities is an important step in treating many diseases and disorders.

Suzanne came to see me because she wanted guidance on how to get her body and digestion back on track. Originally, her persistent acne had prompted her to get medical treatment, which led her to take antibiotics and other pharmaceutical medications for years. This resulted in intestinal imbalances, sugar cravings, weight gain, and depression. Only after seeking out natural medicine did she discover that her acne was caused by a chronic allergy to gluten (a protein found in many grains). By treating the underlying cause of her health problems, she achieved radiant health and vitality—and also gained a new sense of empowerment and confidence in her ability to take care of herself.

The View from the West

Your digestive system uses many processes in making the apple you eat a part of every cell in your body. It all starts when you chew the apple. Enzymes in your mouth immediately begin breaking it down into smaller particles for absorption, while immune cells in your saliva help protect you from abnormal bacteria that might be present. As you swallow each bite of the apple, it travels down your esophagus to your stomach, where the real action begins. Your stomach acid, also known as hydrochloric acid, is the spark that jump-starts the rest of your digestive system. It breaks the apple down into smaller particles, stimulates your pancreas to join in the action, and kills off abnormal bacteria that may be in the food. Stomach acid also enables you to absorb minerals and break down proteins. If your stomach acid is low, you can experience gas, bloating, and an overall feeling of heaviness in your stomach. In addition, low stomach acid can cause poor mineral absorption, which can lead to lowered immunity and poor bone density, among other problems.

Next, the apple—if I can still call it that—is released from your stomach into your small intestine, where a discharge of highly specialized enzymes from your pancreas begins further digestive action. These enzymes break down what is left of your apple into yet smaller particles so that thousands of folds called *villi* and *microvilli*, which are part of the inner wall of your small intestine, can absorb proteins, carbohydrates, fats, vitamins, and minerals from the apple. The small intestine transfers almost all of these elements right through its membrane wall into the bloodstream—or more specifically, the portal vein. The portal vein then takes the digested apple directly to your liver to be processed. From there it is carried by your circulatory system to every cell in your body.

Your small intestine has a difficult and complex job: sorting through everything you eat and separating what should be absorbed from what should be eliminated. If your small intestine is chronically irritated (from yeast, bacteria, parasites, poor digestion, or chemicals) it will allow more toxins and undesirable chemicals to pass into your bloodstream. This can ultimately lead to food allergies, poor liver detoxification, fatigue, skin rashes, autoimmune diseases, and a host of other disorders, including irritable bowel syndrome (IBS) and leaky gut syndrome, which we will explore in this chapter.

The parts of the apple that you don't absorb in your small intestine, such as the fiber, move on to your large intestine (also known as the colon), which removes the water from what is left of your apple. To remain optimally healthy, it is essential that you efficiently absorb what you need from the apple and rid your large intestine of the unabsorbed fiber.

Another important aspect of digestive health has often been overlooked in Western medicine but is extremely important from a natural health perspective. The small and large intestines contain hundreds of different kinds of bacteria, or flora, which can play a critical role in your ability to efficiently process your apple. Some of them, like those found in yogurt, are "friendly" bacteria and enhance your health. They help make vitamins, detoxify chemicals that can cause cancer, and act as part of your immune defense.

Your small and large intestines may also contain flora that are not so friendly, however. These can wreak havoc, causing gas, bloating, diarrhea, constipation, and other symptoms that can severely impair your digestive health. As we will see in this chapter, there are many ways you can reduce your unfriendly flora while at the same time staying on the best of terms with your friendly flora.

The View from the East

In Chinese medicine, diet, the health of the digestive system, and the emotions are all closely linked. Your stomach is healthiest when you provide your body with high-quality nutritious foods on a regular basis, and it is adversely affected by too much thinking and by stress. Worrying can cause your Qi to stagnate in your stomach, resulting in symptoms of belching, stomach pain, and nausea. When your body is well nourished, your mind and your spirit will be as well.

There are many parallels between the views of digestive health in Chinese and Western medicine. In Western medicine, as we've seen, the stomach releases food into the small intestine for absorption of nutrients. In the Chinese view, it is said that the stomach sends food down into the small intestine to be sorted. According to the Western explanation, the stomach releases hydrochloric acid to digest food; according to the Chinese perspective, the stomach "ferments" the food. In Chinese medicine, both the spleen and the stomach play a pivotal role in digestive health. The spleen is in charge of transforming the food and transporting it to every cell in your body. In addition, the spleen and stomach are essential to producing and maintaining Qi—it is said that they literally extract Qi from the food we eat.

The Earth Element

Carol, a mother of two who works as a family therapist, came to see me for problems she was having with her digestion, including chronic constipation and bloating. Even before we met, the melodious sound of her voice in the hallway outside my office suggested that her primary element was Earth. I would later learn that she exhibited many other qualities of the Earth type: a strong, full-figured woman with large lips, she was prone to worry but was always very grounded, compassionate, and empathic.

Carol reported that her digestive system had always been sensitive, but over the past few years her symptoms had become worse. She moved her bowels once every three days, and even then it seemed that she wasn't fully eliminating. Her abdomen appeared distended, and she said that although she hadn't gained weight, she couldn't fit into her old clothes anymore. All she wanted to wear these days was a muumuu.

Carol felt drained emotionally, too. "For the past couple of years," she said, "I've felt like I've given and given to my children, my clients, my friends, my parents, and my husband,

and there's nothing left for me. On my days off I just crash. I don't have the energy to exer-
cise or make healthy food because I'm just too tired."

As a caregiver and nurturer, Carol took care of others but too often at the expense of
herself. She craved sweets and ate them to fill the void she felt from being so exhausted. After
I recommended ways for Carol to create balance in her life and to nurture her digestive sys-
tem, including an intestinal cleanse and aromatherapy, she discovered that she was more pro-
ductive at work and much happier at home. She gained the energy to exercise and eat right,
and her digestive problems disappeared—for the first time in her life!

In Chinese medicine, digestion is represented by the Earth element, which bestows
nourishment on the body, mind, and spirit. The Earth element embodies the concept
of Mother Nature, nurturing you with food and shelter and also with emotional security, comfort, feelings of peace, and a sense of deep fulfillment.

If your predominant element is Earth, you may want to pay very close attention
to the issues outlined in this chapter, because the Earth element plays a particularly
important role in your digestive health, as well as the health of your entire body. Even
if you are not predominantly an Earth type, this chapter will help you make healthy
choices to balance your Earth element and strengthen your digestive health.

If you are an Earth type, you exhibit certain traits and tendencies. First and foremost, you are an especially compassionate and loving person. You are the nurturer,
the mother, the healer, the caretaker, and the supporter. Caring deeply about others,
you tend to welcome people from all walks of life into your world without judgment.
You have an overwhelming sense that everyone can, and should, live together harmoniously, and you thrive in peaceful times. You are a great arbitrator and a strong com-
municator (the primary sense organ of the Earth type is the mouth), and you are apt
to have a rich, melodious voice. With your empathic nature, your warmth, and your
communication skills, you have the capacity to be a very effective counselor. As an
Earth type, you get a great deal of satisfaction from being in nature and having a garden. You feel a strong connection to the earth, and you love to work the soil with your
hands. Like the earth itself, you naturally help sustain growth and life, and you tend
to be deeply concerned about taking care of the planet.

In the Chinese system, the Earth element rules late summer, the time of harvest,
when all the planning and hard work from the previous year come to fruition, and
you are finally able to reap the benefits of your efforts. As an Earth type, you need the
deep sense of well-being and security that comes from bringing home some kind of
a harvest—be it your income, a graduation, or any other tangible symbol of accom-
plishment that you earn through patience and discipline. Without the experience of a
bountiful harvest, you tend to become insecure and feel unsatisfied with your life.

When your Earth element is in balance, you have healthy digestion and your body is readily able to absorb the nourishment you need from your food; this is true for everyone, but especially for Earth types. Having a well-balanced Earth element gives you a strong sense of emotional security, and when you are healthy, you can easily create harmony in your life. You take care of people without draining yourself, maintaining the balance between giving to others and giving to yourself that is essential to keeping healthy. If you are an Earth type, you probably have a strong aversion to being deprived of food, because amid all of life's responsibilities and challenges, eating brings you solace. You tend to have a sweet tooth—the Earth element is associated with sweet flavors—but unfortunately eating too many sweets leads to poor digestion, lowers immunity, and causes blood sugar imbalances. Incorporating sweet vegetables such as yams and cooked carrots into your diet can help curb your cravings for sweets while nourishing your Earth element. Using natural calorie-free herbal sweeteners such as stevia can also satisfy your sugar cravings without jeopardizing your health.

When your Earth element is out of balance, you are very prone to digestive problems because the digestive system is where the Earth element has its most powerful influence. You may also have a tendency to experience food allergies, heartburn, fatigue, premenstrual symptoms, low self-esteem, obsessive worrying, and easy weight gain—which is compounded by your cravings for sweet foods. With your Earth element imbalanced, you are especially susceptible to health problems that are caused by eating dairy products, and your normally melodious voice can become dull, flat, or just the opposite: its musical quality can become exaggerated and excessive.

Imbalances in your Earth element can also cause you to lose touch with your usual sense of healthy boundaries, and you can become excessively needy for love and affection. At the same time, the traits that normally make you a good nurturer may backfire: you can become so sympathetic to other people's needs that you try to take care of them in ways that ultimately prevent them from learning to take care of themselves. You may go far out on a limb in your efforts to "fix" other people's problems, spending so much time attempting to rescue them from their troubles that you only wind up hurting yourself and draining your energy. This can be especially detrimental to your well-being if your life is filled with people who are "takers" rather than "givers." If you are an Earth type, it is especially important for you to be surrounded by loving friends who are as compassionate as you are.

When your Earth element is imbalanced, your attempts to "fix" things are not carefully or even consciously chosen; rather they are impulsive, knee-jerk responses to the needs of others, triggered by your out-of-control feelings on the spur of the moment. Thus when your Earth element is out of balance, you tend toward unhealthy "gut reactions" on both an emotional and a physical level: while your emotions are tangled up in desperately trying to help others, you can suffer from allergic reactions to the food you eat—which are unhealthy "gut reactions" in a literal sense.

As you can see, my patient Carol is a classic Earth type. Her primary physical complaint was problems with her digestive system, which had been shutting down in response to stress. Emotionally, she had become imbalanced, lacking healthy boundaries and taking care of everyone but herself. All her symptoms indicated that she needed to balance her Earth element in order to bring her body back to health.

Are You an Earth Type?

- Are you a nurturer and a caretaker?
- Do you easily empathize with other people's pain?
- Are you deeply compassionate of other people, even strangers?
- Do you tend to welcome all types of people into your life?
- Do you crave sweets?
- When you feel stressed, do you tend to eat?
- Do you gain weight easily?
- Does your voice have a musical quality?
- Are you a natural arbitrator who settles disputes between others quickly and effectively?
- Do you thrive during peaceful times?
- Are you deeply concerned about environmental issues?
- Do you tend to worry about others?
- Do you have trouble saying no when it comes to helping others?
- Do you tend to overextend yourself, even when you're tired?
- Is it difficult for you to maintain boundaries with your coworkers, family, and friends?
- Do you have a lot of digestive problems, especially when under stress?
- Do you feel a great sense of comfort and peace when you are in nature?
- When you are overstressed, do you find yourself feeling needy for love and affection?

If you answered yes to most of these questions, you are very likely an Earth type and should be especially careful about issues that affect your Earth element. Taking the following steps can help you balance your Earth element and create health in your body, mind, and spirit:

Eat regular meals.

Make time each day for peace and quiet and for nurturing yourself.

Create and maintain good boundaries between yourself and others.

Surround yourself with loving and compassionate friends.

Learn to refrain from overextending yourself in trying too hard to fix other people's problems.

Avoid eating too many sweets and dairy products.

Listen to your body; if you are tired, cut back on your commitments and learn to say no to things you really don't have time for.

If you have digestive problems, do an intestinal cleanse.

Identify and eliminate any food allergies you might have.

Get out in nature and bond with Mother Earth.

Celebrate the completion of your projects as if each were a great harvest.

Use the natural methods outlined in this chapter to keep your Earth element in balance, especially during stressful times.

Evaluating Your Digestive Health with Western Medicine

If you have chronic digestive symptoms, it may be because you lack stomach acid, enzymes, or bile, or because you have a yeast overgrowth, imbalanced bacteria, or parasites in your intestines. You may also have irritable bowel syndrome (IBS), which is characterized by abdominal pain and associated with altered bowel movements, possibly resulting from disordered intestinal bacteria and yeast. You may additionally have leaky gut syndrome, a condition in which the intestinal wall becomes significantly more permeable than normal to foods and toxins. If you suffer from any of these, you can successfully treat yourself with natural medicine. Sometimes just making simple adjustments to your diet, supplement regimen, or lifestyle can bring about an enormous difference in your digestive health.

The following questionnaire is designed to help you evaluate the overall health of your digestive system.

CHECKLIST OF SYMPTOMS	√ YES	√ NO	YOUR SYMPTOM CAN BE DUE TO:
Do you experience chronic abdominal gas or bloating?			IBS with an overgrowth of unfriendly yeast, bacteria, or parasites; food allergies, low stomach acid, deficient enzymes, or insufficient bile
Are you constipated (less than one bowel movement a day)?			IBS with an overgrowth of unfriendly yeast or bacteria; insufficient bile, a low-fiber diet, or hypothyroidism
Do you often have diarrhea?			IBS with an overgrowth of unfriendly yeast, bacteria, or parasites; food allergies, deficient enzymes, or insufficient bile
Do you experience intestinal pain when you are under stress?			IBS with or without an overgrowth of unfriendly yeast, bacteria, or parasites
Are your fingernails weak, or do they have pronounced vertical ridges or white spots on them?			Low stomach acid
Do you have bad breath?			IBS, including an overgrowth of unfriendly bacteria; abnormal bacteria in mouth
Do you have frequent vaginal infections?			Overgrowth of yeast in intestines and vagina

CHECKLIST OF SYMPTOMS	√ YES	√ NO	YOUR SYMPTOM CAN BE DUE TO:
Do you have heartburn?			Too much or too little stomach acid, or infection with *H. pylori*
Do you belch a lot?			Low stomach acid, deficient enzymes, or insufficient bile; hiatal hernia; or infection with *H. pylori*
Do you feel as if your food just sits in your stomach after you eat?			Low stomach acid, or eating while under stress
Do you have food allergies?			Low stomach acid that has led to IBS with leaky gut syndrome; an overgrowth of unfriendly yeast, bacteria, or parasites
Do you often experience pain or cramping in your intestines?			IBS with an overgrowth of unfriendly yeast, bacteria, or parasites; food allergies associated with leaky gut syndrome
Do you often experience rectal itching?			IBS with an overgrowth of unfriendly yeast, bacteria, or parasites; food allergies associated with leaky gut syndrome
Do you frequently have undigested food in your stool?			Low stomach acid and deficient enzymes

Add your total number of checks:

Assessing your score: If all your checks are in the "No" column, congratulations! You have taken good care of your digestive health. If you checked "Yes" to six or fewer symptoms, your digestive health may be imbalanced. By following the guidelines in this chapter, you should be able to resolve the conditions that led to your symptoms.

If you checked more than six boxes, you should make your digestive health a high priority. Carefully adhere to the suggestions in this chapter, and consider contacting a naturopathic physician to help you heal your digestive system and order appropriate diagnostic tests.

Are You a Candidate for Candida?

If you suffer from digestive imbalances, you may have an overgrowth of yeast known as *candida*. Women are more likely to have it if they have taken birth control pills or estrogen for many years, multiple rounds of antibiotics, or steroids such as prednisone; or if they eat a diet high in sugar or frequently drink alcohol. In addition to having many of the digestive symptoms in the questionnaire above, if you have intense cravings for sugar and breads, chronic vaginal yeast infections, and chronic yeast infections on your skin or nails (such as athlete's foot or toenail fungus), you may indeed have candida. If you are a likely candida candidate, see your naturopathic physician for laboratory testing and follow the Six-Point Plan beginning on page 186 to heal your digestive system.

COMPREHENSIVE TESTS FOR
DIGESTIVE IMBALANCES

If you suffer from moderate to severe digestive problems (such as frequent, painful abdominal gas and bloating, chronic constipation or diarrhea, or chronic heartburn) and you checked more than six boxes on the questionnaire, it's a good idea to look at why your digestive system isn't functioning optimally. You can have your naturopathic physician order any of the diagnostic tests in the following chart to pinpoint some of the underlying causes of distress. (These tests can determine if you have an overgrowth of intestinal yeast, bacteria, or parasites, and they can reveal why you might be suffering from IBS or leaky gut syndrome.)

Diagnostic Tests

NAME OF TEST	HOW THIS TEST WORKS/WHAT IT TELLS YOU
Complete digestive stool analysis	This test can tell you how well you digest your food and if you have an overgrowth of unfriendly yeast or bacteria, or if you have friendly bacteria.
Intestinal permeability test	You take this test by collecting your urine for six hours after consuming a drink of mannitol and lactulose. If high levels of these compounds are found in your urine, it indicates that you have increased intestinal permeability, or leaky gut syndrome.
Stool test for parasites	This test is usually done after you have taken a laxative to induce diarrhea. You will need to collect at least two or three stool samples to adequately test for parasites.
Blood test for yeast or parasite antibodies	This test can help you determine if you have high levels of immune cells (antibodies) to yeast or parasites.
Helicobacter pylori (*H. pylori*) antibody blood test or breath test	These tests can help you determine if you have an overgrowth of *H. pylori*, bacteria known to cause gastritis (inflammation of the stomach) and ulcers.

Evaluating Your Digestive Health with Chinese Medicine

As we've seen, in Chinese medicine the digestive system is governed by spleen Qi and stomach Qi. If either one of these is in disharmony, a number of digestive symptoms can develop. The most common, known as *spleen Qi deficiency,* can result from mental stress such as excessive studying, from eating too many raw or cold foods (either cold "energetically" or in terms of temperature), or from other poor dietary habits. Symptoms of spleen Qi deficiency include intestinal bloating after eating, fatigue, loose stools, lack of appetite, a pale tongue, and a lack of vitality in the pulse (also known as an "empty" pulse).

Because from the perspective of Chinese medicine the spleen affects so many other systems in the body, the importance of maintaining your spleen Qi with a healthy diet cannot be overstated. When your spleen Qi is strong, your muscles work well and you have an abundance of physical energy and vitality; when it is weak, you feel weary and your muscles can atrophy. Your spleen Qi also keeps your organs in alignment, and it affects your brain. If your spleen Qi is strong, you think clearly and your memory is reliable; if it is weak, your thinking becomes dull and you lack the ability to concentrate.

If your nutritional habits weaken your spleen Qi, you become more susceptible to what Chinese medicine describes as a "damp" condition, which can develop in your body if you live in a wet environment, if you eat an excess of cold, sweet foods like ice cream, or if you take too many pharmaceutical drugs. Excessive dampness, whether in your body or in your environment, can cause lethargy, feelings of stickiness and heaviness, muscle fatigue, puffiness under your eyes, cysts, and nausea. In the intestines, dampness is associated with yeast overgrowth and imbalanced flora and can lead to irritable bowel and leaky gut syndromes. You can prevent a "damp" condition simply by keeping your spleen Qi strong and vital.

In Chinese medicine, if you have an overgrowth of yeast, abnormal bacteria, or parasites in your intestines, you will probably be diagnosed as having either a "damp-cold" or a "damp-heat" condition. If you have a "damp-cold" condition, your tongue will have a sticky, thick white coating on it, and you will have loose, thin stools. Your symptoms may also include a low appetite, cold hands and feet, fatigue, and foggy thinking.

If you have a "damp-heat" condition, your tongue coating will have a sticky yellow coating. Your symptoms may also include loose stools, a low-grade fever, rectal itching, and a bloated feeling in your abdomen. This condition is more likely to occur in a hot, humid climate, and it can be brought on if you have food poisoning from eating contaminated food.

Keeping Your Digestive System Healthy

The Naturally Healthy Diet provides you with the foundation for great digestion. It is exceptionally high in one ingredient that can make an enormous difference in your digestive health—fiber. Fiber can prevent constipation, irritable bowel syndrome, hemorrhoids, and diverticulitis (a condition characterized by small, inflamed pockets in the intestinal wall). It also assists with detoxification by binding with hormones and other chemicals and eliminating them from the digestive system. In addition, fiber can help prevent heart disease, colon and breast cancer, diabetes, and obesity. Unlike other food substances you eat, fiber is not digested; rather, it is processed by bacteria in your intestines. If you have an excess of abnormal bacteria in your intestines, you will produce a lot of gas when you have higher amounts of fiber in your diet. When your intestinal flora are balanced, you can increase your fiber intake without experiencing such unwanted consequences.

There are two kinds of fiber, soluble and insoluble. Each can help you in a different way, and many fruits, vegetables, grains, and beans are good sources of both types. Soluble fiber has been found to enhance heart health by lowering cholesterol.[1] Research has shown that it may have anticancer benefits as well.[2] Foods that are especially good sources of soluble fiber include apples, broccoli, carrots, cooked oatmeal, kidney beans, pinto beans, and psyllium (a seed husk often used in powder form as a fiber supplement). High-fiber foods, such as bran cereal, are primarily insoluble fiber. This kind of fiber helps shorten the time food stays in your digestive system and maintain regularity of bowel movements. Other foods that are especially high in insoluble fiber include pears, spinach, corn, whole wheat bread, spaghetti, lentils, and many types of beans.

How much fiber do you need? Health organizations usually recommend at least 20 to 35 g each day, and many naturopathic physicians recommend upward of 40 g of fiber a day. Most people in the United States, however, consume an average of only 12 g a day. To increase your fiber intake, refer to the "Fiber Content" chart.

Fiber Content of Common Foods

FRUITS	AMOUNT	GRAMS OF FIBER	VEGETABLES	AMOUNT	GRAMS OF FIBER
Apple	1 medium-sized	2.9	**Broccoli**	½ cup	2.0
Apricots (dried)	2 halves	1.7	**Carrots**	1 large	2.9
Banana	1 medium-sized	2.0–3.0	**Spinach**	½ cup cooked	2.0
Artichokes	1 large	4.5	**Celery**	½ cup cooked	3.0
Figs (dried)	3	10.5	**Greens***	½ cup cooked	4.0
Pear	1 large (with skin)	4.5	**Peas**	½ cup fresh or frozen	9.1
Strawberries	½ cup	1.0	**Winter squash**	½ cup baked	3.5
Red raspberries	½ cup	4.6	**Yam**	1 medium-sized (baked, with skin)	6.8
Watermelon	1 thick slice	2.8	**Beets**	½ cup cooked	2.5

GRAINS/CEREALS	AMOUNT	GRAMS OF FIBER	BEANS/NUTS	AMOUNT	GRAMS OF FIBER
Brown rice	½ cup uncooked	5.5	**Almonds**	¼ cup sliced	2.4
White rice	½ cup uncooked	2.0	**Walnuts**	1 tablespoon	1.1
Oatmeal	¾ cup cooked	3.0	**Lima beans**	½ cup cooked	5.8

GRAINS/CEREALS	AMOUNT	GRAMS OF FIBER	BEANS/NUTS	AMOUNT	GRAMS OF FIBER
Whole wheat bran muffins	2	4.6	**Chickpeas**	1 cup cooked	12.0
Bran flake cereal	¾ cup	5.5	**Bean sprouts**	¼ cup raw	0.8
Seven-grain bread	2 slices	6.5	**Pinto beans**	½ cup cooked	5.9
Buckwheat groats	1 cup cooked	9.6	**Brown lentils**	⅔ cup cooked	4.5–5.5
Corn on the cob	1 medium-sized ear	5.0	**Kidney beans**	½ cup cooked	4.5–6.5

*Collard, beet, dandelion, kale, Swiss chard, and turnip greens.

Note: The numbers on this chart are an approximation, based on information from the American Dietetics Association and other sources. Fiber content in foods varies, especially with fruits and vegetables.

Following the Naturally Healthy Diet also includes eating foods that support your digestion from an Eastern perspective. As we have seen, in Chinese medicine foods are classified according to their "energetic" properties, as either "hot," "warming," "neutral," "cooling," or "cold"; you can keep your digestive system healthy by eating a balance of these foods. For example, eating too many "cooling" or "cold" foods can interfere with the function of your spleen Qi and stomach Qi, which work best when you eat foods that are at room temperature or cooked. For a list of foods and their energetic properties in Chinese medicine, see Chapter 1.

As we've seen, you are most prone to digestive problems when your Earth element is out of balance. Reducing stress is a major part of keeping your digestive system healthy, from a Chinese as well as a Western viewpoint. When you are happy and relaxed, your digestive system functions best; your body directs blood toward your stomach, which aids digestion by enhancing the release of the stomach acids and enzymes that help break down food. When you are calm, your intestines move food along at a normal pace and allow you to maintain regularity. When you are stressed, your digestive processes are interrupted and may speed up or slow down. This can lead to stomach pain, heartburn, gastritis, and other symptoms like gas, bloating, constipation, and diarrhea. Under stress you also release stress hormones that direct your blood toward your muscles (in order to deal with whatever is causing the stress) and away from your digestive system. As a result, you may not be able to release enough stomach acid or enzymes to sufficiently stimulate the rest of your digestive system to properly break down and absorb your food.

Let's consider whether stress is a major cause of your digestive symptoms. Do you eat on the run? Do you eat in chaotic environments? Do you wait until you feel starved before you eat? Do you often arrive at the table so tense that you feel you need to "decompress" before you can eat? If your answer to any of these questions is yes, it's time to take control of this important part of your life and make some positive changes. To begin with, create a peaceful eating environment and relaxed mealtimes. If you're ravenous before eating, you're waiting too long; try eating frequent small meals so that you don't end up famished and agitated. Even if you already have good eating habits, you may experience stomach or intestinal symptoms when you are under stress, and you will benefit from exploring techniques that can change your responses to stressful situations.

HERBS, AROMATHERAPY, AND FLOWER ESSENCES TO SUPPORT DIGESTIVE HEALTH

There are numerous plant medicines that can help keep your digestion healthy, especially if you are under stress. Chamomile and peppermint contain essential oils that have long been used to calm an irritated stomach. As aromatherapy, you can use chamomile in your bath, massage it into your skin, or smell it after it has been diffused into the air. Or you can use chamomile and peppermint in their dried herb form to make a tasty tea. Mix equal parts of the herbs and steep in boiled water (one teaspoon of the mixture per each cup of water), and drink as needed; the naturally occurring essential oils in the tea can soothe your stomach and relieve gas, spasms, or cramps in your intestines. Peppermint oil is also available in capsule form. The recommended dose is one to two enteric-coated capsules, taken two to three times a day, to ease digestive problems caused by tension.

Other essential oils that can help relieve intestinal problems due to stress include fennel and cardamom, intestinal antispasmodics that alleviate abdominal bloating, indigestion, and nausea. According to Gabriel Mojay, author of *Aromatherapy for Healing the Spirit,* both of these oils can help to tonify and balance your Earth element and stimulate the flow of Qi in your spleen and stomach. Mojay recommends fennel for digestive problems caused by too much mental stress and by keeping emotions locked inside. Cardamom is also helpful for diarrhea and if you are overwhelmed with worries and nervous exhaustion.

Using flower essences is another way to divert stress away from your stomach and help you cope with the digestive symptoms associated with emotional tension. Vervain is used for intestinal problems arising from stress and overextending yourself. Indian pink is recommended for maintaining calm and staying focused amid stressful chaos. Chamomile, which can be used as a flower essence if you are unable to release emotional tension and have rapidly changing moods and passions, can also help relieve the stress that may be the underlying cause of your symptoms. Flower essences are usually taken under your tongue as pellets or in liquid form as needed.

How to Treat Digestive Imbalances

As we've seen, digestion is essential to overall health and vitality. For many of us, eating healthy food and reducing stress may be all that's needed to keep our Earth element in balance and our digestive systems working at optimum levels. But for others, gastritis (inflammation of the stomach) and stomach ulcers can be major concerns. And for those who have been plagued by lifelong digestive ills, the common symptoms of digestive distress may be signs of a more intractable problem, such as irritable bowel syndrome (IBS).

PUTTING OUT THE FIRE IN YOUR STOMACH

If you've been diagnosed with gastritis or an ulcer, it is imperative that you take the *Helicobacter pylori* antibody blood test or breath test listed on page 177. These tests tell you if you have an overgrowth of *H. pylori,* the type of bacteria behind most cases of gastritis and stomach and peptic ulcers (which occur in the upper part of your small intestine). If the tests reveal you have an overgrowth of *H. pylori,* I highly recommend that you see a naturopathic physician. Medical doctors typically use a combination of drugs, including multiple antibiotics and stomach acid blockers, to destroy *H. pylori.* Antibiotics challenge liver health and destroy friendly bacteria as well. Acid blockers, when used short term, may not be as deleterious to your health, but they should not be used on a long-term basis because they can prevent proper mineral absorption. Naturopathic physicians traditionally use a combination of bismuth salts, antibacterial herbs, and mastic gum to help eliminate *H. pylori.* When *H. pylori* is wiped out, gastritis and stomach ulcers can heal.

Most important, it is not enough to merely eradicate *H. pylori*—you also need to do something to change the environment it thrives in. *H. pylori* grows out of control when you have certain kinds of imbalances in your intestinal environment, including low stomach acid and imbalanced intestinal bacteria. If you are diagnosed with *H. pylori* and have a history of gastritis or stomach ulcers, it is essential that you do an intestinal cleanse to treat the underlying cause of the problem and prevent it from taking hold again. In Point 4, beginning on page 193, you will find my detailed recommendations for doing an intestinal cleanse as part of the Six-Point Plan to Heal Your Digestive System.

Gastritis and ulcers can also be caused by emotional stress, excessive use of nonsteroidal anti-inflammatory drugs, high ingestion of alcohol, prolonged use of steroids, and chemotherapy. All of these conditions can set the stage for gastritis and ulcers by decreasing the amount of protective mucus in your stomach. From a Chinese perspective, gastritis and ulcers can develop if you have an excess of "fire" in your stomach, possibly as a result of having too much stress in your life, which drains your Qi and adversely affects your liver Qi. If your liver Qi becomes stagnant, it can "attack" the stomach, upsetting the natural flow of your digestion. Whatever the cause of gastritis or ulcers, the old naturopathic saying holds true: "To heal, you must first remove the obstacles to your cure."

If you have gastritis or ulcers, you can help put out the fire in your stomach with a diet of soft, soothing, easily digestible foods and herbs (such as the low-fiber version of the diet for nurturing your digestive system, described on page 192). You should avoid all acidic foods and drinks, such as tomatoes, salsa, citrus fruits, vinegar, coffee, sodas, and black tea. Herbs that help heal and soothe your stomach include marshmallow and licorice. These herbs are also great for the treatment of chronic mouth ulcers and canker sores, as well as heartburn—which can result from stomach acids irritating the mucous membrane of your esophagus.

To make marshmallow root tea, see page 100. If you don't have high blood pressure, you can simmer a half-teaspoon of licorice root along with your marshmallow root.

IRRITABLE BOWEL SYNDROME

In the United States, IBS affects one in five adults and three times as many women as men.[3] This condition can significantly affect the quality of a woman's life by limiting her social activities, restricting her ability to take part in sports and recreation, and interfering with her sex life. Seemingly without warning, it can spoil an evening—or an entire vacation! People with IBS often have the added frustration of not knowing what food is triggering their discomfort; their problem seems unpredictable, so all food becomes suspect. They may even develop a tendency to avoid eating altogether.

The term *irritable bowel syndrome* refers to a constellation of symptoms that include intestinal pain, bloating, gas, constipation, and diarrhea. IBS can sometimes mimic symptoms of more life-threatening diseases, so it's important to see your health care provider for a thorough evaluation if you think you have IBS. But many doctors prescribe drugs that simply mask the symptoms associated with the syndrome, seldom addressing the reasons a person might be experiencing them to begin with. IBS can have multiple underlying causes that can be successfully treated through lifestyle changes, diet, and intestinal cleansing. In fact, IBS responds remarkably well to natural medicine.

COMMON CAUSES OF IBS

- Advanced age
- Chronic exposure to drugs or chemicals such as:
  Alcohol
  Antibiotics
  Chemotherapeutic drugs
  Nonsteroidal anti-inflammatory
    drugs
  Oral birth control pills or hormones
  Steroids
- Chronic stress
- Chronic viral infections
- Food allergies
- High-sugar diet
- Intestinal parasites
- Nutritional deficiencies
- Overgrowth of intestinal yeast or abnormal bacteria
- Poor digestion due to low stomach acid, deficient pancreatic enzymes, or insufficient bile
- Weak ileocecal valve

If chronic, IBS can lead to the potentially even more problematic condition known as leaky gut syndrome. This condition develops if the cells that line the wall of the small intestine—which are normally packed closely together—become damaged by the presence of an irritant. Then channels open up between the cells, allowing larger-than-normal molecules of food or chemicals to "leak" through the intestinal wall into the bloodstream. This can ultimately cause a myriad of serious health disorders and immune problems because the body may create antibodies to these compounds. As you can see from the following list, irritable bowel and leaky gut syndromes have been linked to many conditions.

DISEASES AND SYMPTOMS COMMONLY ASSOCIATED WITH IRRITABLE BOWEL AND LEAKY GUT SYNDROMES

- Abdominal pain
- Acne
- Alcoholism
- Allergies
- Arthritis
- Asthma
- Autoimmune diseases:
  Rheumatoid arthritis
  Ankylosing spondylitis
  Myasthenia gravis
  Vasculitis
- Candida (yeast overgrowth)
- Chronic fatigue immuno-deficiency syndrome (CFIDS)
- Constipation
- Diarrhea
- Eczema
- Environmental hypersensitivities
- Fatigue
- Fibromyalgia
- Gluten intolerance (Celiac disease)
- Hives
- Imbalanced bacteria
- Inflammatory bowel disease:
  Ulcerative colitis
  Crohn's disease
- Intestinal bloating, gas, and cramping
- Joint and muscle pain
- Parasite infections
- Psoriasis
- Skin rashes

Most often a leaky gut is the outcome of yeast overgrowth, imbalanced bacteria, or parasites in the intestines. When these organisms thrive in the small intestine, not only can they damage the intestinal wall and cause many of the problems associated with leaky gut syndrome, they can also release toxins that affect the liver, impair the body's natural detoxification mechanisms, and further compromise the immune system.

HOW INTESTINAL FLORA BECOME IMBALANCED

Lehua had been experiencing frequent diarrhea, gas, and bloating for more than a year when she came to see me. It all started after a bout with a parasite, which was treated with a pharmaceutical medication. Her stool tests showed that she had eliminated the parasite, but now she had constant headaches, woke up nauseated every morning, and had been told that she had chronic colitis (inflammation of the wall of her large intestine). The medication prescribed for her colitis caused dangerous side effects, so she had to stop taking it. By the time I saw her, she was extremely tired and afraid to leave the house for fear of not being close to a bathroom. She couldn't exercise, so she had gained weight. She had also been put on anti-depressants. Her life was miserable, but she thought she would just have to live with her condition.

I immediately put Lehua on a program to rebuild her intestinal health. She took herbal medications, changed her diet, and ingested friendly flora. Within only a few weeks, her headaches went away, her energy increased, and her digestion returned to normal.

Lehua's story is an example of how severely imbalanced intestinal flora, when in advanced stages, can lead to life-changing consequences. The pharmaceutical drugs she took eradicated her parasites but were not able to restore her health. Addressing Lehua's problems with natural medicine allowed her to significantly increase the quality of her life.

Why would your flora become imbalanced in the first place? As you've seen, the intestines contain many kinds of flora, some friendly and health-enhancing, and others not so friendly. One of the most common reasons you might have imbalanced flora is a diet high in sugar, which provides extra fuel to any unfriendly residents you may have. Another common reason for imbalanced flora is frequent use of antibiotics and steroids (such as prednisone). Have you ever developed a vaginal infection when taking antibiotics for a bacterial infection elsewhere in your body? The antibiotics can kill off not only the bacteria that are causing your problem, but also the friendly flora that keep yeast from thriving in the mucous membranes of your vagina. When you take antibiotics, the same pattern holds for your intestines: your friendly flora can be devastated. To make matters worse, there are certain unfriendly flora, resistant to antibiotics, that can flourish when you take these drugs.

Incidentally, both a high-sugar diet and the repetitive use of antibiotics also contribute to an imbalance of yeast in the intestines. It is normal to have a small amount of some types of intestinal yeast, but there should not be large colonies of unfriendly yeast expanding and taking over your intestinal territory. Yeast overgrowth, also known as candida, can cause many of the symptoms of IBS.

A structural problem can also contribute to imbalanced intestinal flora: if your ileocecal valve (the valve between your small and large intestines) is weak, bacteria from your large intestine can flood your small intestine, throwing off the balance of the flora in your small intestine. This results in symptoms of gas and bloating and can eventually cause leaky gut syndrome. Your ileocecal valve can become weakened if you have chronic constipation from a low-fiber diet.

Poor digestion can be another cause of imbalanced intestinal flora because of the complicated role digestion plays in breaking food down in preparation for absorption. You are also more susceptible to the development of food allergies when you have poor digestion, and food allergies can wreak even more havoc on a weakened digestive system, resulting in further imbalances in intestinal flora.

Finally, parasites, which you can contract from drinking water, eating food, or swimming in water contaminated with them, can upset your intestinal flora by irritating the lining of your intestines. Chronic parasites often result in frequent diarrhea and intestinal cramps.

The Six-Point Plan to Heal Your Digestive System

As we've seen, intestinal imbalances can result in symptoms not only in the digestive system but throughout the body. They can lead to so many health problems that you may feel overwhelmed at times. But when you discover what is causing your symptoms, you may be surprised to find that many of your health problems, which you had thought were unrelated, have a single root cause. And when you remove that cause, many of your symptoms may disappear simultaneously. Healing your digestive system lifts a burden from your entire body, giving you renewed strength and a great sense of freedom.

Begin the process of healing your digestive system knowing that it can take time to correct your imbalances. Your symptoms did not appear overnight, and fully restoring your digestive health will probably be a gradual process, not a quick fix. The Six-Point Plan that I present here is easy to follow if you take your time; by walking through it at your own pace, you can use it as a road map on your journey to optimum digestive health. It can be used to help you heal from many kinds of common digestive disturbances, including candida, poor digestion, food allergies, IBS, and leaky gut syndrome.

POINT 1: TEST YOURSELF FOR FOOD ALLERGIES

Food allergies are often the result of irritable bowel and leaky gut syndromes. As we've seen, when you have leaky gut syndrome, your intestinal wall becomes less selective about what is allowed to pass through its membrane. Food molecules that normally would not be able to cross your intestinal membrane can now transfer into your bloodstream. When this happens, your immune system correctly perceives the situation as unhealthy and goes into overdrive, naturally creating antibodies to what it considers to be "foreign," and food allergies can result.

Food allergies may be more closely linked to irritable bowel and leaky gut syndromes than we realize, actually increasing our susceptibility to these conditions. Because food allergies can cause changes in, and can irritate, the intestinal lining, they may be part of a complex vicious cycle, not only by being caused by those two syndromes but by playing a role in *causing* them as well. In my practice I've observed that when people with irritable bowel and leaky gut syndromes remove from their diet the foods that they are allergic to, their symptoms often clear up quickly.

The story of my own health crisis, as I related in the Introduction, is a good example of how much you can learn by testing yourself for food allergies. After trying to get by without using my hands for over a year, I was able to begin healing myself when I discovered one of the most important missing pieces to my health puzzle: the relationship between my food allergies and digestive imbalances. But I learned this only after removing, and then reintroducing, certain kinds of food from my diet. After learning to avoid these foods, and by combining dietary changes with detoxification and nutritional supplementation, I was eventually able to restore my health.

You can do your own food allergy test at home using an *elimination-challenge* test. You remove a suspicious food from your diet for a period of time, then eat it again and carefully watch for allergic reactions. This method has the benefit of giving you clear feedback from your body after you eat a food that you may be allergic to.

With my patients, I've found that the best way to do this test is to eliminate from your diet the foods that most commonly cause allergic reactions (along with any other foods you suspect you may be allergic to) for one week, then separately "challenge" each type of food by bringing them back in one at a time. To completely eliminate foods that contain gluten, for example, you will need to avoid eating all grains except rice, millet, amaranth, quinoa, teff, corn, and buckwheat. An allergy to gluten (also known as gluten intolerance or celiac disease) can cause significant digestive problems, intestinal wall inflammation, and malnutrition from poor absorption of nutrients. I've seen many people with autoimmune diseases, such as rheumatoid arthritis, greatly reduce inflammation of their joints when they follow a gluten-free diet. (People with gluten intolerance must avoid all grains that contain gluten for the rest of their lives.)

If you have a food allergy, your allergic reactions generally fall into two categories: they happen right after you eat the food, or they happen in a delayed response typically twenty-four to forty-eight hours later. The immediate type of allergic reaction is usually very apparent when you experience it, but delayed food allergy reactions can be much more difficult to recognize because of this time lapse between consumption of the food and the appearance of the symptoms. Identifying the foods you are allergic to and removing them from your diet requires a serious commitment to your health, and it may mean giving up some of the foods you love; on the other hand, you will probably find that you begin to feel better and that your energy increases noticeably.

You can ask your naturopathic physician to identify your food allergies by ordering a blood test that measures both delayed and immediate antibody reactions to foods. (For example, if your test reveals lots of antibodies to milk, you have a milk allergy.) But I recommend you begin by taking the Food Elimination-Challenge Test, to test yourself for food allergies, because you may find that it tells you everything you need to know about your reactions to foods.

THE FOOD ELIMINATION-CHALLENGE TEST

1. For one week, eat a diet that includes none of the most common food allergens (dairy products, beef, wheat, all grains containing gluten, eggs, corn, peanuts, shellfish, and soy), and also eliminate from your diet any other foods you suspect you are allergic to.
2. After one week, pick one of the foods you have excluded and begin testing it by eating it three to four times that day. Test one you most miss in your diet first. That way, if you have no adverse reaction, you will be eating it that much sooner.
3. For two to three days, watch for any symptoms of an adverse reaction. (Allergic reactions to food can include any of the symptoms listed in the "Conditions and Symptoms" chart.)
4. After three days, test another one of the excluded foods by adding it to your diet. It is important to test foods one at a time in order to be sure which ones you are reacting to. For instance, if you started testing a suspect food on Saturday, don't begin testing a different one until Tuesday. Continue to carefully "challenge" the foods that were eliminated from your diet until you've discovered which ones cause symptoms.

Once you've successfully identified any foods that you may be allergic to, begin to *exclude them from your diet* so that you give your digestion the opportunity to heal. With these problematical foods no longer in your diet, you can now take the proactive steps in the rest of the Six-Point Plan. Continue to exclude the foods to which you are allergic for at least three months. If you can fully heal your digestive system, you may find that you no longer have allergic reactions to many of the foods in question and can eventually begin eating them again.

CONDITIONS AND SYMPTOMS COMMONLY ASSOCIATED WITH FOOD ALLERGIES

Achy, weak muscles or tendons	Insomnia
Anxiety	Intense cravings for food
Apathy	Irregular heartbeat
Asthma	Itchy ears
Canker sores	Joint pains
Chronic swollen lymph nodes	Migraines
Coughing	Mood swings
Dark circles under the eyes	Mucus in your sinuses or lungs
Depression	Postnasal drip
Diarrhea	Psoriasis
Dizziness	Puffy eyes
Ear infections	Rashes
Eczema	Rectal itching
Fatigue after eating certain foods	Ringing in your ears
Foggy thinking	Sore throat
Gas and bloating in your intestines	Sweating in excess
Hay fever	Swelling in your tongue or lips
Headaches	Urgent and frequent urination
Hives	Water retention in your hands or feet
Hyperactivity	Watery eyes or blurred vision

POINT 2: TAKE SUPPLEMENTS AND HERBS IF YOU HAVE LOW STOMACH ACID, DEFICIENT ENZYMES, OR INSUFFICIENT BILE

Once you've completed Point 1, you can apply the next four points in your Six-Point Plan all together. By making these four points work for you concurrently, you will speed up the process of healing your digestive system.

In Point 2 you can assist your digestion if you have low stomach acid, deficient pancreatic enzymes, or insufficient bile. The questionnaire on page 175 can help you make this determination.

If you do have low amounts of any of these three digestive aids, your symptoms may give you some indication as to which is the culprit. Symptoms of low stomach acid include a feeling that food just sits in your stomach, belching, heartburn, intestinal bloating, and weak fingernails with ridges on them. Deficient pancreatic enzymes can result in gas and bloating after meals. Symptoms of insufficient bile can include dry skin, constipation, digestive bloating, and diarrhea or indigestion after you eat a fatty meal.

Deficiencies of stomach acid, enzymes, or bile can cause numerous digestive problems, including IBS, but many of them can easily be corrected with supplementation. Some of my patients have digestive problems when they are under lots of stress, and often they respond well to digestive aids taken only during these times. Other patients have more chronic symptoms, and their digestion is considerably improved by taking supplements on a regular basis with meals.

To increase your stomach acid, you can drink a small amount of lemon water or diluted apple cider vinegar; stir one teaspoon of either fresh-squeezed lemon juice or apple cider vinegar into one-half cup of warm water, and drink before meals. You can also supplement your diet with betaine hydrochloric acid (betaine HCL), which is comparable to the stomach acid that your body produces. I recommend that you take betaine HCL in the form of capsules (rather than tablets), which can be purchased at a health food store, and that you work with your naturopathic physician while taking it. Most naturopaths will advise that you start by taking a low dose (one pill, or ten "grains") with at least six ounces of water, always with your meals. If you have any adverse reaction, such as stomach pain or heartburn, stop taking it and use lemon water or diluted apple cider vinegar instead. You shouldn't take betaine HCL if you have gastritis or a stomach ulcer.

"What? *Increase* my stomach acid to treat my heartburn?"

You may be surprised to learn that *low* stomach acid can cause the symptoms of heartburn—exactly the opposite of what you've probably been told. Many conventional Western doctors believe that heartburn comes only from high stomach acid, and as a rule they recommend antacids (or stomach acid blockers, as they are often called) for reducing heartburn, because they lower the acids in your stomach.

With some of my patients, I have found this belief to be valid—they require antacids to treat their heartburn. But many of my patients who have been on antacids actually experience *less* heartburn when they take a stomach acid *supplement* with their meals. In many cases, they increase their stomach acid, and—presto!—their heartburn disappears.

Stomach acid supplements may be especially effective for reducing heartburn symptoms due to eating while under stress, or eating too quickly. Simply changing these behaviors can decrease symptoms of heartburn. But if your life is such that you often have to eat quickly or while under unavoidable stress, taking stomach acid with meals may significantly reduce heartburn. I advise that you do this under the guidance of a naturopathic physician.

I recommend that you take an antacid only if necessary. Take it for a short time only, not every day (and certainly not with each meal), and always use a natural rather than a synthetic antacid. Taking an antacid on a long-term basis, especially a synthetic one like Prevacid, can result in numerous nutritional deficiencies and symptoms of irritable bowel and leaky gut syndrome.

Before you assume that an antacid will help you with heartburn, try the remedies I've suggested to increase your stomach acid and see if that corrects your problem. You don't want to lower your stomach acid if you don't have to, because you need it for good digestion. This is a classic case of the ancient Hippocratic dictum "First, do no harm": you may be able to take care of your heartburn without doing anything harmful, and unnecessary, to your body. Most people find that their symptoms of heartburn disappear once they get their digestive system back on track.

If you need a natural antacid for heartburn, I recommend an orange peel extract called Heartburn Free that contains d-limonene (see Appendix B for details); take one pill every other day for twenty days, then one pill for relief as needed. (You should not use this product if you have a stomach ulcer.)

If your levels of digestive enzymes are deficient, you can significantly enhance your digestion by taking additional digestive enzymes. When you purchase digestive enzyme supplements, you will see many words on the container that end with the suffix *-ase,* including protease (which breaks down proteins), lipase (which breaks down fats), and amylase, sucrase, cellulase, and maltase (which break down carbohydrates). You should buy enzyme supplements with at least an 8X or 10X strength and take one to two pills, always at mealtimes, to enhance your digestion. (If you have gastritis or a stomach ulcer, you shouldn't use digestive enzymes.)

As with stomach acid, your digestive enzymes can be low as a result of stress, so remember that reducing the stress in your life will also help increase your enzyme level. Genetically, many people of Asian or Native American ancestry can lack the enzyme lactase, which digests lactose, or milk sugar. If you lack this enzyme and you ingest dairy products, you can experience intense gas, bloating, and loose stools. To remedy this situation, purchase only lactose-free milk or use lactase enzymes when you are ingesting dairy products.

If you have poor digestion due to an insufficient amount of bile, supplementing with bile salts can help. Bile emulsifies fats in your diet, and bile deficiency may result in poor digestion of fats and fat-soluble vitamins. If you've had your gallbladder removed, you tend to have a lack of bile when you need it most—your gallbladder normally stores bile and releases it to help you digest fats when you eat a fatty meal. Many enzyme supplements also contain bile salts. Look for formulas containing 50 to100 mg of bile salts per pill, and take one to two pills with fatty meals.

If you have a history of chronically low stomach acid, deficient pancreatic enzymes, or insufficient bile, you will also benefit from doing an intestinal cleanse as outlined in Point 4. This is because when you have these imbalances, you are more likely to have an overgrowth of undesirable bacteria in your intestines, which could result in IBS and leaky gut syndrome.[4]

POINT 3: NURTURE YOUR DIGESTIVE SYSTEM WITH HEALTHY FOOD

The Naturally Healthy Diet (outlined in Chapter 1) will nourish your digestive system and support your spleen Qi and stomach Qi. But if your digestion is out of balance or you are prone to chronic intestinal problems, you will need to fine-tune your diet to further improve your digestive health. The following dietary recommendations for treating IBS can also help resolve digestive problems not commonly associated with IBS, such as painless diarrhea or constipation without cramping.

Some foods are soothing to your intestines because they are easily digested; others, which contain a lot of fiber, encourage healthy digestion by increasing regularity. If you suffer from certain symptoms commonly associated with IBS, such as loose stools with excessive gas, cramping, and bloating, I recommend that you give your tender intestines a break from raw or high-fiber foods, which can be irritating to your digestive system, and eat a low-fiber diet for one to two weeks. You will probably begin to feel much better as you initially decrease your consumption of fiber and raw foods. After reducing your fiber and treating imbalances in your intestinal flora, you will soon be able to tolerate increased fiber.

A low-fiber diet includes easily digested complex carbohydrates such as *well-cooked* brown or basmati rice, squash, yams, and cream-of-rice hot cereal. If you are not allergic to wheat, you can eat yeast-free bread and pasta.

Your diet can also include fish, lean poultry, and eggs that are poached or hard-boiled. For vegetable dishes I suggest cooked peas and steamed vegetables such as zucchini, cauliflower, broccoli, carrots, and green beans. Limiting your fiber intake includes avoiding beans and soy products, which also cause gas. Nuts are hard to digest and should also be avoided. You should refrain from eating dairy products, which are high in milk sugar. Avoiding dairy products when you have IBS is also recommended in Chinese medicine: IBS is considered a "damp" condition that will only become worse when you eat "damp" foods, like dairy products.

For your low-fiber diet I also recommend soups, because they are easy to digest and a convenient way to ingest cooked vegetables. From a Chinese medicine perspective, soups are also beneficial to digestion. The best way to nourish your spleen Qi and stomach Qi is by eating your food warm or at room temperature.

If you suffer primarily from constipation with gas and intestinal bloating—a different pattern of symptoms commonly associated with IBS—it's best to start increasing fiber in your diet. As we saw earlier in this chapter, fiber is an essential part of keeping your digestion healthy. It also plays an important role in helping you heal from many digestive problems.

To increase fiber, eat more grains such as brown rice, rolled oats, quinoa, amaranth, millet, and buckwheat groats. Include salads and one piece of low-glycemic fruit, such as an apple, in your diet every day. Make vegetable juices that include *all* of the vegetables' high-quality fiber by using a blender rather than a juicer. (With a juicer, you discard the fiber that can be so good for you.) You can also increase your fiber by eating beans in small quantities. Soak dried beans in water overnight in the refrigerator before cooking; this makes them much easier to digest. Avoid beans altogether if you experience excessive gas after eating them.

Whether you are eating a low- or high-fiber diet, you should avoid foods that can promote yeast growth. These include fermented foods and yeast-containing products such as breads made with yeast, baked goods, some B vitamins made from yeast, vinegars, beer, pickles, and sauerkraut. Also included are mushrooms, malted products such as barley malt (found in many drinks and cereals), and high-carbohydrate foods like corn, potatoes, and tapioca.

For either fiber-modified diet, you can use ginger, fennel, and cinnamon to make your food more flavorful while supporting your digestion. In Chinese medicine, these herbs are known for their ability to strengthen spleen Qi and stomach Qi and eliminate "damp-cold" conditions that can compromise digestive health. In addition, because they are classified as "warm" herbs, they can stimulate digestion and relieve gas pains. (They can have these effects according to Western medicine as well.) You can use these herbs as teas or add them to your favorite dishes.

Point 4: Use Natural Medicines and Intestinal Cleansing To Balance Your Digestive System

You can additionally improve your digestive health by taking natural medicines to help eliminate unwanted yeast, bacteria, and parasites. I've used the herbs in the "Natural Medicines to Evict Unfriendly Residents" chart with great success to treat patients with IBS due to these three issues. Garlic is a potent way of treating all three, and the most economical. It's also the safest, and it can be used by expecting and breast-feeding mothers. (The other natural medicines listed on the chart should not be used by pregnant and lactating mothers.) But if you are experiencing an excess of gas, garlic could initially exacerbate your symptoms.

When you take these medicines to treat an intestinal imbalance, I suggest you start out slowly and increase your dose gradually. This will help prevent a "die-off reaction": if you kill off your abnormal intestinal inhabitants too quickly, it will cause them to release toxins that create mayhem in your liver and overwhelm your body's detoxification systems. A die-off reaction can result in fatigue and headaches and on the whole make you feel much worse before you begin to feel better. If you experience these symptoms, cut back on the dose of your medicine, drink lots of water, and exercise to help your body eliminate the toxins. In no time, you'll feel better and can begin increasing the dose of your medicine again, slowly building up to the recommended level.

If you have IBS and your symptoms are only mild, you will probably need to take one of the following natural medicines for a minimum of three weeks in order to eradicate your unfriendly intestinal guests. For moderate to severe IBS symptoms, you will most likely need to take it for four weeks or more. If you've had laboratory testing, the chart can help you target whichever yeast, bacteria, or parasites were found; your naturopathic physician can help you devise a specific plan based on the results of your stool test.

Natural Medicines to Evict Unfriendly Residents

HERB	ANTIYEAST PROPERTIES	ANTIBACTERIAL PROPERTIES	ANTIPARASITIC PROPERTIES	HOW TO TAKE THIS HERB	DOSE
Garlic	√	√	√	Week 1: Take 1 clove a day or 1 tablet 2 times a day. Weeks 2–4: Take 1–2 cloves a day or 1 tablet 2–3 times a day with food. *Note:* Garlic can cause an increase in gas and bloating and may cause heartburn in some people. Garlic is safe during pregnancy and lactation.	1 medium-sized clove of raw garlic, or a 900-mg tablet (containing 5,000 mcg allicin)
Oregano Oil	√	√		Week 1: Take 1 pill two times a day with food. Weeks 2–4: Take 1 pill 3 times a day with food. *Note:* Do not use during pregnancy and lactation.	Standardized extract of oregano oil containing 50 mg per pill
Berberine	√	√	√	Week 1: Take 1 pill 2 times a day with food. Week 2: Take 1 pill 3 times a day with food. Weeks 3–4: Take 2 pills 2 times a day with food. *Note:* Do not use during pregnancy and lactation.	Standardized extract of berberine containing 200 mg per pill

HERB	ANTIYEAST PROPERTIES	ANTIBACTERIAL PROPERTIES	ANTIPARASITIC PROPERTIES	HOW TO TAKE THIS HERB	DOSE
Olive Leaf Extract	√	√		Week 1: Take 1 pill 2 times a day. Weeks 2–4: Take 1 pill 3 times a day. *Note:* Olive leaf extract can also stimulate immune cells to fight infection and has potent antioxidant properties. Do not use during pregnancy and lactation.	500 mg per pill containing 15 percent olive leaf extract

Source: See the various sources in note 5.

While you are taking natural medicines, I highly recommend that you do an intestinal cleanse for a minimum of two weeks and a maximum of four weeks. Your cleanse will improve the function of your digestive system and help further eradicate unfriendly flora. It will also help your body deal with a potential die-off reaction due to the release of toxins caused by killing off the unfriendly flora, and at the same time help eliminate those toxins from your body. Many people lose weight doing an intestinal cleanse, and often my patients report that they feel great while they are cleansing. If you don't need to lose weight, be sure you get enough calories during your cleanse.

From a Chinese medicine perspective, an intestinal cleanse is a way to clear "dampness" from the intestines. While you are doing your intestinal cleanse, you may notice that the coating of your tongue changes. It can initially become thick, with a yellow or white tint, but as you move through your cleanse it may turn thinner and clearer. According to Chinese medicine, this indicates that you are detoxifying, successfully eliminating "dampness" from your body, strengthening your spleen Qi and stomach Qi, and balancing your Earth element.

Start your intestinal cleanse when your digestive system is able to handle a high-fiber diet. During the cleanse you will drink a series of shakes made up of finely ground psyllium husk, bentonite clay (available at a health food store), and a hypoallergenic rice-based protein powder. (See Appendix B for resources.) The psyllium will accelerate your intestinal transit time (the time it takes for food to pass through your body), and the bentonite clay will help remove toxins from your intestines that are released from killing off yeast, bacteria, or parasites. In the unlikely event that you are allergic to rice, consider using a whey protein powder or none at all. You can also add unsweetened soy milk, oat milk, or almond milk to your shakes. During your cleanse, continue to avoid all known food allergens and any foods you suspect you may be allergic to.

How to Take Cleansing Shakes

Days 1–3: Put 1 teaspoon of finely ground psyllium, ½ teaspoon of bentonite clay, and 1–2 tablespoons of protein powder in your blender. Add 2 cups of water, unsweetened soymilk, or other nondairy milk, and blend. Take this shake once a day, thirty minutes before you eat breakfast. (If you find that it fills you up and you don't need to eat your breakfast or anything else for a few hours, that's okay.)

Days 4–6: If you are tolerating your shakes well, continue to use the same recipe as in days 1–3, but increase the number of shakes. Take one shake in the morning thirty minutes before breakfast and one shake in the evening thirty minutes before dinner.

Days 7–9: If you are tolerating your shakes well, continue taking them twice a day as you did in days 4–6, but increase the dose of bentonite and psyllium. Take 2 teaspoons of psyllium and 1 teaspoon of bentonite with each shake. You should increase your dose of psyllium and bentonite only if you are feeling good at the lower dose, and passing 1–2 well-formed bowel movements every day without straining.

Day 10 to the end of your cleanse: If you're tolerating your shakes well, increase the number to three a day. Take your third shake thirty minutes before lunchtime if you have access to a blender. If not, take your shake thirty minutes before dinner and another one before bed. You can also increase your dose of psyllium to 3 teaspoons (one tablespoon) per shake. But you should not increase your dose of bentonite; it can be constipating in higher doses, which could negate some of the positive effects of your cleanse.

When you are nearing the end of your cleanse, slowly decrease the number of shakes you are taking. For instance, if you've been taking three shakes a day, cut back to two shakes a day for two days, and then cut back further to one shake a day, in the morning only, for a few more days as your cleanse winds down.

(If you enjoyed the beneficial effects of your shakes, you can continue having them after your cleanse. Have one every morning thirty minutes before breakfast, or as your breakfast. Use the same amount of protein powder, and use 1–3 teaspoons of psyllium, but discontinue the bentonite clay.)

After each shake, drink at least eight ounces of water to "chase" it. Drinking plenty of water during your cleanse will help your body flush out toxins. If you have a history of chronic constipation, be cautious with your use of bentonite clay because it can cause constipation. If you don't have a minimum of one bowel movement a day while on your cleanse, decrease your dose of bentonite clay or eliminate it from your shakes altogether.

If you experience a lot of bloating after you begin your cleanse, you may not be tolerating the fiber in your shakes very well. In that case, decrease the amount of psyllium, eliminate the bentonite, and take only one shake a day until your body has adjusted to the increase in fiber. When you no longer experience bloating, you can increase the number of shakes and continue with the rest of your cleanse.

POINT 5: CULTIVATE FRIENDLY FLORA IN YOUR INTESTINES

With Point 4 of your Six-Point Plan, you are ousting a whole population of unfriendly visitors from your intestines. But even while you are busy cleaning house, you can start bringing in some new, friendly flora. You ingest friendly flora routinely if you eat yogurt or drink acidophilus milk, but these aren't your best options if you are treating IBS or have an allergy to dairy products. The good news is that you can take dairy-free supplements that are full of the friendly flora known as acidophilus. There are many different kinds of acidophilus; two of the most commonly prescribed are lactobacillus and bifidobacterium bifidis. Studies have found that an abundance of these flora in the intestines and other mucous membranes, such as those in the vagina, can help prevent the growth of yeast.[6] In addition, friendly flora play many other helpful roles in the intestines, like breaking down toxic substances found in food, boosting the intestine's immune defense, and maintaining a healthy pH balance. They can also prevent the growth of abnormal bacteria such as *H. pylori,* salmonella, and undesirable strains of *E. coli.*[7]

You can find acidophilus supplements at a health food store. Most acidophilus products contain fructooligosaccharides (which may be referred to as FOS on the package label), special sugars that feed friendly flora and will not pose any problem to your intestinal health. Always buy high-quality acidophilus that has been refrigerated, and be sure to keep it in the refrigerator after your purchase.

I recommend you take a minimum of two billion acidophilus organisms a day. (This may seem like a large number, but normally you have much greater amounts in your digestive system.) Take the acidophilus at least two hours away from your antiyeast, antibacterial, and antiparasitic herbs; you may find that it's easiest at night before bed. Continue supplementing your diet with this amount of acidophilus until you've completed your intestinal cleanse. Then take at least one billion acidophilus organisms a day for two additional months. If you are ever required to take an antibiotic, be sure to take at least two billion high-quality acidophilus organisms at the same time and every day for at least two weeks afterward. This will help prevent the antibiotics from killing off your friendly flora.

POINT 6: REINTRODUCE SOME OF THE FOODS YOU WERE ALLERGIC TO

Once you've healed your digestive problems with Points 1 through 5, you can begin reintroducing the foods you discovered you were allergic to in Point 1. In most cases, my patients have been able to tolerate many foods they were allergic to after avoiding them for three months; others have found that they needed to avoid them for longer periods. When reintroducing foods, I recommend you begin with those that caused you the mildest reactions and proceed gradually to those that were more problematic.

To reintroduce a food, eat it at one meal and watch for any adverse symptoms for the next two to three days. Do not confuse the issue by reintroducing other foods you may be allergic to during this period. If you have no allergic symptoms, incorporate the food back into your diet on a limited basis, eating it no more than three or four times a week. You are more likely to have an allergic reaction to a food that you eat every day; with a "rotation diet" you vary your diet every day by rotating the foods you eat, so you avoid being exposed to the same allergen day after day, breaking the cycle of chronic exposure that can lead to a food allergy. (If you chose to have your naturopathic physician order a blood test to identify your food allergies, you may have received a rotation diet plan, which often accompanies the test results.)

In the event that, when you reintroduce a food, you find that you still have an adverse reaction, exclude it from your diet for another three months, then try reintroducing it again. If you are still reactive to the food, avoid it for an entire year before you try again. If after a year you *still* have symptoms, you could very well have a "fixed" allergy due to your genetic makeup. This means that you may never be able to eat the offending food without having symptoms.

With many food allergies that result from irritable bowel and leaky gut syndromes, you are likely to find that when you reintroduce a food after at least three months, you no longer have an adverse reaction. This can be a delightful experience: my patients often use words like "liberated" and "empowered" to describe how they feel after reintroducing foods that previously caused problems. If you've been through years of allergic reactions and perhaps resigned yourself to living with your condition for the rest of your life, there's nothing quite like being able to eat and enjoy foods you were formerly allergic to—and be absolutely symptom free.

Your Digestive Health: Final Thoughts

You can nurture your digestive health gently and effectively with the methods we've explored in this chapter. And when you've completely healed your digestive system and put in a whole new garden of friendly flora, you can maintain healthy digestion with the Naturally Healthy Diet (outlined in Chapter 1).

Your digestive system is vital to your overall health because it supports all the other systems in your body. Fully nourishing your digestive health makes it that much easier for you to create bountiful health throughout your body, mind, and spirit and to reap the harvest of a lifetime of optimal well-being.

Remember that healthy digestion is a gift of the Earth, deeply rooted in your Earth element; if you are an Earth type, pay close attention to your Earth qualities and especially your need to preserve balance in your life, both physically and emotionally. Your body, in its wisdom, wants wellness; when you've fully restored the integrity of your digestive health, it will maintain itself naturally as long as you continue making healthy choices every day.

The Essence of Chapter 6

- Keep your Earth element in balance to maintain your digestive health.
- Support your digestive system every day with the Naturally Healthy Diet.
- Eat a high-fiber diet to maintain good digestive health.
- Decrease stress in your life and soothe your digestive system with aromatherapy, herbs, and flower essences.
- Treat the "fire" in your stomach if you have gastritis or ulcers.
- Follow the Six-Point Plan to help your body recover from yeast overgrowth, imbalanced bacteria, parasites, poor digestion, food allergies, IBS, and leaky gut syndrome.
- Remember that every time you sit down for a meal you are nourishing your body, mind, and spirit.

Chapter 7

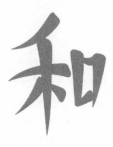

Harmony

Orchestrating Your Hormonal Dance

"From the very beginning of your life, your hormones govern much of who you are."

—MARLA AHLGRIMM AND JOHN KELLS, *The HRT Solution*

*C*andace was in her late thirties and beginning to experience overwhelming fatigue and premenstrual symptoms. "I felt like I was living in a fog all day," she said, "and my dreams to pursue a degree in psychotherapy seemed out of the question. I was just too tired, and in the days before my periods my mood swings dominated my life." Her symptoms were obvious signs of imbalance in her hormonal system. Careful questioning and hormone testing indicated low progesterone and low thyroid function.

"When I sought out natural medicine," Candace recalls, "I was frustrated and at the end of my tether. I was surprised that with a few simple supplements to support my hormonal system, I could feel so much better in such a short period of time. My symptoms had definitely been trying to get me to give my body what it was crying out for! I'm happy to say that I'm now in my second year of a masters program and fully capable of keeping up with the workload."

Your Hormones

Your hormones, from puberty to menopause and beyond, dramatically shape your health and the quality of your life. They work together in a choreographed dance that determines your sex characteristics, influences your menstrual cycle, fertility, and libido, and affects your levels of energy, drive, and vigor. They can also determine the way you feel, your moods, your behavior, your personality, and even your destiny. When your hormones are out of balance, you can experience food cravings, weight gain, fatigue, depression, irritability, and irregular, painful periods. Many women acutely feel the transitions of their hormones throughout their menstrual cycles. You may also have exaggerated and disruptive symptoms before and during menopause.

If you are in this stage of your life, you may be feeling a great deal of confusion about whether to take replacement hormones. Only a few years ago medical doctors were recommending and prescribing hormone replacement therapy (HRT)—consisting of estrogen and progesterone—to prevent heart disease; today this is virtually unheard of, now that studies have shown that HRT can actually increase the risk of heart disease. Research continues to reveal the possible adverse effects of HRT, yet at the same time many women benefit from taking hormones. You will discover in the pages that follow information to help you make the best decisions about creating a healthy hormonal balance.

Hormones other than estrogen and progesterone can play significant roles in how your body looks and feels at every stage of life. Your thyroid and adrenal glands both release hormones that give you energy. When these are in ample supply, you tend to look and feel great. But if they are deficient, you need extra sleep, you gain weight more easily, you can feel depressed, and your menstrual cycle is affected.

As you've discovered, diet and lifestyle can have a profound influence on your body; your hormonal system is no exception. A diet high in sugar can lead to an excessive level of insulin, a hormone released by the pancreas. Over time this can wreak havoc, increasing your risk of obesity, heart disease, and diabetes. Or if you are under stress for prolonged periods of time, your hormones end up doing an erratic, poorly timed dance that can leave you feeling tired, irritable, and depressed. In this chapter, we will explore many ways that you can use natural medicine to create and maintain a healthy hormonal balance throughout your life.

The View from the West

The hormonal system, also known as the endocrine system, controls many important physiological functions in the body. It is made up of a number of glands, including the pituitary gland, ovaries, thyroid gland, adrenal glands, and pancreas, which work together in a complex way that is essential to health. Hormones are substances released from these glands that have an effect somewhere else in the body. The primary hormones include ovarian hormones (estrogen, progesterone, and testosterone), pituitary hormones (follicle-stimulating hormone, luteinizing hormone, and growth hormone), thyroid hormones, and adrenal hormones. All of these hormones are chemical messengers that play a major role in the body's inner workings. Their release is controlled by a master gland in the brain called the hypothalamus; their mission is to reach their destination, stimulate specific cells, and then travel to the liver to be broken down and eliminated from your body. If any part of this process fails, a hormone imbalance can result. An imbalance can be due to too little or too much hormone being released from a gland, too many hormones in the diet, or poor breakdown of the hormone in the liver.

The View from the East

Thousands of years ago practitioners of Chinese medicine developed their own understanding of the menstrual cycle, menopause, and hormone imbalances. While there is no exact description of hormones in Chinese medicine, they function in a manner similar to the flow of Qi, Blood, yin, and yang. The closest Chinese counterpart is the notion of kidney Essence, the foundational substance that allows for growth, development, and reproduction.

According to Chinese medicine, the progression from youth to menopause occurs in seven-year intervals. When you are seven years old, your kidney Essence becomes abundant; at roughly fourteen years of age, you begin your entry into womanhood with your first period, or your "Heavenly Water"; when you reach twenty-one, your kidney Essence is at its peak; at twenty-eight your body is at its maximum strength; when you are thirty-five, your kidney Essence begins to wane; at forty-two, your face and hair begin to reflect the wisdom of your years; and when you are forty-nine, your Heavenly Water slows and you begin menopause.

Evaluating Your Hormones, West and East

The most important way of gathering information about your hormones is by looking at their effects on your body. For instance, if you are in perimenopause (the period of time prior to menopause when your hormones are changing) you will experience symptoms telling you if your body is not transitioning smoothly. Or if you have low thyroid hormone or exhausted adrenal glands, you will have telltale symptoms that your body is struggling to feel normal. Laboratory tests, including blood, saliva, and urine tests, can also be ordered to evaluate your hormones.

If you have a hormone imbalance, your Chinese medical diagnosis is apt to be highly individualized, based on the quality of your symptoms, and it can be difficult to make an exact correlation between your Western and your Chinese diagnosis. For example, two women who have premenstrual syndrome may be described as having the same disorder in Western terms, but in Chinese medicine they would most likely be given different treatments if they have different symptoms. For purposes of this chapter, I will describe some common symptom patterns and make correlations between Western and Chinese medicine to help you balance your hormones and your Qi.

Creating Hormonal Health

The Naturally Healthy Lifestyle and Diet (outlined in Chapter 1) will provide the foundation you need to keep your hormones balanced. When your hormones are imbalanced, returning to the basics of good health will help bring your body back to optimal wellness. In addition, you will find a number of other solutions that can help you re-create excellent hormonal health.

THE MENSTRUAL CYCLE: YOUR DANCE WITH THE MOON

Understanding the menstrual cycle from both West and East is key to creating hormonal health. The menstrual cycle is complex; many hormones, glands, and organs are involved in this dynamic monthly process, which can greatly influence your thoughts and your emotions. As your hormones fluctuate throughout the month, they allow you to explore and honor different aspects of yourself. According to Dr. Christiane Northrup, author of *Women's Bodies, Women's Wisdom,* "The ebb and flow of dreams, creativity, and hormones associated with different parts of the cycle offer us a profound opportunity to deepen our connection with our inner knowing."[1] She describes the ways a woman's intuition and consciousness change as she moves through her cycle: the phase between the beginning of her period and ovulation is a time of inspiration, when she tends to be more extroverted and outgoing; at midcycle, when she ovulates and is most fertile, she is at the peak of her creativity; after ovulation, her energy begins to turn inward and she becomes more quiet and reflective. As Dr. Northrup points out, during this time after ovulation a woman has more direct access to her unconscious desires and needs, and the feelings and emotions that arise can offer guidance to the deeper issues in her life.[2]

Physiologically, the menstrual cycle has four distinct phases that give rise to these changes in consciousness: the period, when you are shedding your endometrium (the lining of your uterus); the follicular phase, when you are building a new lining in your uterus in preparation for a fertilized egg; ovulation, when you release an egg from your ovary; and finally the luteal phase, when the lining of the uterus continues to build until your hormone levels drop. The cycle begins again when you shed the lining in your next period.

Your menstrual cycle, which typically lasts twenty-eight days, shows how deeply you are connected with the natural world. The cycle was observed in many ancient cultures as a woman's connection to the earth and the moon; in fact the words *menstruation* and *month* derive from the same root as *moon*. Many women's menstrual cycles parallel the moon's phases.[3] (Hence some women refer to their period as their "moon.")

As your hormones wax and wane each month during your dance with the moon, your pituitary hormones (follicle-stimulating hormone and luteinizing hormone) and your ovarian hormones (estrogen and progesterone) play especially important roles. The function of each of these in your cycle is as follows:

Follicle-stimulating Hormone (FSH). FSH is released by the pituitary gland when estrogen levels are low, right before your period starts. It stimulates your ovarian follicles, which contain your eggs, to grow and develop.

Luteinizing Hormone (LH). LH is released by the pituitary gland during the follicular phase of your cycle (between your period and ovulation) in response to low levels of estrogen. A surge of LH is released right before you ovulate, to stimulate the release of estrogen and progesterone from your ovaries.

Estrogen. Estrogen is released throughout your cycle, primarily from your ovaries in response to FSH. It stimulates estrogen-sensitive cells in breast tissue and prepares the lining of the uterus for a fertilized egg. Some estrogen also comes from the adrenal glands, fat and muscle cells, and hair follicles. You need estrogen for normal female development, fertility, pregnancy, bone health, mental health, skin health, and vulvar and vaginal health. But when estrogen is not in balance with other hormones or when it is poorly eliminated from the body, it can be harmful. Too much estrogen can lead to symptoms of premenstrual syndrome, heavy bleeding, and increased risks of breast and uterine cancer. Too little estrogen can result in hot flashes, dry skin, poor bone density, and depression.

Progesterone. Progesterone is released by the ovaries at ovulation and also by the adrenal glands. This hormone is responsible for maintaining the lining of the uterus, supporting a pregnancy, and regulating the menstrual cycle by keeping estrogen in balance. When released by the adrenal glands, progesterone also serves as a precursor to estrogen, testosterone, and other hormones.

HEAVENLY WATER

In traditional Chinese medicine, when a girl begins to menstruate around age fourteen, it is commonly said that her Heavenly Water has arrived. "Menstrual blood is not blood," according to Chinese scholar Fu Qing Zhu (1607–84), "but Heavenly Water, originating within the Kidneys."[4] If a girl is healthy, her Heavenly Water—sometimes referred to as her "Dew of Heaven"—will continue to ebb and flow on a monthly basis as she evolves into womanhood and until she eventually reaches menopause, or "the cessation of Heavenly Water."

According to Chinese medicine, Heavenly Water forms when the kidney Essence overflows; in order to have a menstrual cycle, a women has to have a surplus of Blood and kidney Essence. Kidney Qi governs the entire monthly cycle, although the Qi of other organs, including the spleen, heart, and liver, is also intimately involved in the menstrual cycle. The Chinese consider it normal for a woman to have a cycle that ranges from twenty-six to thirty-two days in length, and to menstruate for four to seven days.

Dr. Northrup's description of "the ebb and flow" of intuition and consciousness through the menstrual cycle parallels the Chinese view of the changes of yin and yang and the Five Elements throughout this period. For much of the follicular phase of your cycle (the phase from your period until ovulation), which Dr. Northrup describes as the time when you feel more outgoing and open to inspiration, your yang Qi—your outward, expansive energy—dominates your quiet, inward yin Qi. This also overlaps the time when, in Chinese medicine, your Wood element is said to be preparing your uterus for the possibility of pregnancy. You may remember that your Wood element represents springtime, outward growth, an extroverted personality, and creativity.

When you ovulate, your yang begins to rise abruptly, and your yin continues to rise, suggesting that you are entering the peak of your energy and vitality. In Chinese medicine, this time in your cycle corresponds to the Fire element, which represents love and the zenith of your charisma, libido, and sexual attractiveness.

After ovulation you enter the luteal phase of your cycle, which lasts from ovulation until your period. According to Chinese medicine, in the early part of this phase yin Qi only slightly dominates yang Qi—and then in the later part yang Qi rapidly declines a few days before your period starts. In Chinese medicine, much of the luteal phase—when yin and yang energy are becoming almost equal—reflects the Earth element, which provides nourishment to the uterus in case there is a developing embryo. If you are not pregnant, your yang energy drops rapidly before your period, during the part of the luteal phase governed by your Metal element. Your Metal element, which corresponds with the breaking down of the uterine lining, represents the fall, the end of the growing season and a time of preparation for coming winter.

During most of your period, yin Qi dominates yang Qi. In Chinese medicine, during this phase of the cycle the Water element allows for the release of Heavenly Water, cleansing the uterus so that another menstrual cycle can begin. In the cycle of the seasons, the Water element represents winter, the time of quiet preparation for regeneration and springtime.

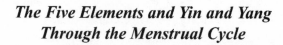

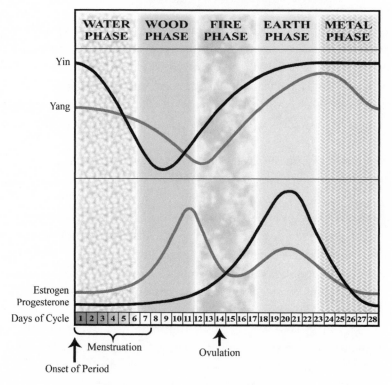

MENSTRUAL IMBALANCES

Uncomfortable symptoms associated with the menstrual cycle, such as premenstrual syndrome (PMS), irregular cycles, or menstrual cramps, are signs that your hormones are not in balance. In conventional Western medicine, the most common solution to these imbalances is birth control pills, synthetic hormones that shut down the production of the pituitary and ovarian hormones. They suppress ovulation by making the body "think" that it's pregnant all the time. Obviously, taking birth control pills does nothing whatsoever to correct the underlying cause of a hormone imbalance.

As we've seen, in natural medicine symptoms are your body's way of trying to get your attention and tell you that something is out of balance. Let's take a closer look at PMS, irregular cycles, and menstrual cramps and at what you can do to relieve them naturally.

DARKNESS BEFORE THE MOON

Trisha told me that during the week before her period she turned into Dr. Jekyll and Mrs. Hyde. "I had no idea why my life felt like it was falling apart before every period," she said, "I actually felt like I was going crazy. Not only did I have bloating, breast tenderness, and swelling, but I would turn into a raging, crying, impossible person. One minute I'd be blaming others, then the next I'd be desperate for love and affection." She felt like her body was out of control and explained that her boyfriend would avoid her during this time.

Trisha had been experiencing premenstrual symptoms due to an excess of estrogen. I recommended that she change her diet, increase her exercise, and take supplements to help her liver break down estrogens more efficiently. After a few regular menstrual cycles Trisha said, "I didn't realize that PMS was not 'normal' until I finally sought out help. Thank God I learned what I needed to do to change those dramatic body and mood swings!"

The emotional and physical drama that can occur before a period is like the darkness before the moon rises. Many women dread this time because of the symptoms of premenstrual syndrome, which represent a hormonal imbalance. Symptoms of PMS can occur anytime within the fourteen days prior to menstruation and usually disappear within the first few days of the period. By some estimates, more than 150 different symptoms are associated with PMS.[5] Some of the most common include:

PHYSICAL SYMPTOMS OF PMS	EMOTIONAL SYMPTOMS OF PMS
Bloating	Irritability
Abdominal distension	Inability to cope with stress
Breast and nipple pain	Anger
Enlarged or lumpy breasts	Anxiety
Fatigue	Tearfulness
Fluid retention	Forgetfulness
Food cravings	Foggy thinking
Acne	Confusion
Constipation or diarrhea	Depression
Insomnia	Mood swings
Vertigo	Nervous tension

PHYSICAL SYMPTOMS OF PMS	EMOTIONAL SYMPTOMS OF PMS
Altered libido	Frustration
Herpes outbreaks	Low self-esteem
Pelvic discomfort	Personality changes
Decreased immunity	
Vaginal infections	
Backaches	

To treat PMS, it's important to investigate the underlying causes. The most common causes are an imbalance in estrogen and progesterone, decreased serotonin levels, poor elimination of hormones, low thyroid gland function, excessive stress leading to adrenal gland fatigue, and the standard American diet.

Most PMS symptoms are signs of estrogen dominance, low progesterone, or both. Estrogen dominance means that there is more estrogen than progesterone in circulation in the second half (the luteal phase) of the menstrual cycle. Low progesterone can occur when your ovaries don't produce enough progesterone after ovulation. Symptoms that commonly occur when you have PMS due to these hormone imbalances include breast swelling and tenderness before your periods, heavy periods, or irregular periods. Most women who experience PMS will benefit from having their naturopathic physician test their hormone levels on day 21 of their cycle to determine if they have too much estrogen or too little progesterone. I recommend a saliva hormone test or a twenty-four-hour urine collection test.

One reason you may experience estrogen dominance is that your environment is saturated with chemicals and pesticides that can mimic estrogen in your body. You can ingest these chemicals and pesticides through your diet or be exposed to them through other means. You could also have high levels of estrogen because of poor breakdown and elimination of hormones, especially estrogen, through your liver and intestines. Or it may be that your liver is so busy fending off the toxins of modern life—including alcohol, food colorings and additives, hair dyes, and chemicals found in cosmetics and shampoos—that they have "congested" your liver, resulting in elevated levels of estrogen in your body. In addition, if you are chronically constipated or have abnormal bacteria in your intestines, you may actually reabsorb estrogen that would otherwise have been removed from your body through your stool. Finally, you may have higher levels of estrogen if your body doesn't produce enough progesterone. (This is most commonly seen in perimenopausal women.)

Another cause of PMS is low serotonin levels during the second half, or luteal phase, of the menstrual cycle. Serotonin is the "feel-good" brain chemical that has a profound effect on sleep and mood. According to Deborah Sichel, M.D., and Jeanne Watson Driscoll, M.S., R.N., authors of *Women's Moods,* estrogen and serotonin interact with cell receptors in the brain that increase your sense of well-being. When your estrogen level drops before your period, serotonin levels can drop as well, resulting in the feelings of depression many women experience with PMS.[6] Often women with PMS are prescribed a selective serotonin reuptake inhibitor (SSRI) like Prozac or Zoloft, which are commonly used to treat depression by increasing serotonin levels. The good news is that you can address these underlying hormonal or biochemical imbalances that cause PMS without resorting to drugs.

The most effective strategy for healing from PMS is to incorporate the following changes into your life, some of which you've already discovered in earlier chapters.

- Follow the Naturally Healthy Diet.
- Avoid caffeine.
- Exercise regularly.
- Decrease stress in your life.
- Do the liver cleanse outlined in Chapter 4.
- Take a multivitamin every day.
- Take 100 mg of vitamin B_6 every day.
- Take 1,200 mg of calcium and 600 mg of magnesium every day.
- If you experience depression with your PMS, take 900 mg of the herb St. John's wort (be aware that this herb can interfere with some prescription medications) and 1,000 mg of the amino acid L-tyrosine every day.

If your level of progesterone is low, consider taking chaste tree berry, an herb with progesteronelike effects. (See page 219 for a description of how to take this herb.) You can also take natural progesterone during the second half (the luteal phase) of your menstrual cycle; for most women, I recommend about 25 mg a day, taken sublingually (under the tongue) or as a transdermal cream, from midcycle until the beginning of menstruation. You can buy progesterone in either of these forms over the counter. (See Appendix B for details.) For a dose more specific to your needs, or to have natural progesterone capsules prescribed, consult your naturopathic physician. (Some women respond better to oral progesterone capsules than to creams or sublingual progesterone.)

To assess if your PMS is due to low thyroid or adrenal gland function, you can take the questionnaires included later in this chapter.

MENDING IRREGULAR MOON CYCLES

After Diana was told a hysterectomy would be the best option to control her heavy menstrual bleeding, she came to see me for another opinion. "I knew that heavy periods could come with menopause," she said, "but I never imagined that a hysterectomy could be part of it, too."

I asked Diana to take some blood tests to check her thyroid function and to take her basal body temperature for seven mornings and report back me. Her blood tests came back within normal range, but her basal body temperature was extremely low. She also had a number of other symptoms suggesting low thyroid hormones, including constipation, dry skin, and hair loss. I immediately started her on natural thyroid medicine. After a month Diana said, "It was like a miracle! My bleeding stopped and my menstrual cycles returned to normal. The surgery would have been all for nothing."

Estrogen and progesterone follow characteristic patterns through each menstrual cycle and play important roles in keeping your cycles, and your periods, regular. Irregular menstrual cycles (either too short or too long) and irregular periods (either too light or too heavy) are signs that your hormones may be imbalanced. As we've seen, both estrogen and progesterone are affected by diet, exercise, stress, and other hormones.

Diet affects your menstrual cycles because it provides you with cholesterol, the building block your body needs to make hormones. Exercise can also be an important factor. When women are too thin—either because of their diet or from too much exercise—they may be unable to produce enough hormones to have normal menstruation. Unfortunately, women who don't menstruate during their reproductive years are at a higher risk for osteoporosis later in life because female hormones are important bone builders. On the other hand, women who have too much body fat may produce excessive estrogen in their fat cells, resulting in heavy and abnormal bleeding.

As you know, stress can be a menace to every system in your body. Chronic, unrelenting stress profoundly affects your hormone balance. It can result in irregular menstruation by causing you to ovulate early, late, or not at all. Ovulation is necessary for producing progesterone, which is important in maintaining a normal menstrual cycle. One of the most common forms of stress affecting the menstrual cycle is travel; often a woman's period comes early or late after a long, stressful trip.

As we will see, other hormones from the thyroid and adrenal glands play important roles in menstrual cycles. If you have low thyroid hormones, abnormal periods can result. My patient Diana had low thyroid function (which was not evident on her blood tests) that caused her to have excessively heavy periods. By correcting her thyroid hormone imbalance, she had more energy, her menstrual cycle became regular, and she was able to avoid unnecessary surgery. Adrenal hormones can also cause irregular menstrual cycles. These glands release hormones that help you cope with stress, but an excess release of adrenal hormones can throw off your cycle.

Women who have heavy bleeding with their periods may also have low levels of progesterone and too much estrogen. When estrogen is not balanced by progesterone, the uterine lining can become unusually thick and result in heavy periods. If a woman doesn't have a period for a long time because of low levels of progesterone, her "unopposed" estrogen (estrogen that is no longer balanced by progesterone) continues to stimulate her uterine lining and can cause abnormal precancerous cells and even endometrial cancer to develop. Other causes of irregular cycles, irregular periods, and heavy menstrual bleeding include uterine fibroids, polyps in the endometrium (the uterine lining), inflammation of the endometrium, blood clotting disorders, and cervical cancer. If you have missed your period, it may be because you are pregnant or because you have a hormone imbalance or condition that goes beyond the scope of this book, such as high prolactin levels (hyperprolactinemia) or polycystic ovarian syndrome. As you can see, many factors are involved in irregular menstruation, and treatment varies depending on your diagnosis. If you have irregular cycles or irregular periods, make sure you have adequate nutrition and reduce your stress level. If your problem persists, I recommend that you see your health care provider for diagnostic tests and a complete treatment plan.

Overcoming Painful Moons

In Western medicine, menstrual cramps are often considered a "normal" part of a woman's monthly period unless they are especially severe. As a naturopathic physician and practitioner of Chinese medicine, I disagree. Menstrual cramps that interfere with your quality of life and compel you to ingest anti-inflammatory drugs every month are not normal. Monthly cramps are a sign that there is an underlying problem. In my practice, I've had a great deal of success in working with women who experience menstrual cramps.

Some women experience menstrual cramps because they have a problem such as an ovarian cyst, scar tissue from a previous surgery, uterine fibroids, or pelvic inflammatory disease. If these disorders have been ruled out and you still find yourself reaching for Midol every month, there are many things you can do to alleviate your cramps with natural medicine. Most of my suggestions are good not only for making menstruation painless but for enhancing your quality of life.

One young woman who came to see me was suffering from unusually painful menstrual cramps. Her medical doctor wanted her to undergo a laparoscopic surgical procedure to investigate whether she had endometriosis, a condition in which endometrial tissue (which normally grows only inside the uterus) grows outside the uterus and causes pelvic pain. During her initial office visit I learned that she ate a standard American diet—lots of saturated fat in animal meats, few fruits and vegetables, and an inordinate amount of white breads and sugar. She also rarely exercised. I recommended that she change her diet and start exercising regularly, and I prescribed nutritional supplements to support her body and decrease her menstrual cramps. The results after only a month: no more menstrual cramps—and no invasive surgery!

If you suffer from menstrual cramps, I recommend the following for prevention and treatment.

- Follow the Naturally Healthy Diet, take a daily multivitamin, and get regular exercise.
- Increase your intake of "friendly" fats from fish and flax oils; these fats decrease inflammation in the body, which can reduce menstrual cramps.
- Be sure you are taking at least 400 i.u. of vitamin E, 1,000 mg of calcium, and 500 mg of magnesium each day. If your cramps are acute, take an additional 300 mg of magnesium at the onset of your period, and continue to take this additional amount for the first three days of your period. (Note: Taking too much magnesium can cause diarrhea.)
- Drink ginger tea, which can reduce inflammation and decrease spasms in the uterus. I recommend that you drink a strong cup of ginger tea as soon as your period begins, and drink at least three cups a day on the days you would normally expect cramps.
- Take crampbark, an herb that is an excellent uterine relaxant and antispasmodic. As a tincture, the recommended dose is half a teaspoon every two or three hours; in capsule form, take 300 mg three times a day. To take crampbark as a tea, mix three tablespoons of the herb in three cups of water, simmer on low heat for ten minutes, strain, and drink one cup (hot or cold) three times a day. You can make a large batch of tea and keep it in the refrigerator for later use. Note: Feel free to mix crampbark tea and ginger tea together.

MENSTRUAL IMBALANCES: THE VIEW FROM THE EAST

From a Chinese medicine point of view, imbalances in the menstrual cycle occur if there are chronic imbalances in the flow of Qi and Blood. The liver is in charge of maintaining the flow of Qi and Blood; if they are deficient, or excessive, or not moving freely, menstrual problems and symptoms such as breast pain, headaches, menstrual cramps, PMS, and irregular periods can result.

Other organs that are responsible for normal menstruation in Chinese medicine include the spleen and kidneys. If your spleen Qi is weak, you can experience sugar cravings, digestive disturbances, and fluid retention; you may also experience lengthened menstrual cycles, or skip your period entirely. Deficient kidney Qi can cause you to become infertile because your kidneys are responsible for ovulation.

One of the best Chinese herbal formulas for treating stagnant liver Qi is Free and Easy Wanderer, also known as Xiao Yao Wan. It is especially helpful in the treatment of PMS because of its ability to move Qi, nourish Blood, and noticeably improve a woman's mood. In fact, Free and Easy Wanderer can bring so much relief that one of my teachers, a cardiologist and acupuncturist from China, calls this formula "women's happy pills."

If you have menstrual imbalances associated with emotions such as frustration and irritability, I recommend you take Free and Easy Wanderer. (See Appendix B for more information.) For all menstrual imbalances, I recommend that you take the following steps to help maintain the flow of your Qi and Blood and to strengthen your spleen and kidney Qi:

- Eat warm, cooked foods to nourish your spleen Qi.
- Avoid eating an excess of dairy products and sugar, which weaken your spleen Qi.
- Avoid caffeine and alcohol because of their Qi-depleting effects on your liver, kidneys, and spleen.
- Eliminate excess salt in your diet because it can weaken your kidney Qi.
- Exercise regularly and decrease stress to help your liver keep your Qi and Blood freely moving.

Using the Five Elements to keep your elements in balance can help prevent menstrual problems, especially if you are a Wood or Earth type, because both of these types tend to have more difficulties with their cycles. If you are a Wood type, you are prone to PMS symptoms that include severe headaches, emotional swings, intense menstrual cramps, heavy bleeding, abnormally frequent periods, or missed periods. If you are an Earth type, your PMS symptoms are apt to include food cravings (for sweets in particular), water retention, breast swelling and bloating, and feelings of lethargy before your period. See Chapter 4 if you are a Wood type and Chapter 6 if you are an Earth type for additional ways to relieve your symptoms. If you implement these recommendations and you still have symptoms of PMS, irregular menstruation, or menstrual cramps, I recommend that you see a practitioner of Chinese medicine.

Perimenopause to Menopause and Beyond

During perimenopause, your hormones are waxing and waning as your body makes the gradual transition from a fertile, menstruating woman to a menopausal woman. In some ways, the transition of perimenopause is similar to adolescence. As Dr. Susan Love, author of *Dr. Susan Love's Hormone Book,* points out, "With the exception of hot flashes, the symptoms of perimenopausal women [are] closer to those of adolescents entering puberty than to those of postmenopausal women."[7] In both adolescence and perimenopause your hormones and menstrual periods fluctuate, but in adolescence your menstrual cycles become more regular with time while in perimenopause they tend to become less regular until they cease altogether.

Women can begin experiencing the changes of perimenopause prior to their forties, although some women don't experience them until their late forties or early fifties. Perimenopause can last up to eight years before menopause begins; menopause is defined as your last period plus one year without a period. The most common signs of perimenopause are alterations in menstrual cycles, such as lighter or heavier periods, skipped periods, or cycles that are longer or shorter in length. There can also be changes in body temperature, sleep patterns, and mood.

During perimenopause women can experience a hot flash at any time of the day or night. Hot flashes are sensations of mild to intense heat, lasting from a few seconds to a few minutes, which cause some women to break out in a sweat. Some women refer to them as "power surges"; many of my patients have told me that when they have a hot flash, they feel a strong wave of energy race through them and an intense connection with their bodies. Others seem to have a very different experience; one woman described feeling so irritated by her hot flashes that she wanted to jump out of her skin.

Hot flashes at night, which are often accompanied by night sweats, can disturb a woman's sleep patterns, leading to a loss of sleep. Changes in hormones themselves can also result in insomnia, which can ultimately cause alterations in mood and behavior. In perimenopause a decrease in estrogen levels during your cycle can reduce your level of the mood-enhancing neurotransmitter serotonin.

Not all women experience these symptoms. Although I sometimes use the term *symptoms* for the problems and discomforts that women may face during perimenopause and menopause, I hesitate to do so. The word suggests an underlying illness or condition that needs to be treated. The truth is that when you are in perimenopause or menopause, whether you have physical difficulties or not, you are going through a completely natural transition; you are not sick, and there is nothing fundamentally wrong with you. I've had many patients come into my office wondering what they "should do" now that they are often skipping periods. Except for the changes in their menstrual cycles, they feel completely healthy. In fact, they *are* completely healthy; they are simply experiencing the transition from perimenopause to menopause and beyond.

In Western medicine, menopause is often thought of in terms of a lack of estrogen—even as a kind of "disease" of estrogen deficiency—but the view from the East offers a refreshing alternative. In Chinese medicine, the transition into menopause is perceived as a normal, healthy process. If a woman arrives at menopause well nourished and with abundant kidney Essence, she will have few, if any, symptoms. But if she arrives exhausted, with her kidney Essence depleted, she will be more likely to have hot flashes, insomnia, erratic mood changes, or other difficulties.

The Chinese system holds that perimenopause and menopause give you the opportunity to direct your energy toward your spirit. From puberty until you reach menopause, every month your body is producing Blood for your menstrual flow, or Heavenly Water. If this process continued indefinitely, you would exhaust your kidney Essence, which could lead to premature aging and weakness. In perimenopause your body, in its wisdom, initiates a change to slow down the aging process and prevent the loss of Blood and kidney Essence. Instead of constantly sending Qi downward from your heart to your uterus to enable you to bear and nourish children, in perimenopause your body begins to reverse the flow of Qi upward, from your uterus to your heart, to nourish and uplift your spirit.

This view sees menopause not as a loss of youth but as a time of great potential and joy. As a menopausal woman, your energy is freed up for your self-empowerment, allowing you greater access to spiritual knowledge. You are becoming the wise woman, what Chinese medicine authority Bob Flaws describes as "the mother of her community and a fountain of wisdom."[8]

If you experience symptoms during perimenopause or menopause, there are many things that you can do from the standpoint of both Western and Chinese medicine to make your transition easier.

Tests to Evaluate Your Hormones

To find out if you would benefit from hormones, I recommend that you have your hormones tested. There are many ways to do this. I routinely order a test to assess my patients' levels of estrogen, progesterone, testosterone, and other hormones. If a woman is still menstruating, I recommend doing the test on day 21 of her cycle (counting from the first day of her previous period) in order to adequately evaluate her progesterone levels.

I've found that the most accurate hormone tests are saliva tests and twenty-four-hour urine collection tests. Some laboratories offer salivary hormone testing that spans the entire menstrual cycle. This is particularly helpful if you have irregular cycles, because it provides information on what your hormones are doing throughout your cycle, rather than just on one day. (See Appendix C for information on laboratories for hormone testing.)

I generally don't order blood tests to evaluate women's hormone levels, because hormones in the blood are bound to proteins (albumin and sex-hormone-binding globulins) that prevent blood tests from being as reliable. Tests that measure the free, unbound hormones in your saliva, or the amounts of hormones in your urine, give you a clearer assessment of your hormone levels.

HORMONE REPLACEMENT THERAPY

In conventional Western medicine, doctors have traditionally prescribed HRT to women during perimenopause and menopause. For many years, HRT was widely considered a safe, health-promoting therapy that kept women from experiencing the highs and lows of their hormonal changes. To some, HRT seemed nothing less than miraculous. While on it, women said that they looked better, they didn't wrinkle, their vaginal tissues stayed moist, and they felt "forever young."

The honeymoon ended in the summer of 2002 when the Women's Health Initiative study reported that Premarin (estrogen derived from the urine of pregnant horses) and Provera (synthetic progesterone) increased the risk of heart disease, strokes, and breast cancer.[9] In fact, the study had to be halted due to the serious ethical issues involved in continuing to keep women on hormones that could be so harmful to their health. Referring to Premarin, gynecologist Dr. Susan Hendrix voiced the concerns of many women when she told the *New York Times* that "it's pretty astounding to go from a year ago thinking this is one of the most benign drugs to a 180-degree turn in the opposite direction."[10]

Another study, published in the *Journal of the American Medical Association,* found that postmenopausal women who took Premarin and Provera had twice the risk of developing Alzheimer's disease—a progressive disorder resulting in loss of memory and brain function—compared with women who didn't take these drugs.[11] These findings have generated a great deal of fear about the side effects of HRT.

Since these studies made national headlines, many women have chosen, with or without their physician's advice, to discontinue conventional HRT. As a result, some have experienced the roller-coaster effects of sudden drops in estrogen—such as hot flashes, irritability, and night sweats. To remedy these symptoms, a number of these women gave up and went back onto conventional HRT; others sought out different alternatives.

To clear up the controversy and confusion surrounding HRT, you will find it helpful to become familiar with two key distinctions. First, the hormones used in HRT can be either "bioidentical" or "nonbioidentical." Hormones that are bioidentical (short for "biologically identical") have the exact biochemical structure as the hormones that your own body produces. Nonbioidentical hormones, in contrast, have a different biochemical structure than your body's own hormones.

Second, the hormones a woman takes in HRT can be either natural or synthetic. That is, they can be derived from natural plant or animal sources, or they can be synthesized in a laboratory. (Natural hormones are sometimes referred to as "semisynthetic" because they are derived from natural sources but involve some degree of laboratory manipulation.)

The important thing to remember about HRT is that you can minimize side effects by choosing hormones that are *both bioidentical and natural*. They are considered safer than those typically prescribed in conventional HRT, which often involves the use of hormones that are either synthetic or nonbioidentical. In fact, long before the results of the Women's Health Initiative study were publicized, many naturopathic physicians were prescribing hormones that were bioidentical and natural.

For some women, HRT can significantly increase the quality of life during perimenopause and menopause. But each woman has individual needs and must decide for herself whether the risks are worth the benefits.

One compelling alternative to conventional HRT is bioidentical natural hormones (estrogen, progesterone, or testosterone) derived from hormonelike substances in soybeans or wild yams. I've found that they can often be taken to alleviate symptoms in much lower doses than those traditionally used in conventional HRT. To minimize potential side effects, I recommend that women take them in the lowest possible dose, for the shortest duration of time necessary, and for a maximum of five years. Let's take a closer look at how they can help you through your transition.

BIOIDENTICAL NATURAL ESTROGEN

Bioidentical natural estrogen replacement therapy utilizes hormones consisting of estradiol, estrone, and estriol, the three primary estrogens that are naturally produced in a woman's body. Two commonly prescribed hormone replacement preparations called Triest and Biest consist of small amounts of estradiol (the strongest-acting estrogen) and estrone (which is slightly weaker than estradiol) and larger amounts of estriol (which is one-fourth the strength of estradiol). This ratio of strong-to-weak estrogens is significant, because it means these preparations give you a lower overall amount of estrogen than other hormone replacement preparations. Numerous studies on estrogen replacement therapy and its potential side effects have made it clear that the higher the dose of estrogen you take and the longer you take it, the higher your risk of developing breast cancer, gallstones, endometrial cancer, and other problems associated with estrogen use. Triest usually consists of 10 percent estradiol, 10 percent estrone, and 80 percent estriol, and Biest typically contains 20 percent estradiol and 80 percent estriol. Your physician can adjust these amounts to best suit you by ordering your hormones through a compounding pharmacy, a type of pharmacy that specializes in preparing hormone prescriptions (allowing you to receive exactly the amounts you need).

There are other estrogen products available through gynecologists, including Estrace, Estraderm, Vivelle, Climara, and Fempatch, that are bioidentical but synthetic. They may have more side effects than Triest and Biest because they consist of 100 percent estradiol or estrone.

Triest and Biest may be safer than nonbioidentical hormones such as Premarin because of the ways they interact with DNA. According to Dr. Tori Hudson, leading naturopathic physician and author of *The Women's Encyclopedia of Natural Medicine,* "A nonbioidentical hormone may act like a constant environmental toxin to the genetic material within the cell."[12] Premarin is known to contain more than two hundred different compounds that are foreign to human cells—some are horse hormones!—and many of them may alter your cell metabolism in a way that sets the stage for cancer. Although it is not yet known if Triest and Biest have this effect, they are believed to be safer not only because they are bioidentical and natural but because they are weaker than other estrogen preparations.

BIOIDENTICAL NATURAL PROGESTERONE

Bioidentical natural progesterone appears to be far superior to Provera, a nonbioidentical synthetic progesterone, in almost every way. It has a different chemical structure altogether and fewer side effects. According to a 2001 study published in the journal *Medical Hypothesis,* natural progesterone may be safer than synthetic progesterone.[13] When used correctly, bioidentical natural progesterone can ease perimenopausal and menopausal symptoms, decrease symptoms of premenstrual syndrome, regulate a woman's menstrual cycle, and decrease heavy menstrual bleeding. It can also protect you from uterine cancer in the event that you are on estrogen replacement therapy, have an effect on your moods, and make you feel calmer, more balanced, and better able to sleep. But if used in excess, bioidentical natural progesterone can have side effects that include depression, nausea, acne, headaches, vertigo, drowsiness, and irregular menstrual bleeding.

BIOIDENTICAL NATURAL TESTOSTERONE

Bioidentical natural testosterone can decrease hot flashes and increase sex drive. (It's common for women in perimenopause and menopause to experience lowered sex drive and decreased ability to achieve orgasm.) It can be taken in pill form or applied as a cream. Some women have benefited from applying bioidentical natural testosterone directly onto their clitoris to increase sexual sensitivity. I recommend that a woman's dose not exceed 5 mg a day because too much could result in undesirable side effects, including facial hair growth, hair loss, acne, and aggressive behavior. You will need a prescription for bioidentical natural testosterone, which can be filled through a compounding pharmacy.

NATURAL ALTERNATIVES TO HRT

Many women choose to move through their hormonal transition without using any form of HRT; others who are on HRT still experience some symptoms associated with their hormonal transition. In either case, the following natural remedies can help. If you have hot flashes, night sweats, erratic mood changes, or other symptoms, I recommend that you use these plants, foods, and homeopathic medicines to alleviate them.

PHYTOESTROGENS

Phytoestrogens are natural substances found in plants that can have estrogenlike effects on your body. Although they contain no estrogen, they interact with your cell receptors in much the same way that your body's own estrogen does. But they don't increase your estrogen levels. Foods that contain phytoestrogens include soy, alfalfa, apples, asparagus, barley, carrots, cherries, corn, fennel, oats, pears, peas, pomegranates, rice bran, rye, sunflower seeds, sweet potatoes, squash, and wheat germ. The herbs black cohosh and red clover are also potent phytoestrogens with a long history of use in the treatment of midlife symptoms.

Black Cohosh. This herb can help relieve the night sweats, hot flashes, vaginal atrophy, and depression associated with perimenopause and menopause. According to a number of studies, black cohosh is safe and can be taken for months at a time, until you no longer need it for controlling your change-of-life symptoms. But one animal study suggested that black cohosh can increase the spread of breast cancer. Until further studies are done, avoid black cohosh if you have a history of breast cancer. The recommended dose is 80 mg twice a day.

Red Clover. Red clover can be consumed as a tea, eaten in a salad as red clover sprouts, or taken as an herb in a standardized extract of 40 mg of total isoflavones a day. A cautionary note: The jury isn't in yet on whether this herb is safe for women who have had breast cancer. If you don't have a history of breast cancer, it is considered safe to use red clover for several months at a time, until your body has gone through its hormonal transition.

PLANT CONSTITUENTS WITH PROGESTERONELIKE EFFECTS

These "phyto-progesterones" have long been used in natural medicine to help women through their perimenopause, especially when they have irregular menstrual cycles. Phyto-progesterones don't actually contain progesterone, but they may have effects that indirectly favor the production of progesterone. The most commonly used phyto-progesterone is chaste tree berry, which has traditionally been used to help regulate women's menstrual cycles and treat PMS; it can also be used to ease midlife symptoms. Chaste tree berry is a good choice for women who have a deficiency of progesterone but don't want to take hormones. It works by signaling your pituitary gland to release a hormone that stimulates your ovaries. The recommended dose is 175 mg of the standardized powdered extract, or 40 drops of the liquid extract, a day.

HOMEOPATHIC MEDICINES

Homeopathic medicines are prescribed for their "energetic" properties, according to a patient's unique physical and emotional symptoms. (See Appendix A for more information.) They are often recommended for the imbalances some woman experience in midlife. While many homeopathic remedies can help, the following are three of the most commonly prescribed remedies for perimenopausal and menopausal symptoms. For most women, the usual recommended dose is 200c taken once a day for three days, or a lower dose of 30c taken once a day for two weeks. (If your condition doesn't improve with these doses, see your naturopathic physician for a consultation.) Note: Homeopathic medicines are safe to take if you have had breast cancer.

Sepia. Sepia is used to help women who have hot flashes, night sweats, and PMS. On an emotional level, it is recommended if you feel irritable, overwhelmed, indifferent, disconnected from your friends and family, and prone to weeping without knowing why, or have a tendency to make sarcastic remarks yet feel remorseful about them later.

Pulsatilla. Pulsatilla is recommended for hot flashes, PMS, abnormal menstruation, and migraines associated with your period. Women who respond best to this remedy often have cravings for cream, butter, and cold foods like ice cream. On an emotional level, pulsatilla is recommended if you feel insecure, timid, or needy for consolation or have changeable moods that can go from being agitated one moment to weepy the next.

Lachesis. Lachesis is recommended if you are aggravated by heat, have hot flashes that especially affect your face, migraines that tend to be on the left side, or headaches before your period starts. It is used if your perimenopausal symptoms are worse before your period and better as soon as your menstrual flow begins, and worse from suppressed sexual expression. Lachesis is also used for emotional changes that occur during PMS, such as jealousy, depression, and irritability.

OTHER NATURAL ALTERNATIVES TO HRT FROM CHINESE MEDICINE

In Chinese medicine, balancing your Qi is the most important step you can take to keep yourself healthy during perimenopause and menopause. According to the Chinese view, HRT depletes and weakens a woman's vital energy by resisting the natural order of change. Giovanni Maciocia, a leader in the field of traditional Chinese medicine, points out that Western methods of treating menopausal symptoms with HRT deceive the pituitary gland into reacting as if normal ovulation is continuing. This causes a disruption in the natural flow of Qi during the hormonal transition.

According to Chinese medicine, a woman can experience uncomfortable perimenopausal and menopausal symptoms if her kidney Essence and Blood are depleted before her body makes its transition. The lack of Essence and Blood causes yang Qi to flare upward, resulting in hot flashes and insomnia. This heat can accumulate in the liver, lungs, and heart, causing migraines, headaches, hypertension, ringing in the ears, palpitations, restlessness, anxiety, and other problems. Without sufficient yin energy to nourish a woman's tissues, dry skin, lack of vaginal secretions, and vaginal and vulvar thinning can result. Many of these symptoms are quelled by eating a diet consisting of yin or "cooling" and "cold" foods, and avoiding yang or "warming" and "hot" foods. (For a listing of foods from a Chinese perspective, see Chapter 1.)

As we've seen, in Chinese medicine an understanding of the Five Element system can be an important aspect of maintaining your health, allowing you to make choices that will keep your dominant element balanced. Each of the Five Element types may show strong tendencies during perimenopause or menopause. Remember that these are the most likely trouble areas for each type, potential weaknesses to watch out for. You can prevent these symptoms by keeping your dominant element well balanced.

- **If you are a Metal type:** You are vulnerable to problems related to dry skin, including vaginal dryness, during your midlife transition. On an emotional level, you are prone to become overly critical or judgmental if your Metal element is not in balance.

- **If you are a Water type:** You tend to have bladder problems, such as incontinence or bladder infections during your transition. If your element is imbalanced, you are apt to have insomnia and sexual problems. (You can become obsessed with sex, or lack any interest at all.)

- **If you are a Wood type:** You are especially prone to problems with your menstrual cycles during your transition. If your Wood element is out of balance, you tend to have irregular menstrual cycles, including heavy or exceptionally light periods.

- **If you are a Fire type:** You are especially likely to experience hot flashes during menopause; you may also tend to have erratic mood swings and an irregular heartbeat. Throughout your transition, you are apt to have insomnia if your element is imbalanced.

- **If you are an Earth type:** You have a tendency to gain weight during your transition and to experience water retention and bloating. You are also subject to excessive worrying and headaches if your element is not in balance.

There are a number of traditional Chinese herbal formulas that can help to balance the hormonal system during perimenopause and menopause. Most include the herb dong quai, also known as Chinese angelica. In Chinese herbal medicine, dong quai is used in combination with other herbs to alleviate hot flashes, PMS, irregular menstrual bleeding, and menstrual cramps. An herbal formula containing dong quai developed in Shanghai, known as Two Immortals Decoction (Er Xian Tang), works effectively in treating perimenopausal and menopausal symptoms. You can obtain this herbal formula through a practitioner of Chinese medicine. Dong quai should not be used if you have heavy menstrual bleeding because it can cause further bleeding.

So far we've explored your key female hormones, and how you can keep them balanced. Now you will discover how four other important performers in your hormonal dance affect your health.

Your Thyroid: Maintaining Your Vitality

When Jackie came to see me, she was overweight and experiencing severe fatigue, despite drinking copious amounts of caffeine. My first thought was that her thyroid hormones must be the culprit. "After months of dieting and not losing a pound," she said, "I decided something must be wrong. I was experiencing other symptoms like dry skin and hair loss, and I started having severe headaches for the first time in my life. I had blood tests done to see if there was something wrong, but my medical doctor said that everything looked normal.

"When I went to see Dr. Steelsmith, she had me fill out her questionnaire pertaining to low thyroid symptoms. I remember answering all the questions and feeling like maybe there was a solution to my problems after all." Jackie was right; since starting natural thyroid medicine, she has lost weight, is back to her energetic self again, and has had a resolution of a number of her other symptoms as well.

The thyroid gland, a small butterfly-shaped organ located in your neck just below your Adam's apple, releases hormones that can have a profound influence on your energy and vitality. When you have adequate levels of thyroid hormones, your body functions efficiently. If your thyroid releases excessive amounts of hormones, however, you can experience weight loss, a rapid heartbeat, and anxiety. Low levels of thyroid hormones, or hypothyroidism, can slow down the metabolism of every cell in your body. Women are more commonly diagnosed with thyroid disorders than men, and in my practice I commonly see patients with symptoms of low thyroid hormones, including fatigue, depression, weight gain, irregular menstrual cycles, severe perimenopausal symptoms, insomnia, aversion to cold weather, constipation, premenstrual syndrome, headaches, and migraines.

Excessive amounts of thyroid hormones can easily be diagnosed with blood tests, but low thyroid hormones can be more difficult to assess, and blood tests, although helpful, are not the most accurate way to diagnose the disorder. As a result, many women end up suffering from the symptoms of chronically low thyroid hormones for years before being properly diagnosed and treated. As Richard and Karilee Shames, the authors of *Thyroid Power,* point out, "The standard lab tests are unable to identify the millions of borderline low thyroid sufferers. Inadequate testing results in inaccurate diagnosis . . . The thyroid tests used today are just not sensitive enough to identify mild thyroid failure."[14] When a diagnosis cannot be made, most women simply accept their weight gain, depression, constipation, fatigue, and other symptoms as natural conditions of aging.

The good news is that early in 2003 the American Association of Clinical Endocrinologists released new guidelines that narrow the acceptable range for normal thyroid hormone levels. These new guidelines are helping many women get appropriate treatment for low thyroid function. But some women still have low thyroid levels even though their blood tests look normal, a condition known as *subclinical hypothyroidism*. It's important to realize that although your thyroid may consistently appear to be normal on standard laboratory tests, you may still be living with a deficiency of thyroid hormones.

The thyroid gland releases hormones in response to signals from the pituitary gland. If your levels of thyroid hormones are low, your pituitary tells your thyroid to secrete more of the inactive form of thyroid hormone, known as T-4. Once T-4 is released, it must be converted into T-3, the active form of thyroid hormone, which can increase your metabolism. The liver plays an important role in converting T-4 to T-3.

One theory regarding subclinical hypothyroidism is that some women have problems converting T-4 to T-3. This may be due to impaired liver function resulting from nutritional deficiencies, or environmental factors such as excessive mercury exposure. Some women may also have low thyroid function because of a history of autoimmune thyroiditis (inflammation of the thyroid gland), which can occur if a woman's immune system makes immune cells that attack her own thyroid tissue. Initially, women with this condition may experience a hyperthyroid state (excessive thyroid hormones), which eventually turns into a hypothyroid state (low thyroid hormones). Because this condition can come on slowly and the symptoms are often similar to those of other conditions, thyroid imbalances can be overlooked for years.

DO YOU HAVE LOW THYROID FUNCTION (HYPOTHYROIDISM)?

How do you know if you have low thyroid hormones? The following questionnaire will give you an overall idea of your thyroid status and your likelihood of having low thyroid hormones.

	√ **YES**	√ **NO**
Do you have chronically cold hands and feet?		
Do you have an aversion to cold weather?		
Do you have poor circulation?		
Do you have heart palpitations?		
Do you gain weight easily?		
Do you have difficulty losing weight, or have you gained weight even though you exercise and eat well?		

	√ **YES**	√ **NO**
Do you have high cholesterol levels even though you exercise and eat well?		
Do you have trouble getting up in the morning?		
Have you lost the outer one-third of your eyebrows?		
When you wake up, are your eyelids or your entire face puffy?		
Are you tired most of the time, even though you get enough sleep?		
Do you have trouble sleeping at night, even though you feel exhausted all day long?		
Do you drink a lot of caffeine in order to just feel "normal"?		
Do you often feel mentally sluggish and/or unable to focus?		
Do you have joint and muscle pains unrelated to exercise?		
Do you have dry skin?		
Is your hair dry and brittle?		
Is your hair falling out?		
Do you have allergies?		
Do you have frequent headaches or migraines?		
Do you have digestive complaints?		
Do you have chronic constipation?		
Do you have chronic hives?		
Do you tend to retain fluid and have chronic swelling in your tissues?		
Do have frequent periods of depression?		
Do you experience anxiety that can become severe enough that you feel panicked?		
Do you suffer from low blood sugar?		
Is your sex drive unusually low?		
Do you suffer, or in the past have you frequently suffered, from unusually acute PMS?		
Do you have, or in the past have you frequently had, irregular menstrual cycles?		
Have you had repeated miscarriages?		
Have you had infertility?		
Do you have, or in the past have you frequently had, unusually heavy periods?		
If you are experiencing perimenopause or menopause, do you have significant symptoms that are not relieved when you take HRT?		
Have you ever had an injury to your neck, such as whiplash?		
Have you ever been exposed to the environmental chemicals chlorine, fluoride, mercury, or lead in significant amounts?		
Do you have lowered immunity?		
Has anyone in your immediate family been diagnosed with a thyroid disorder?		

Add your total number of checks in each column:

If you answered no to every question, congratulations! You most likely have sufficient levels of thyroid hormones.

If you answered yes to 8 questions or fewer, your thyroid is probably not the cause of your symptoms, although it may still be involved. I recommend that you take your basal body temperature, as described below; if your reading indicates your temperature is normal, it is unlikely that your thyroid is a primary health issue.

If you answered yes to between 8 and 16 questions, you may have a thyroid problem. I recommend that you take your basal body temperature and have a blood test, as described below, to help you determine if your thyroid gland is underfunctioning. (It may be that your symptoms aren't directly related to your thyroid gland; you may have a problem with your liver's ability to process thyroid hormones, an adrenal problem, or other hormone imbalance.)

If you answered yes to 16 or more questions, your thyroid is most likely involved in your myriad symptoms. I highly recommend that you learn as much as you can about your thyroid status by taking your basal body temperature and having a blood test.

When your thyroid hormones are low, your metabolism slows down, and your body temperature drops. Though it is not the only means of assessing your thyroid function, your basal body temperature will give you an important clue about the health of your thyroid. Your basal body temperature is defined as the temperature of your body when it is at rest.

To take your basal body temperature, use a basal thermometer (available at most drugstores), which is calibrated to read smaller temperature changes than a regular thermometer. Take your temperature first thing in the morning, before you get out of bed, by putting your thermometer in your armpit for at least ten minutes. Try to remain as still as possible when you take your temperature. If you are premenopausal, take your basal temperature for three consecutive mornings on the second, third, and fourth days of your menstrual cycle. (The first day of your menstrual cycle is when your period starts.) If you are no longer having periods, you can take your basal body temperature for at least ten consecutive days, at any time during the month, to assess your thyroid status. Normally, your basal temperature is between 97.8 and 98.2 degrees Fahrenheit, but if you have low thyroid function it will consistently fall below 97.8 degrees. (Note: An infection in your body can throw off your results; wait until your condition is resolved before taking your basal body temperature.)

You may also be able to gather additional information about your thyroid status by taking a blood test. Ask your physician to order a *thyroid panel*—a blood test that measures various thyroid hormones, including thyroid stimulating hormone (TSH) and T-3 and T-4 hormones. It's also a good idea to have a thyroid antibody blood test. The presence of antibodies to your thyroid gland may indicate Hashimoto's thyroiditis, an autoimmune thyroid condition that can cause hypothyroidism.

HOW TO TREAT LOW THYROID FUNCTION

There are numerous ways to help get your thyroid back on track naturally. If your blood tests reveal that you have low thyroid function, you may need a prescription for natural thyroid medication. Natural thyroid preparations contain T-4 (the inactive form of thyroid hormone) and T-3 (the active form of thyroid hormone).

In conventional Western medicine, hypothyroidism is typically treated with synthetic thyroid medications, such as Synthroid, which are made with levothyroxine and only contain T-4. These kinds of medications seem to work for some people who are able to take them without side effects. But many of my patients on synthetic thyroid medications containing only T-4 have complained that they still have lots of hypothyroid symptoms. This may be because they don't effectively convert the T-4 into T-3, resulting in very little active thyroid hormone actually getting into their cells to increase their metabolism. (A study published in the *New England Journal of Medicine* in 1999 showed that patients who took T-4 plus T-3 had greater improvements in mood and brain function than when they took T-4 alone.)[15] In these cases, I recommend that patients take natural thyroid medication on a trial basis. Many of my patients who don't respond well to synthetic thyroid medication see a decrease of their hypothyroid symptoms when they use natural thyroid medication.

If your blood tests look normal but your basal body temperature is low and you answered yes to sixteen or more questions on the thyroid questionnaire, you could have subclinical hypothyroidism and should see your naturopathic physician for guidance. You may need nutritional support for your thyroid gland and may find that your symptoms improve when you take natural thyroid medication.

If your blood tests look normal and your basal body temperature is normal, but you answered yes to sixteen or more questions on the thyroid questionnaire, you may still need to consider taking nutritional support for your thyroid gland. You should also assess your adrenal function (which we'll look at in the following pages), your liver function (see Chapter 4), and the health of your immune system (see Chapter 2) to ensure that you are taking the best measures to ensure your vitality.

In any case, if you need nutritional support for your thyroid gland there are a number of ways to give it the extra boost it needs to function optimally.

Iodine. Iodine is an essential mineral in your body's ability to make thyroid hormones. If you are iodine-deficient, you can develop a goiter—a benign thyroid tumor. Iodized salt, seafood, and seaweed (particularly kelp) contain a lot of iodine. The RDA for females over eleven years of age is 150 mcg a day; pregnant women should take 175 mcg a day, and breast-feeding mothers should take 200 mcg a day. Check to see if your multivitamin contains the RDA of iodine, or you can take it as a dietary supplement to make sure you are getting a sufficient amount.

Tyrosine. Tyrosine is an amino acid that is a natural component of thyroid hormones. Your body can make tyrosine from the amino acid phenylalanine, which is normally found in sufficient amounts in the diet. But if you have low thyroid function, you may benefit from taking tyrosine as a supplement in low doses. I recommend you take 500 mg of tyrosine twice a day.

Minerals. Minerals are important in the synthesis of thyroid hormones. Both zinc and selenium are essential in the conversion of T-4 to T-3.[16] Taking a good multivitamin containing 40 mg of zinc and 200 mcg of selenium can enhance your thyroid function.

Diet. Your diet can also interfere with your thyroid health; if you have hypothyroidism, you should avoid eating excessive amounts of foods known as *goitrogens,* which can block an enzyme necessary for proper thyroid function. These include soybeans, peanuts, brussels sprouts, broccoli, cabbage, turnips, mustard, millet, walnuts, almonds, cassava root (tapioca), and pine nuts. The good news is that cooking these foods can destroy the compounds that have adverse effects on the thyroid.

The cause of hypothyroidism is complex. Some women have a hypothyroid condition because of their genetic makeup, while many others may have it as a result of excessive exposure to environmental contaminants such as fluoride, lead, and other toxins.

As the Shameses note in *Thyroid Power,* high levels of exposure to fluoride may be contributing to the epidemic of low thyroid conditions in the United States. They point out that fluoride, which is "currently touted as harmless enough to be put in the water supply, has been used in the past as a powerful medication to slow down overactive thyroid activity."[17] To avoid exposing yourself to excessive levels of fluoride, I recommend that you use a reverse osmosis water filter for your tap water and avoid using fluoridated toothpaste. (For more information on the deleterious effects of fluoride, see Appendix B.)

Dr. Walter Crinnion, naturopathic physician and expert in the field of environmental medicine, has found that a number of environmental toxins including lead, dioxins, and PCBs (polychlorobiphenyls) can interfere with normal thyroid function and regulation.[18] Mercury, which is found in seafood in varying amounts, can interfere with thyroid function by binding up selenium, a mineral that is essential for the conversion of T-4 to T-3. These chemicals are ubiquitous in our environment and are found in high concentrations in those who are chronically exposed. If you have concerns about your exposure to fluoride, lead, and other toxins, see Chapter 3 (to learn how to remove these compounds from your water) and Chapter 4 (to start a liver detoxification program).

LOW THYROID FUNCTION: THE VIEW FROM THE EAST

What can Chinese medicine tell us about the causes of low thyroid function? There is no exact equivalent in traditional Chinese medicine for thyroid hormones; however, the symptoms of low thyroid are perceived as a deficiency of Qi and yang. The signs of a Qi and yang deficiency include many of the symptoms that Western medicine attributes to low thyroid conditions, such as fatigue, cold hands and feet, and easy weight gain.

In Chinese medicine, treating a Qi and yang deficiency means eating foods that support spleen Qi (including warm or cooked foods that are easily digested), decreasing stress, increasing exercise, and taking herbs that enhance spleen Qi and yang energy. Ginger is one of the best herbs for this purpose. You can use ginger as a tea, or as a flavoring in your food, to nourish your digestive system and warm up your entire body. In traditional Chinese medicine, Qi and yang deficiencies are also treated with combinations of herbs; if you have a low thyroid condition, consult a trained Chinese herbalist to have a formula made specifically for your symptoms.

According to the Five Element system in Chinese medicine, Earth types have the strongest tendency to develop what Western medicine calls hypothyroidism. The Earth element rules the spleen and the stomach, the two organs responsible for making Blood, which is critical to healthy thyroid function. When the spleen and stomach aren't able to make enough Blood, Qi and yang deficiency can result. One reason women develop hypothyroidism is that they have a tendency to become Blood-deficient. This is because Blood can be depleted during menstruation, pregnancy, and lactation. Women can also become Blood-deficient if they eat an excess of foods that impair spleen Qi and stomach Qi (these include sugar, white bread, pasta, and cold, uncooked foods). In addition, a stressful lifestyle that causes anxiety, tension, and anger adversely affects a woman's liver Qi, which in turn can further deplete her spleen Qi and stomach Qi, resulting in deficient Blood, Qi, and yang. If you have low thyroid function, it's important to support your Earth element. See Chapter 6 to discover how to keep your Earth element in balance.

Your Adrenals: Getting Your Drive Back

When Cindy finally came to see me, it was after two years of trying many branches of Western medicine to treat her intense anxiety. Her gynecologist had given her hormones and a psychiatrist had put her on a few different antidepressants, but none of them helped. In fact, she said they only made her symptoms worse.

I asked Cindy to write down everything she had eaten for the previous few days. After looking over her diet diary, I told her, "You're not eating anything!" I explained that almost everything she was eating consisted of simple carbohydrates laden with hidden sugars, and that her diet was very low in protein—all of which could contribute to anxiety. Cindy said she was shocked to hear this, because this was the one area of her health that she was sure she had under control. She believed that her low-fat vegan diet was good for her.

I gave Cindy a list of foods to eat, and after ordering tests to make sure she didn't have diabetes, I asked her to take an adrenal test. When the results came back, she was surprised to learn that her stress hormones were exceptionally high. "After a few months of changing my diet by eating more protein and less sugar, and taking supplements to support my adrenal glands," she said, "I got my life back!"

The adrenal glands, which are located on top of your kidneys, are responsible for releasing hormones that provide you with the drive to accomplish what you want in life. The adrenal hormones are involved in your body's growth, development, cardiovascular function, and immunity. They also help you cope with fear and stress. In our evolutionary history, the adrenal glands played a role in our survival. If a tiger is chasing you, your adrenal glands release adrenaline, a stress hormone that helps you flee from danger. Or if a tiger is stalking you slowly, day after day, your adrenal glands constantly release cortisol, a hormone that helps you cope with longer term stress. If your lifestyle today makes you feel as if you are either being repeatedly chased or continually stalked by a tiger, your adrenal glands respond by producing more stress hormones, which eventually become depleted. Long-term consequences of excessive adrenal stress include osteoporosis, premature aging, depression, insomnia, fatigue, decreased immune function, and insulin resistance (which we will explore later in this chapter).

Your adrenal hormones help control your blood pressure, blood sugar level, and body fluid balance. They also assist with the conversion of your thyroid hormones to the active form. When you have an underfunctioning adrenal gland, your symptoms can include low blood pressure, imbalances in your blood sugar level—especially hypoglycemia—and fluid retention in your tissues. If you have hypothyroidism, low adrenal function can make it more difficult for you to feel optimal even on thyroid medication.

You can assess your adrenal function by answering the following questionnaire.

Do You Have Low Adrenal Gland Function?

	√ YES	√ NO
Do you frequently experience excessive fatigue?		
Is your tolerance for stress significantly decreased?		
Do you feel like you are always "running behind the bus"?		
Are you frequently anxious?		
Are you easily irritated?		
Do you have mild depression?		
Do you have chronic allergies resulting in hay fever, asthma, and hives?		
Do you have low blood pressure?		
Do you bruise easily?		
Do you have brittle fingernails?		
Do you have dark streaks on your fingernails?		
Do you have thin, dry skin?		
Do you crave salt?		
Do you crave sugar?		
Do you have low blood sugar (hypoglycemia)?		
Do you have to eat frequent meals in order to feel "normal"?		
Do you find that your body cannot tolerate alcohol well?		
Do you suffer from frequent headaches?		
Do you have difficulty concentrating?		
Do you easily become light-headed?		
Do you experience dizziness with a change in body position (for instance, when standing up from a sitting position)?		
Do you have insomnia?		
Do you often feel nervous and agitated, especially when you are hungry?		
Do you suffer from lowered immunity and frequent infections?		
Do you have excessive sweating in your underarms and in the palms of your hands?		
Add your total number of checks in each column:		

If you answered no to every question, congratulations! You most likely don't have low adrenal gland function. If you answered yes to one to ten questions, your adrenal health may be compromised, and if you answered yes to ten or more questions there is a good chance that your adrenal glands are stressed. The more questions you answered yes to, the more aggressive you need to be in supporting your adrenal health.

Most conventional Western doctors assess adrenal gland function by ordering tests that measure the amount of cortisol in a single blood draw or in a twenty-four-hour urine collection. While these tests may determine whether you suffer from a severe adrenal gland deficiency or excess, they don't tell you if your adrenal gland is functioning marginally. For a more precise assessment of your adrenal function, your naturopathic physician can order a saliva test called an adrenal stress index (ASI). The test measures the amount of cortisol you have in your body at four different times of day. Saliva testing is the preferred method because it measures the amount of cortisol readily available for your cells to use.

In addition to adrenaline and cortisol, your adrenal glands produce a cascade of hormones including estrogen, progesterone, testosterone, and DHEA. These hormones are derived from cholesterol and converted into the adrenal hormone pregnenolone, which is referred to as the "mother" hormone because your body converts it into all of your other adrenal hormones (except adrenaline). Both pregnenolone and DHEA can be tested in order to assess your adrenal function. An ASI test can also measure your level of DHEA and determine if your adrenal glands would benefit from pregnenolone or DHEA supplementation.

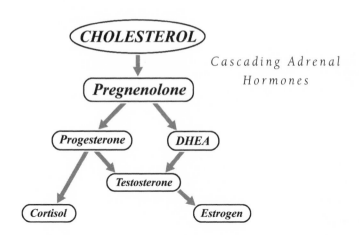

Cascading Adrenal Hormones

HOW TO SUPPORT YOUR ADRENAL GLANDS

As we've seen, if you are constantly experiencing stress, your adrenal glands are apt to go into overdrive until they are "exhausted" and less able to respond. Low energy, depression, decreased immunity, low blood pressure, hypoglycemia, and a host of other symptoms can result. To support your adrenal glands, eat the Naturally Healthy Diet (outlined in Chapter 1). When you skip meals or eat a diet too high in sugar and "white" carbohydrates, such as white bread and white rice, you stress your adrenal glands. It is essential—especially if you have low adrenal function that manifests as low blood sugar (hypoglycemia)—that your diet include adequate protein and fat.

Exercise rejuvenates your adrenal glands. Studies have routinely shown that moderate exercise can decrease stress hormones. Along with exercise, frequent rest and relaxation can promote adrenal health because they give you a chance to recuperate from daily stress.

Nutritional supplementation can also enhance adrenal function. For patients with symptoms of adrenal exhaustion, I recommend vitamin C and pantothenic acid.

Vitamin C. This is an important supplement for adrenal exhaustion because you lose a lot of this nutrient in your urine when you experience acute and chronic stress. Vitamin C is also essential in the manufacture of adrenal hormones. I recommend that you take at least 1,000 mg twice a day if you have low adrenal function.

Pantothenic Acid. Pantothenic acid, or vitamin B$_5$, plays an essential role in the manufacture of adrenal hormones. Foods high in pantothenic acid include whole grains, legumes, broccoli, cauliflower, salmon, sweet potatoes, and tomatoes. The recommended dose for adrenal support is 250 mg twice a day.

In addition to nutritional supplementation, supplemental adrenal hormones can help your adrenal glands mend from years of stress. The two most important hormones for this purpose are dehydroepiandrosterone (DHEA) and pregnenolone.

DHEA. DHEA, the most abundant hormone in your body, counterbalances cortisol and acts as a precursor to other hormones, including estrogen and testosterone.[19] DHEA keeps your muscles strong, enhances your immunity, increases your libido, and improves your mood and quality of life. When you are in your twenties your level of DHEA is much higher than when you are in your forties. (As you may have experienced, when you are in your twenties, you can push yourself to the limit and bounce back much more easily than when you are in your thirties or forties.) It's normal for your DHEA level to drop as you get older, and when you are under chronic stress, DHEA is the first adrenal hormone in your body to decrease. DHEA supplements can give your adrenal glands the extra boost they need while you are implementing dietary and lifestyle changes that support your adrenal glands regularly.

How do you know if you should take supplemental DHEA? It's important to take an ASI test to determine your body's DHEA level first, and then take only the smallest amount of DHEA needed to supplement your adrenal function. Most women need only a low dose of DHEA; I rarely recommend more than 10 mg daily. Side effects of taking too much DHEA include many of the symptoms of excessive testosterone ingestion, such as acne, facial hair growth, and oily skin. Remember, your aim is to create hormonal balance; taking too much of any one hormone, or taking hormones that you don't need, can wreak hormonal havoc and disrupt your health and well-being.

Pregnenolone. Pregnenolone, which is found in high concentrations in the brain, not only helps you cope with stress but improves your memory and concentration.[20] If you are under stress for a long period of time, your level of pregnenolone drops (and subsequently so do all of your other adrenal hormones). You feel tired, unable to cope with stress, and lacking in your usual energy and enthusiasm. Other signs of decreased pregnenolone include low blood pressure, cravings for salty foods, joint pain, frequent urination, and a loss of underarm and pubic hair.

If your ASI test results indicate that your pregnenolone level is low, you can take up to 50 mg a day to support your adrenal glands while you are modifying your lifestyle and improving your diet. It is important that you work with your naturopathic physician to assess your level of pregnenolone, before and after you take supplements. Again, your goal is to create hormonal balance; taking an excess of any hormone, or taking hormones you don't need, can adversely affect your overall health.

YOUR ADRENAL HEALTH: THE VIEW FROM THE EAST

At first glance, Chinese medicine appears to have no exact parallel to the Western view of your adrenal glands and their functions. But on closer inspection, most of the symptoms associated with an exhausted adrenal gland in Western naturopathic medicine are very similar, if not identical, to the symptoms that Chinese medicine attributes to deficiencies of kidney Qi, kidney yin, or kidney yang. In fact, the herbal medicines recommended in the West to promote adrenal health also support kidney Qi, kidney yin, or kidney yang in the Chinese system.

Ginseng is one of the most important Chinese herbal medicines for coping with stress, and according to Western medicine, ginseng can lower your level of the stress hormone cortisol. In Chapter 2 we saw the immunity-enhancing effects of Siberian ginseng; in Chapter 3 we saw that Chinese ginseng can increase the libido. Both of these types of ginseng, which are used in traditional Chinese medicine, can also give your adrenal glands a boost by supporting your kidney Qi and kidney yang.

Another type of ginseng, American ginseng, which grows wild in North America, also has properties that support kidney Qi and kidney yin. It replenishes fluids, so American ginseng is a better choice for women who live in warmer climates or who have too much "heat" or yang energy.

The Different Faces of Ginseng

HERB	CHINESE ENERGETIC PROPERTIES AND THERAPEUTIC BENEFITS	RECOMMENDED DOSE FOR ADRENAL SUPPORT
Siberian ginseng	This "warming" herb is excellent for treating fatigue and low immunity and for decreasing the effects of stress.	Take 200 mg, containing a standardized extract of 0.5 percent eleutheroside E, 2–3 times a day.
Chinese ginseng	This "warming" herb is used to balance energy during times of stress. It increases your mental alertness (yet doesn't overstimulate) and has a long history as an aphrodisiac.	Take 100 mg, standardized to contain 4 percent total ginsenosides, twice a day.
American ginseng	A "cooling" herb that can help you cope with stress; it is especially recommended for women with fatigue associated with anxiety, agitation, and insomnia.	Take 200 mg in capsules standardized to contain 7 percent saponin or ginsenoside content, twice a day. (American ginseng should not be used if you have diarrhea or a high fever.)

Your adrenal health is also supported by keeping your dominant element balanced to promote your kidney Qi, kidney yin, and kidney yang; in turn, supporting your adrenal health helps you keep your dominant element in balance. The syndrome known in Western natural medicine as "adrenal fatigue" can affect each of the Five Element types in distinct ways. Let's take a closer look at the relationship between the Five Elements and adrenal health, and the ways that each is most likely to be affected by adrenal stress.

If you are a Metal type, you have a tendency to exhaust your adrenal glands when you maintain too much rigidity and discipline in your life. For all of your creativity and impressive accomplishments, you are apt to lose sight of your ability to let go, kick back, relax, and just have a good time. When your adrenal glands are fatigued, you are most likely to manifest skin rashes and respiratory symptoms.

If you are a Water type, you are most vulnerable to poor adrenal function if your lifestyle doesn't honor the needs of your true self—the inner voice that yearns to spend quiet time contemplating deep issues and nurturing your spiritual needs. If you suffer from adrenal fatigue, you tend to have diminished sex drive, increased urination, chronic low-grade urinary infections, and a lack of stamina and willpower.

If you are a Wood type, the key issue affecting adrenal health is your unique capacity for hard work. You are apt to push yourself strenuously until you burn out, resulting in adrenal fatigue. When this happens, you have a tendency to develop allergies, muscle spasms, unstable blood pressure, and a dependency on caffeine. On an emotional level, you can become despondent, anxious, and frustrated.

If you are a Fire type, when your adrenal glands are stressed your characteristic exuberance and passion for life become replaced, initially, by an excess of agitated energy; if the stress to your adrenal glands is chronic, you eventually become completely exhausted. Fire types with poor adrenal function often have symptoms of low blood pressure and heart palpitations.

Finally, if you are an Earth type, when your adrenal glands are underfunctioning, you tend to have symptoms of low blood sugar resulting in anxiety and fatigue. You crave sweets and eat sugar in order to feel "normal," but the quick rise in blood sugar backfires, creating a sugar seesaw; one moment you are high on sugar, and the next your energy drops quickly, causing even greater sugar cravings. Your generous, compassionate nature can become distracted, or even thwarted, by these ups and downs.

Your Pancreas: Insulin and Your Weight

Kristie came to see me because she'd gained fifteen pounds in the previous eighteen months, and her blood work showed high cholesterol and high triglycerides. "I love to eat bread, potatoes, pasta, and just about anything that is sweet," she said. "In fact, if I could, I'd just live on these foods. But during the past few years I haven't been able to lose the weight I've gained, even though I didn't eat a lot of fat."

Once Kristie discovered that the starchy foods in her diet were causing her to gain weight, it was as if a light went on in her life. It took time, but eating more protein and quality fat, and fewer carbohydrates, made a big difference and she started losing weight. "Now I'm comfortable in my body," she says, "and the extra bonus is that I also have more energy."

If you are overweight, you probably don't think of your pancreas as playing an important role in weight gain. But the pancreas, a gland located in the abdomen, releases the hormone insulin, which can indeed influence body weight. The good news is that, in most cases, the decisions you make every day about what to eat can help your pancreas function most efficiently to keep you at your optimal weight.

Insulin is released in response to the presence of sugar in your bloodstream; you need insulin to shuttle sugar from your blood into cells throughout the body. If you eat excessive amounts of sugar, or high-glycemic foods that convert quickly to sugar (for a list of high-glycemic foods, see Chapter 1), your pancreas releases a lot of insulin to help move the sugar out of your bloodstream into your cells. But if your cells are constantly bombarded with high levels of insulin and sugar, they set up a defense system to prevent absorbing any more sugar. This is called insulin resistance, metabolic syndrome, or Syndrome X; if this condition develops, sugar that would normally be used for energy inside your cells is stored as fat instead. The result is weight gain, especially around the abdomen, resulting in an "apple-shaped" figure—one of the classic signs of Syndrome X (though not everyone with this figure has the syndrome). Insulin resistance can be one of the most important factors affecting health; over time a person with chronic insulin resistance is not only apt to gain weight but is at higher risk for heart disease and type 2 diabetes.

According to the American Association of Clinical Endocrinologists, insulin resistance affects one in three American adults.[21] This is not surprising, since the U.S. surgeon general has reported that 61 percent of Americans are significantly overweight, and that Americans spend more money on fast foods, which are high in sugar, than on movies, books, magazines, newspapers, videos, and recorded music combined.

TESTS TO MEASURE INSULIN RESISTANCE

Signs that you may have insulin resistance can be seen on blood tests. For instance, insulin resistance is associated with high levels of total cholesterol, low HDL (favorable) cholesterol, high LDL (unfavorable) cholesterol, or high triglycerides. Other tests will give you additional evidence of insulin resistance, such as a fasting blood glucose (sugar) test, an oral glucose tolerance test (a more accurate indicator), and a measurement of insulin after a twelve-hour fast.

PREVENTING AND TREATING INSULIN RESISTANCE

Insulin resistance does not develop overnight; it's a gradually acquired condition. But there are many things you can do to prevent and to treat it. You can begin by following the Naturally Healthy Diet (outlined in Chapter 1), which is low in sugar and high-glycemic carbohydrates, and by incorporating regular exercise and stress management into your life. I've seen many patients with insulin resistance turn their health around with these simple yet profoundly effective lifestyle changes.

Surprisingly, a low-fat, low-protein diet can increase your risk of developing insulin resistance if it contains an excess of high-glycemic carbohydrates. Many women have told me that after being on a low-fat vegetarian diet for a few months, they were alarmed to find that instead of losing weight, they had gained ten or fifteen pounds! This almost certainly happened because their diet caused their blood sugar levels to rise rapidly after meals. As a result they developed insulin resistance, which caused them to gain weight—a frustrating scenario, since these women thought they would surely lose weight by carefully avoiding fat in their diet.

In addition, if you are under chronic stress and your adrenal glands release a lot of cortisol (stress hormone), your cells can become more resistant to insulin.[22] You are more likely to develop insulin resistance if you don't get enough exercise because regular exercise is important in managing your blood sugar level (it helps maintain the sensitivity of your cells to insulin). It also helps your body use sugars more efficiently and handle stress better. Finally, research shows that postmenopausal women who choose HRT are at higher risk for insulin resistance.[23] If you take HRT, you need to be especially careful about your diet, stress levels, and exercise to prevent insulin resistance.

If you develop insulin resistance, the following supplements can help your body regulate your blood sugar more effectively.

Chromium. Chromium helps control blood sugar levels by working closely with insulin in transporting sugar into the cells. Chromium has gained a reputation for aiding weight loss, though it is less well known that it does this by improving the cells' sensitivity to insulin. The recommended dose is 500 mg twice a day.

Biotin. Biotin is an important nutrient in the treatment of insulin resistance because it enhances the sensitivity of cells to insulin. One of the B vitamins, biotin is found in many foods, including chicken, cooked eggs, saltwater fish, milk, cheese, soybeans, whole wheat, and rice bran, and it is also synthesized by intestinal bacteria. To help treat insulin resistance, I recommend that you supplement your diet with 5 mg of biotin twice a day. It is a very safe nutrient with no known side effects.

INSULIN RESISTANCE: THE VIEW FROM THE EAST

In Chinese medicine, the condition known in the West as insulin resistance is considered a deficiency of spleen Qi (which is associated with an imbalanced Earth element), and a deficiency of kidney Qi (associated with an imbalanced Water element). These deficiencies occur because an excess of sweets and fats in the diet makes the spleen work harder, which causes heat to accumulate. In its efforts to cool the heat, kidney yin, which is a type of kidney Qi, eventually becomes depleted.

The dietary treatment for this condition in Chinese medicine is remarkably similar to the Western treatment for insulin resistance: eat a healthy diet (which includes low-glycemic carbohydrates, adequate protein, and fat) and eat regular meals. In addition, Chinese medicine recommends herbal formulas for building spleen Qi and kidney yin; these formulas can also help people who suffer from what Western medicine describes as a blood sugar imbalance resulting in insulin resistance. Specific herbal formulas can be obtained from a practitioner of Chinese medicine.

Growth Hormone: Fountain of Youth or Health Risk?

Supplemental growth hormone (GH) has been touted as the latest elixir of youth, able to turn back the biological clock and make people feel younger. When you are young, your pituitary gland releases natural growth hormone in large quantities for normal growth and development, but as you age, your body releases less of it. Supplemental GH, which is sometimes taken by people in hopes of preventing the aging process, has become controversial.

Proponents of supplemental GH claim that it can increase muscle tone, enhance immunity, strengthen bones, and promote a healthy heart. They assert that without GH people age faster and have droopier eyelids, deeper wrinkles, more flaccid muscles, lower immunity, an increased tendency to gain weight, and a greater likelihood of depression and low self-esteem. Everything you read about GH sounds very appealing, except the price. (It's prohibitively expensive.) Unfortunately, even though some claims made about GH may have some merit, there's another side to the story.

Supplemental GH may increase your risk of cancer and other serious disorders. A review published in the *Journal of Endocrinology* in 1999 states that GH elevates levels of insulinlike growth factor (IGF-1), which may increase the risk of breast cancer in women and prostate cancer in men.[24] GH may also increase your risk of developing insulin resistance, diabetes, hypertension, atherosclerosis, abnormal growth of bones and internal organs (including the heart, liver, and kidneys), and other health conditions. Until more information is available and more studies are conducted on the long-term effects of supplemental GH, I don't recommend that you take it unless it is medically necessary. (It is sometimes prescribed for specific health conditions.)

You can naturally enhance your level of growth hormone with an exercise program. Exercise stimulates the pituitary gland to secrete more growth hormone, without ever producing too much. This is the perfect choice for maintaining your normal growth hormone level: it's natural, effective, and free.

Orchestrating Your Hormonal Dance: Final Thoughts

Your hormones can influence every aspect of your health. Waxing and waning in an elegant choreographed performance, they shape your growth and development and connect you with nature's rhythms. If you have hormonal imbalances, you may need to see your naturopathic physician for further advice specific to your concerns, but everyone can take steps to help coordinate their hormonal dance. In my daily practice, I continually see women create harmony in their lives by addressing the underlying sources of hormonal imbalances and choosing natural medicine to restore health. With the methods that we've explored in this chapter, you can nourish your hormonal health throughout your life.

The Essence of Chapter 7

- Make your hormonal health a top priority.
- Become familiar with changes in your consciousness as you move through the phases of your menstrual cycle, as well as the role of the Five Elements and how they affect your Qi.
- Treat the underlying causes of PMS, irregular menstrual cycles, and painful periods with natural medicine.
- Take steps to maintain the flow of Qi and Blood to prevent imbalances in your menstrual cycle.
- If you decide to take HRT, take natural bioidentical HRT in the lowest possible dose for the shortest duration of time.
- Use herbs and homeopathic medicines to help you through your hormonal transition from perimenopause to menopause and beyond.
- Eat "cooling" or "cold" foods to help ease your midlife symptoms.
- Assess your thyroid and adrenal glands, and take natural medicines if you need to help them work optimally.
- Prevent and treat insulin resistance with your diet, lifestyle choices, and natural medicine.
- Exercise to naturally increase growth hormone.

Chapter 8

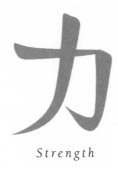

Strength

Building Healthy Bones for Life

*"Hope sleeps in our bones like a bear
waiting for spring to rise and walk."*
—MARGE PIERCY, *Stone, Paper, Knife*

*T*ARA CAME *to see me for information on preventing osteoporosis. During her initial visit she described how she'd felt a few weeks earlier when receiving the results of her first bone density test. "I nearly panicked," she said. "The report seemed to indicate that within five years I would have osteoporosis! I'm only forty-nine years old, but my dreams of travel and independence dissolved as I looked at the scientific evidence that doomed my future." She told me that her medical doctor was pushing her to take Premarin and Fosamax (a drug for rebuilding bones), but she decided to look into different forms of treatment.*

I showed Tara the correct way to read her test results and explained that bone density was not the only factor in bone health. I outlined the reasons women lose bone mass and explained how to build it back. Together we worked out a plan that included natural hormones, regular weight-bearing exercise, and nutritional supplements. I recommended that Tara take minerals—calcium and magnesium—and prescribed stomach acid pills to help with their absorption. After only a few weeks, she reported that the digestive problems she'd been experiencing for years were dramatically reduced.

I've seen Tara as a patient for a number of years since then, and she has had regular bone density tests. "In the years since starting natural medicine," she now says, "my bone loss has stabilized, and I'm thrilled. I've learned how to take responsibility for my health. It's about choice—not about medicating myself in order to sustain unhealthy habits."

Your Bones

There is something profound about our relationship to our bones. When we are deeply certain of something, we say we feel it "in our bones," or that our natural tendencies and characteristics are "bred in the bone." Not only do your bones protect your internal organs and hold your body upright, but they also store precious minerals that serve you in innumerable ways.

Until recently, many of us took our bones for granted as a reliable and powerful part of our bodies. But within the past several years osteoporosis—the condition of having porous, low-density bones that are capable of spontaneously breaking and crumbling—has become a household word. Now osteoporosis is considered by the National Institutes of Health (NIH) to be a major public health threat. In the United States today ten million people are estimated to have the disease, of whom eight million are women. The NIH also estimates that 34 million more people may have low bone mass, placing them at increased risk for osteoporosis.[1] With a heightened awareness of this condition, many women are now eager to know what they can do to preserve their bone health.

Bone mass is defined as the amount of bone in the body, and bone density as the amount of bone in a given area. In recent years several tests have emerged to measure bone density, and new pharmaceutical drugs that have been developed to prevent and treat osteoporosis have been heavily promoted. But along with this lavish attention on osteoporosis, Western medicine has all too often portrayed menopause—during which bone loss intensifies—as an ominous precursor to the inevitable onset of delicate bones. This has created a great deal of unnecessary apprehension, as many women have come to imagine a future limited by fragility and pain.

The new tests tell you only part of the story, and the drugs may have long-term side effects that we won't know of for many years to come. But as we will see in this chapter, there's no need for fear; osteoporosis is certainly not an inevitable outcome of menopause. The risk of getting osteoporosis can increase with age, but there are a number of other factors that elevate your risk. Thankfully, many of them are dietary and lifestyle factors that you can control, helping to prevent the condition. And even if you do develop osteoporosis, natural treatments exist to help prevent a fracture.

Osteoarthritis, a bone-related condition and the most common form of joint disease, is another problem that can plague women as they get older. In the United States osteoarthritis affects more than twenty million people and is more common in women after age forty-five.[2] Conventional Western doctors typically prescribe countless anti-inflammatory medications to decrease the pain and swelling associated with osteoarthritis, but these drugs are not without side effects. Again, there are many natural medicines from both the Western and the Eastern traditions that you can use to decrease pain and reverse or slow the progression of this disease.

According to Chinese medicine, bones are supported by kidney Qi. If you squander your kidney Qi and kidney Essence early in life, your bones can become weak and brittle, resulting in osteoporosis or osteoarthritis as you age. But as long as you support your overall health, your bones will be strong and healthy.

The View from the West

Your bones are healthy if they have good strength, density, and quality. (The "quality" of bones refers to their architecture and integrity on a cellular level.) While following the Naturally Healthy Lifestyle can help keep bones healthy, many women—due to personal history, aging, or less-than-optimal lifestyle habits—are at risk for osteoporosis, especially beginning at menopause. This is because chronically low levels of hormones at the onset of menopause, particularly estrogen, progesterone, and testosterone, can result in bone loss.

Hormones stimulate the cells that build bone and inhibit the cells that destroy bone, thereby playing a major role, along with diet and exercise, in establishing bone mass and bone quality. When the cells that build new bone work more slowly than the cells that destroy old bone, bones become less dense. For younger women, a short-term lower level of hormones isn't usually a problem, and it's common for women during pregnancy or lactation to show decreased bone mass, which then rebounds when normal menstrual cycles have resumed. But if you have a prolonged hormonal imbalance, you can develop thin, porous bones that are at a higher risk for fracture later in life.

Osteoporosis is defined as a disease characterized by low bone mass and low bone quality, with an increase in bone fragility and susceptibility to fracture. *Severe osteoporosis* is defined as established osteoporosis plus one or more fractures due to fragile bones.[3]

Women may be diagnosed with a related condition called *osteopenia*, defined as low bone mass or a moderate increase in facture risk. But a diagnosis of this condition shouldn't trigger panic. In my practice, I see many women in their forties who've been diagnosed with osteopenia. Many of these women are frightened by the prospect of becoming handicapped because of their low bone mass. I explain to these women that their new "diagnosis" is a baseline measurement of their bone mass and recommend that they repeat the test in one to two years to evaluate whether bone loss is occurring. I explain that this test doesn't measure bone quality or bone strength, which are also important for bone health. Often bone density tests motivate women to start making lifestyle changes that support their bone health.

The Western approach to bone health continues to evolve, and new drugs are being formulated to treat low bone density. No one knows, however, if they could lead to serious consequences later in life. The bottom line is that no drug can replace a lifetime of healthy habits.

Risk Factors for Osteoporosis

- A family history of osteoporosis, especially in a first-degree relative, such as a mother, grandmother, or sister
- A history of anorexia nervosa
- An early menopause
- An abnormal cessation of menstruation prior to menopause
- A low intake of calcium throughout life
- Cigarette smoking
- Excessive consumption of alcohol

- An inactive lifestyle
- A history of using corticosteroids and anticonvulsant drugs
- A small body frame
- Low bone mass
- A personal history of bone fracture after age fifty
- Being female
- Advanced age
- Being Caucasian or Asian

Source: National Institutes of Health: Osteoporosis and Related Bone Diseases National Resource Center.

OSTEOARTHRITIS

Why is it that some women's joints wear out long before their time? The reason may be stress on the joints, an acid-forming diet, excess weight, genetics, or a combination of factors. Osteoarthritis, the degeneration of the cartilage on the surface of the joints, usually results from chronic overuse. Cartilage is important for the smooth-gliding action of joints throughout their range of motion; it also provides joints with a "shock absorber" to buffer bones from stress. If you have osteoarthritis, the wearing-down of your cartilage results in inflammation and pain. As osteoarthritis progresses, bone spurs can develop on the edges of a joint, or small pieces of bone or cartilage can break off and float inside the joint space, leading to more joint pain. The joints most commonly affected by osteoarthritis are the knees, hips, spine, and hands, although any joint can be affected. If you are overweight, there is more stress on your weight-bearing joints, such as your knees and hips, so you are more susceptible in these areas.

For many years, osteoarthritis was considered simply an uncomfortable part of aging that could not be reversed. But research now indicates that there may be a genetic predisposition in 25 to 30 percent of osteoarthritis cases and that joint cartilage can mend itself, given the right tools.[4] Through exercise, diet, and natural medicines, there's a lot you can do to prevent osteoarthritis and to treat it if you already have it. Even if you are genetically predisposed to the disease, you may be able to reduce the likelihood of activating the genes that put you at risk—and literally change your genetic destiny.

The View from the East

Osteoporosis, viewed from a Chinese medicine perspective, is primarily due to a decline in kidney Essence and kidney Qi. Kidney Essence (ancestral Qi, and the basis of kidney Qi) forms your bones when you are in the womb and continues to nourish them as you develop from infancy through adulthood. Kidney Essence and kidney Qi become deficient as part of the natural aging process, but if stress or illness causes you to age more quickly, they become prematurely depleted—for example, if you squander them by continually pushing your body and mind to the limit while providing yourself with very little rest and rejuvenation. If your kidney Essence is depleted early in life, your bones become brittle and weak, and if your kidney Qi is deficient, you can experience fatigue and stiff, aching joints and bones. In contrast, when your kidney Essence and kidney Qi are abundant, you have strong and healthy bones throughout your life. (See Chapter 3 for more information on how to maintain your kidney Essence and kidney Qi.)

Your susceptibility to osteoporosis may also depend on your type, according to the Five Elements of Chinese medicine. People who are Metal types are the least likely to develop osteoporosis, but as we will see they are more prone to other bone-related problems, such as osteoarthritis. If you are a Water type, you are more apt to develop problems with your bones because your kidney Qi "rules" them. (The kidneys are the primary organ of the Water type.) When your Water element is chronically imbalanced, you are at higher risk for developing osteoporosis.

Wood types may develop osteoporosis because they are always on the go and often don't know when to stop. If you are a Wood type, your tendency to neglect your needs and work yourself to the breaking point causes excessive release of bone-depleting stress hormones that can result in brittle bones. It is as if you are no longer supple and able to bend freely with the wind, but instead are dehydrated, stiff, and easily snapped by the slightest pressure.

If you are a Fire type, you may be prone to osteoporosis if your anxious tendencies go unabated. Too much high-strung energy causes the release of excessive adrenaline, which can ultimately decrease your bone density. If your Fire element is out of balance, too much Fire flaring upward will consume your yin, resulting in dry bones.

If you are an Earth type, you are vulnerable to osteoporosis if you exhaust your energy trying to take care of everyone else while neglecting yourself. Ultimately, a lack of self-nurturing can lead to a deficiency of spleen Qi, which manifests as poor digestion, resulting in poor mineral absorption and weak, fragile bones.

As we have seen, all of the Five Elements work together to keep you healthy and balanced. If one element is deficient due to a stressful lifestyle, other elements will become imbalanced as well. Regardless of your dominant element, if you prematurely exhaust your Qi, you can be at higher risk for developing osteoporosis.

OSTEOARTHRITIS AND CHINESE MEDICINE

The condition we call osteoarthritis in Western medicine is known in Chinese medicine as "wind dampness disease" or "wind visiting joints." It is caused by deficient Wei Qi (defensive Qi), which allows "wind cold" or "dampness" to invade the joints and cause an obstruction of Qi. If your Qi is unable to flow through a joint, you experience joint pain, swelling, and eventually heat in the affected joint.

According to the Five Element system, Metal, Water, and Wood types are the most likely to develop osteoarthritis. If you are a Metal type, you are especially prone to osteoarthritis because, when your health is out of balance, you characteristically become mentally as well as physically inflexible. Eventually this rigidity can manifest as chronic joint pain and stiffness. You can prevent joint pain by keeping your Metal element well balanced.

As we've seen, your kidney Qi rules your bones, and your kidneys have a strong connection with your Water element. If you are a Water type, you are particularly susceptible to imbalances in your joints when your kidney Qi is depleted. To keep your Water element balanced and your joints in healthy condition, nourish your kidney Qi and Essence. (See Chapter 3.)

It's not unusual for Wood types to become afflicted by the wear and tear associated with osteoarthritis. If you are a Wood type, you are inclined to push your body so hard in pursuit of your goals that you can overwork your joints in the process. These tendencies can be ignored when Wood types are young, but as they get into their forties and beyond, they often show signs of osteoarthritis. To help keep your joints healthy, pace yourself and be sure to take time to replenish your energy.

Fire types are less apt to have osteoarthritis than the other types, but they are not entirely exempt. If you are a Fire type, you tend to be passionate about the things you love, but if you become overexcited, your heart Qi can become chronically depleted;

this can result in deficient kidney Qi, which in turn can lead to osteoarthritis. It is essential for you to rekindle your vital energy and nourish your Qi after your enthusiasm dies down.

If you are an Earth type, you can be subject to osteoarthritis because you tend to have weak joints that don't hold up well under continued stress. You are also prone to osteoarthritis because you are susceptible to "damp" conditions in your joints. Your sensitivity to "dampness" extends to your environment as well; you may even be able to predict the weather—especially damp weather—because you can "feel it" in your bones. To help prevent osteoarthritis, keep your Earth element in balance. (See Chapter 6.)

Tests to Evaluate Your Bones

One of the best ways to evaluate the density of your bones is with a dual energy bone densitometry, or DEXA, test, which uses a special type of X-ray taken of your hip and lower spine. A DEXA test gives you a T-score, which is a measurement of your bone density compared with that of women who are at peak bone density (in their twenties and early thirties). Treatment and diagnosis of osteoporosis is based on the T-score, but the T-score doesn't reflect your total bone health, which also includes your bone quality and strength. In addition, your DEXA test results may be misleading: critics of the test have raised concerns that the bone density standards established by the World Health Organization don't take into account ethnic diversity and the various sizes of women's frames.

An international osteoporosis journal has suggested that, as a result, today's acceptable ranges for normal bone density may lead many women to be falsely diagnosed with low bone density.[5] A diagnosis of osteoporosis is only 2.5 standard deviations lower than the bone density of healthy young women. According to Dr. Susan Love, author of *Dr. Susan Love's Menopause and Hormone Book,* "The level of bone density that defines osteoporosis has been set rather high, with the result that most older women will fall into the 'disease' category—which is very nice for the people in the business of treating disease."[6]

It's important to remember, when interpreting your DEXA test results, that the test does not determine if bone loss is slow, progressive, or static. Repeat tests every two to three years are needed in order to get a clearer picture. In addition, a DEXA test may also result in false readings, indicating that a woman's bone density is better than it actually is; this can occur when she has calcium deposits in her hip or spine associated with osteoarthritis.

Despite the drawbacks, a DEXA test can provide you with valuable information if the results are interpreted within the context of its limitations. When I read a woman's DEXA test results, I always take into account her body size, frame, and lifestyle. In order to get the best results, I recommend that women with low bone density have repeat DEXA tests at the same facility, if possible, in order to be tested on the same type of machine. Keep in mind that the error rate of this test is 1 to 2 percent, so a bone density loss of this amount may be due to error rather than actual bone loss.[7]

Medical convention says to wait until you are about fifty years old to have a DEXA test, but I recommend that you get one when you've reached peak bone density (by about age thirty) or if you have many of the risk factors for osteoporosis on page 243. This will give you a baseline and enable you to track your bone density over the years. (If you are past age thirty and haven't yet had a DEXA test done, I suggest that you get one and repeat it every five years. If you are menopausal and at risk for osteoporosis, you should repeat the test every one to two years.)

Your physician can order a DEXA test for you. If your insurance doesn't cover the cost, you will have to pay for it out of pocket (about $200 to $250). As you review your DEXA test results with your physician, remember that your bone density is only one aspect of your bone health. Whether you have many of the risk factors for osteoporosis or not, I recommend that you actively participate in a bone-building program. In my daily practice, one of my goals is to help each woman I see achieve optimal bone health well into her senior years. A woman may choose to take hormones, or even bone-building drugs, in her effort to maintain healthy bones. But I cannot stress enough that no hormone or drug will take the place of a healthy lifestyle and diet.

Bone Density Classifications

A DEXA test T-score represents your bone density compared with the average bone density of healthy young women.

Normal Bone Density: Your T-score is **-1.0 or greater** on a DEXA test.

Osteopenia: Low bone mass or a moderate increase in fracture risk. You have osteopenia if your T-score is **between -1.0 and -2.5** on a DEXA test.

Osteoporosis: You have osteoporosis if your T-score is **-2.5 or less** on a DEXA test.

Severe Osteoporosis: Established osteoporosis plus one or more fractures due to fragile bones.

Source: World Health Organization, WHO Technical Report, Series 843, Geneva, 1994.

In addition to DEXA testing, you can also evaluate your bones with a Pyrilinks urine test, which measures the fragments of collagen that collect in urine when bone breaks down. The Pyrilinks test is especially useful for assessing your amount of bone loss while you are implementing your bone-building program or other therapy. (With a DEXA test, you have to wait up to two years to see if the changes you've made in your diet and lifestyle have improved your bone density.) I recommend that you take this test to get a baseline before you start a bone-building program. After four to six weeks on your program, take the test again to see if the amount of your bone loss has decreased. I've used this test to monitor the success of many women with whom I've worked—women who have taken low-dose natural hormones, nutritional supplements, and exercised regularly to prevent osteoporosis. The test costs about $40 to $60 and can be ordered through your health care provider.

If you live in a northern region, or if you don't regularly expose your skin to the sun, it's a good idea to measure your vitamin D level. Vitamin D is essential for healthy bones because it plays a key role in telling your body to absorb calcium if the calcium level in your blood is low. Exposure to the sun's ultraviolet rays triggers vitamin D synthesis, which decreases with age. You can ask your physician to order a blood test that measures 25-hydroxyvitamin D, the form of vitamin D that's made in your liver after your skin has been exposed to ultraviolet light. Dr. Michael Holick, chief of endocrinology, nutrition, and diabetes at Boston University Medical Center, recommends that a woman's vitamin D level be at least 20 ng per ml on her blood test, which is above what most commercial medical laboratories consider normal.[8] It is recommended that you have the test done in midwinter, when the angle of the sun doesn't provide as much ultraviolet radiation for you to make vitamin D. (If you live in a southern region and are able to expose your arms and legs to the sun for at least fifteen minutes a day throughout the year, you probably have adequate amounts of vitamin D in your body.) If your test results show that your vitamin D level is low, take a daily vitamin D supplement along with calcium, as recommended in the following pages.

Osteoarthritis announces its presence much more loudly than osteoporosis, and your body will let you know if you're afflicted. This condition is characterized by stiffness in a joint after getting out of bed or sitting for a long time, swelling, tenderness, or pain in one or more joints, and a "crunching" feeling or the sensation of bone-rubbing-on-bone when you move a joint. An X-ray can help determine how much joint damage you have, but X-rays are often unable to show early stages of osteoarthritis. CT scans are sometimes used to diagnose osteoarthritis because they provide more detailed information.

EVALUATING YOUR BONES FROM THE EAST

In Chinese medicine, the strength and integrity of bones are evaluated both by symptoms and by the quality of kidney Qi and kidney Essence. As we saw in Chapter 3, kidneys can become deficient in yin, yang, or Essence.

If you suffer from achy bones and a sore back, and you also have excessive mental strain and feelings of being agitated and tired at the same time, you probably have a deficiency of kidney yin. If you have a sensation of being "cold in your bones," soreness in your back, and weak legs, you most likely have a deficiency of kidney yang. (In Chinese medicine, feeling "cold in your bones" is different from having "achy bones." It is a distinct sensation of being chilled in the joints, especially the knees, and is usually accompanied by stiffness.) If your bones are fragile, or you have weak knees and legs, loose teeth, and prematurely gray hair, you probably have a deficiency of kidney Essence. If you experience any of these symptoms, your bones will benefit greatly from following the guidelines outlined in this chapter, which strengthen your bones and balance your kidney yin, kidney yang, and kidney Essence.

The Naturally Healthy Lifestyle for Your Bones

Your bones are dynamic living tissues that are in a constant state of building and transforming. Inside your bones are cells that build bone (osteoblasts), and cells that destroy old bone (osteoclasts). When you exercise, you prompt the cells that build your bones to work harder, resulting in increased bone mass and bone density.

Your bones go through many stages during your lifetime. Nature intended your bones to build strength and mass during the first third of your life, and you have built 98 percent of your bone mass by age twenty. Your bones reach their maximum density somewhere between age thirty and thirty-five, after which you lose a small amount of bone until menopause, and then bone loss accelerates for about five years. From five years after menopause until about age seventy, the rate of bone loss slows down but can still happen at a rate of one to two percent per year.[9]

The loss of bone that occurs before and after menopause is a natural process. If you've built enough bone during the first third of your life, you can afford to lose some bone mass and still have good bone health through your senior years. If you continue to stress your bones with regular weight-bearing exercise, and supply them with the nutrition they need, you can maintain your bone health for life.

EXERCISE FOR YOUR BONES

By making your muscles work hard, especially against resistance, you stimulate your bone-building cells (osteoblasts) to lay down new bone. You can build healthy bones for life with regular exercise, and it's never too late—or too early—to start. The exercise you did when you were young can still have a profound impact on how dense your bones are as an adult. This is why it is so important to encourage young girls to play sports and also to achieve a healthy weight that maintains their menstrual cycles in their teenage years; regular menstrual cycles mean adequate levels of hormones that ensure strong, healthy bones.

Any exercise that works against gravity can build bone, but some types of exercise build bone faster than others. Swimming is a great cardiovascular exercise and it can have some effect on your bone density, but not as much as exercises that stress your bones and muscles like weight lifting and jogging. Miriam Nelson, Ph.D., author of *Strong Women, Strong Bones,* has reported that postmenopausal women who lifted weights for one year increased their bone density by one percent, while a group of women who didn't do any exercise lost about two percent of their bone density. She also found that the women who lifted weights increased their scores on a balance test by 14 percent; loss of balance is one of the major causes of hip fractures in older women.

Having strong muscles not only helps create strong bones, it also tones your body, makes you feel and look great, gives you more energy and vitality, and increases your sense of well-being. You feel empowered when you have more capable muscles— picking up a heavy object doesn't seem so daunting and you don't need to wait for a more able-bodied person to do it for you. You also spare yourself the many back, neck, and body aches that come from being out of shape. When I started lifting weights about six years ago, I was amazed by the difference it made in my life. As a child I was always athletic, as a teenager I was active in sports, and from age nineteen to thirty I taught aerobics classes. But nothing compared to the increases in strength that I gained in just a few months of lifting weights. In fact, after only a year of consistent weight lifting I was able to carry a sixty-pound pack up Mount Rainier! I never would have been able to do that with aerobics alone. Including weight lifting in your bone-building program will give you the fastest and greatest improvements in your strength and bone density.

Here's how to get started with weight lifting. First, buy gym clothes that you're comfortable in. Wear something flexible but not loose. (Extra material gets in the way.) Second, get a good pair of athletic shoes. Third, buy some low-weight dumbbells (three to five pounds), ankle weights, or resistance tubes, and use them to build your bones at home. There are a number of videos that you can buy that will show you how to lift weights safely, slowly, and methodically. Dr. Nelson has easy-to-follow videos geared to women at all stages of physical fitness. (See Appendix B for details.) You don't have to lift a lot of weight to achieve an increase in strength and bone density—most women choose to use lighter weights and do many repetitions rather than heavier weights with few repetitions. This can also help to spare your joints and prevent injury.

Be sure to work out your arms, chest, abdomen, back, buttocks, and legs at least three times a week. You can mix exercises using weights with those that don't require

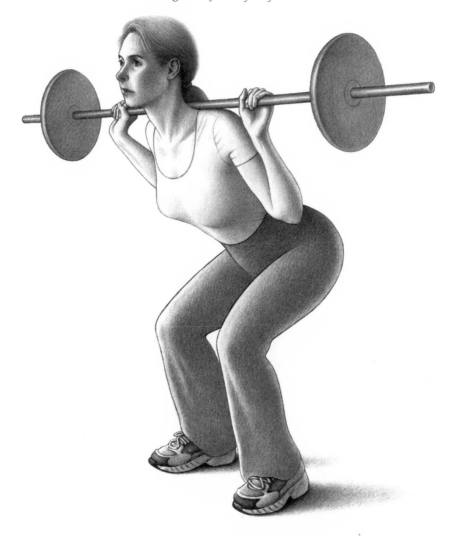

weights: basic biceps and triceps exercises strengthen your arms, push-ups build muscles in your chest, stomach crunches enhance the strength of your abdominal muscles, and squats and leg lifts build muscles in your buttocks and legs. On the whole, your spine gets stronger when you strengthen your abdomen and do upper-body exercises. Some exercises, such as squats, involve multiple muscle groups and give you a great overall body workout.

If you've never lifted weights before, you are in for a treat. Within just a few weeks, you will begin to feel positive changes in your body that you might not have thought possible. Once you start your program, you'll want to continue because it feels so good to be strong. Many of my patients told me that they simply didn't have time to exercise—but once they started, they were hooked and somehow they found the time!

Another option is to join a gym and hire a trainer. A trainer can help you create a program that will give you all the benefits of weight lifting and minimize your potential for injury. Work with a trainer for at least two months, once or twice a week, and check in with him or her once every two or three months afterward.

Along with weight lifting, I recommend that you protect your bone health with exercises that improve your balance, such as Tai Chi and yoga. Throughout China, groups of people are commonly seen early in the morning in the parks practicing the graceful motions of Tai Chi exercises. No doubt this practice contributes to the low incidence of osteoporosis in Chinese women. Studies have found that Tai Chi can be a great exercise for promoting a sense of balance in seniors; it also increases flexibility and engenders a peaceful state of mind. You will probably find classes in Tai Chi offered at your local community center or health club.

Yoga can also improve your balance as well as your flexibility. If you join a yoga class, choose one that's appropriate for your level of experience; some types of yoga are much more physically demanding than others. For deep relaxation along with increased flexibility, strength, and balance, I recommend hatha yoga. If you're looking for something more challenging, try Iyengar or Bikram yoga.

Exercise can be one of the best ways to prevent and treat osteoarthritis—if you choose the right kind. It's important to avoid exercises that put too much repetitive wear and tear on your joints. Several years ago I began to experience joint pain in my knees. I had been running nearly every day for about six years, and I'd also taken up step aerobics classes, which involved a great deal of turning and twisting of my knees. After a few months of pain, I had to face the fact that these forms of exercise were creating too much stress on my knee joints. I realized that I'd have to change my exercise routine if I want to have fully functional knees when I'm fifty, so I started working out on an elliptical trainer at the gym, lifting weights, and doing yoga more frequently. Since making these changes, I haven't had any knee pain; what might have developed into osteoarthritis was avoided with a simple change of lifestyle.

If you already have osteoarthritis, nothing can take the place of exercise to help you feel great and maintain your joint health. Listen to your body's signals: slow down, or stop and rest, if your joints hurt, and don't do exercises that exacerbate your symptoms. To work out your heart and cardiovascular system, do more joint-friendly exercises like swimming or pedaling a stationary bike. If you lift weights, use lighter weights and techniques that put as little stress as possible on your joints. And start a stretching or yoga class—it will do wonders to increase your range of motion.

FOOD FOR YOUR BONES

One of the great things about the Naturally Healthy Diet is that, time and again, the foods that are good for one aspect of your health prove to be beneficial to every part of your body. Bone health is no exception. For instance, essential fatty acids—the omega 3 fats found in flax oil, which we know are good for your heart—turn out to be good for your bones as well. And conversely, eating too much salt, which is known to increase hypertension, is detrimental to your bone health because it makes your kidneys spill calcium into your urine. The Naturally Healthy Diet gives your bones the basic fuel they need to be strong and vital throughout your life. There are, however, a few extra bone-building diet tips that will further help you maintain strong bones.

The following list highlights foods and drinks that can directly contribute to your bone health, and those that you should avoid. Most bone-healthy foods and drinks are rich in the nutrients your body needs to build bones; those that deplete your bone health typically do so by pulling minerals out of your bones or inhibiting your assimilation of minerals.

BONE-BUILDING DIETARY CHOICES	BONE-DEPLETING DIETARY CHOICES
Adequate protein	Too much or too little protein
Dairy products	Excessive amounts of sugar and refined carbohydrates
Fruits and vegetables, especially leafy greens (such as kale, collard greens, bok choy, Swiss chard, and spinach)	Excessive amounts of sodium
	Too much or too little fiber
Whole soy foods	Caffeinated drinks
Low-mercury fish, especially with bones (such as sardines)	Chocolate
	Alcoholic beverages
Fats found in fish oil, evening primrose oil, and flax oil	Sodas high in phosphoric acid

Many holistic health care practitioners are critical of relying on dairy products as a source of calcium. They argue that "milk is for baby cows," not for humans, and that because it contains high levels of protein, it could cause an acidic pH in your body, resulting in increased calcium loss from your bones. But all the research I've reviewed shows that dairy products are a good source of calcium. While it's true that excess protein consumption can be detrimental to bone health, too little protein can contribute to osteoporosis.[10]

If you have no adverse reactions to dairy products, such as increased mucus production, they can provide you with a source of calcium that is easily absorbed. In fact, specific proteins in dairy products, including whey protein, have been found to stimulate the cells that lay down new bone (osteoblasts) and suppress the cells that pull calcium out of bone (osteoclasts).[11] Lactulose, another compound found in dairy products, enhances calcium absorption.[12] The debate about dairy products will continue, but the bottom line is that they are valuable, calcium-rich foods that can help prevent osteoporosis. If you choose to eat dairy as a source of calcium, purchase organic products.

If you are allergic to dairy products, increase your intake of other foods high in calcium, such as tofu made with calcium sulfate, cooked spinach and other leafy greens, almonds, hazelnuts, raisins, oranges, mangoes, dried apricots, and fish that include the bones (like sardines). One of the easiest ways to ingest calcium is to include calcium-fortified drinks, such as soy milk or orange juice, in your diet.

Fruits and vegetables are loaded with minerals that are essential to keeping your bones healthy throughout your life. (Leafy vegetables are an especially good source of the bone-building powerhouse vitamin K.) A study published in the *American Journal of Clinical Nutrition* found that women who consumed high amounts of fruit during childhood had higher bone density in their hipbones than women who didn't.[13] This may be explained by the fact that fruits help to create a more alkaline pH, which is important in conserving minerals that keep bones strong. Another study supported the hypothesis that "alkaline-producing dietary components, specifically potassium, magnesium, and fruits and vegetables, contribute to maintenance of bone mineral density."[14]

Soy has been much praised for its ability to help Asian women weather the tides of perimenopause, and it may also be partly responsible for their decreased incidence of osteoporosis. Soy is thought to be especially effective for preserving minerals in bones, since the proteins in soy don't create an acidic pH as readily as other forms of protein do.[15] Another bonus to eating soy products is that they contain genistein, a potent bone-building compound.[16]

Balancing the fiber in your diet is important for your bone health. Eating an excess of fiber can be harmful to your bones because it can impair the absorption of minerals in your food. (If you take fiber supplements, be sure to take extra minerals as well—at a different time of day than you take your fiber.) On the other hand, having insufficient fiber in your diet can be bone-depleting. For example, eating too many refined carbohydrates, which contain very little fiber, can unnaturally raise your blood sugar level, create a more acidic pH, and draw minerals out of your body.

Fish is a very bone-healthy source of protein, quality fats, and (if eaten with the bones) calcium. In China, an entire fish, bones and all, is often added to soups and stews to increase the mineral content of the broth. The essential fats in fish have also been found to enhance bone health; studies have shown that when animals are fed a diet lacking essential fats, they develop osteoporosis. It appears that these important fats can influence mineral absorption and have a positive impact on bone density and metabolism. The essential fats that were found to have the most favorable effect on bone health include those in fish oil and evening primrose oil.[17]

To maximize your bone health, I recommend that you limit your intake of bone-depleting foods and drinks. Excesses of protein, sugar, refined carbohydrates, sodium, caffeinated beverages, chocolate, alcohol, and sodas can all impair your bone density by robbing your body of the minerals you need to have strong and healthy bones, and they can also adversely affect every other system in your body. It's okay to indulge in these kinds of foods and beverages once in a while—for example, when you are having dessert at a party. But don't eat as if every meal were a holiday feast.

As long as you eat a diet that provides your body with the tools it needs to create and maintain your bone density, you are building healthy bones for life.

PREVENTING AND TREATING OSTEOARTHRITIS WITH YOUR DIET

Maria told me that her arthritic symptoms started fifteen years ago. Back then her medical doctors prescribed anti-inflammatory drugs and told her that she would have to limit her activities due to the pain in her knees, hips, and feet. She said that for five years she took the anti-inflammatory medications even though she was always concerned about their side effects. Then she discovered fasting. "After four days on a vegetable juice fast," she said, "all my joint pain went away. This was a great discovery, but I knew that I couldn't eat only vegetables the rest of my life. I had to find answers."

When Maria first came to see me, I ordered several tests and found that she had abnormal intestinal flora and leaky gut syndrome resulting in multiple food allergies. I prescribed a month-long intestinal cleanse to heal her intestines. After her cleanse she continued to eat a healthier diet and follow other guidelines that I recommended to keep her bones healthy. Today, she says, "not only did this cleanse eliminate the pain, but many years later I'm still very athletic and free of joint pain. Now I can eat any food in moderation, and don't have to take anti-inflammatory drugs!"

Diet may be an important factor in preventing osteoarthritis because it appears to play a key role in the development of the condition. Dr. Norman Childers, Ph.D., of Rutgers University found that when some people with osteoarthritis avoided tomatoes, white potatoes, eggplant, and peppers (which are all in the nightshade family), they had a decrease in their joint pain.[18] If you suffer from osteoarthritis, you may need to remove these foods from your diet for several months before you begin to experience a decrease in symptoms; on the other hand, many of my patients who stopped eating these foods experienced noticeable relief in their osteoarthritis symptoms within only a few weeks.

I've also observed that when people eat a diet that is predominately acid-forming, they have increased joint pain, and when they eat a more alkaline-forming diet, their pain is decreased. (See Chapter 3 for more information on acid-forming and alkaline-forming foods.) It's not exactly clear why an acid-forming diet would increase joint pain, but it appears that the more acid-forming your diet is, the more calcium is pulled out of your bones. This mobilization of calcium may increase inflammation in your joints and initiate the formation of bone spurs. If you have osteoarthritis, I highly recommend that you decrease acid-forming foods in your diet and increase mineral-rich foods. You don't have to eliminate all acid-forming foods, just make sure that you are eating plenty of the alkaline-forming foods that are an essential part of your Naturally Healthy Diet.

Your diet can also affect your joints if you have food allergies and imbalanced intestinal flora. In Chapter 6 we saw how digestive health is critical to the health of the whole body; the joints are a good example of this. My patient Maria experienced a dramatic improvement in her health and cured her joint pain when she did an intestinal cleanse and changed her diet.

VITAMIN AND MINERAL SUPPLEMENTS FOR YOUR BONES

Many women today who are concerned about preventing osteoporosis take vitamin and mineral supplements in addition to eating a diet that supports healthy bones. By increasing your intake of certain nutrients, you guarantee that your body has the essential components it needs to build or maintain strong bones. Most of the research on supplements for bone health is centered on calcium and vitamin D, but many other vitamins and minerals are also important for bone health. Dr. Jonathan Wright, a well-known nutritionally oriented medical doctor, recommends additional doses of certain nutrients to help prevent and treat osteoporosis. The "Supplements for Bones" chart, which outlines the most important vitamin and mineral supplements for bone health, includes Dr. Wright's recommendations. Some of the nutrients listed are found in your multivitamin, but others you will need to take separately. Since most cases of osteoporosis occur in older women who may not assimilate their nutrients well, doses higher than those found in your multivitamin are often recommended to ensure absorption and help treat osteoporosis.

Calcium is one of the most important bone-building supplements you can take because it is the primary mineral that bones are made of. Your body needs to maintain a certain level of calcium in the blood at all times for the healthy function of the heart and other systems. If your diet doesn't supply you with enough calcium, or if you don't absorb your calcium very well due to low stomach acid or a vitamin D deficiency, your body in its wisdom will maintain your blood calcium level by taking calcium out of your bones. While in the short run your bones can absorb the loss, if it's

Supplements for Bones

NUTRIENT	PREVENTING OSTEOPOROSIS*	TREATING OSTEOPOROSIS*	HOW THIS NUTRIENT SUPPORTS YOUR BONE HEALTH
Calcium	1,200–1,500 mg	1,200–1,500 mg	Is the primary mineral that forms bones
Magnesium	500–800 mg	500–800 mg	Assists with normal calcium metabolism
Vitamin B_6	50 mg	50 mg	Can lower homocysteine level and may play a role in the manufacture of structural proteins in bone
Vitamin B_{12}	300 mcg	300 mcg	Can lower homocysteine level
Vitamin C	1,000 mg	1,000 mg	Is important in forming structural proteins in bone
Vitamin D	400 i.u.	800 i.u.	Signals intestines to absorb calcium when blood calcium level is low
Vitamin K_1†	300 mcg	5–10 mg	Is important for the production of osteocalcin, a protein that provides structure to bone tissue
Vitamin K_2†	Amount varies with the individual	45 mg	Prevents bone loss, reduces fracture risk, and improves bone density
Boron	2 mg	3–6 mg	Enhances the conversion of vitamin D to its active form
Folic Acid	800 mcg	1–3 mg	Reduces homocysteine level
Manganese	20 mg	20 mg	Is essential for the production of compounds that allow calcification to occur in bones
Zinc	40 mg	40 mg	Is necessary for the formation of osteoblasts and osteoclasts; enhances the action of vitamin D
Copper	2–3 mg	2–3 mg	Is important in the formation of connective tissue; helps maintain bone strength
Silicon	50 mg	100 mg	Is involved in the calcification of bone; plays a role in forming cartilage
Strontium	500 mcg	500–700 mg	Is involved in bone building and bone remodeling

*Daily doses recommended.

†Do not use vitamin K if you are on a blood-thinning drug such as warfarin or Coumadin. I don't recommend taking high doses of both forms of vitamin K at the same time. Ask your naturopathic physician for advice.

happening all the time your bones will become depleted of calcium, possibly resulting in the thinning of your bones (osteopenia), and eventually osteoporosis.

Calcium does not work in isolation to build or maintain your bones; it needs the support of other nutrients. The vitamins and minerals listed in the "Supplements for Bones" chart all work together to ensure that the bones are healthy. Some help lower the level of homocysteine, a compound that can increase the risk of osteoporosis, while others help your bones by stimulating proteins that play a role in bone remodeling.

The question of which calcium supplement is the best has been the subject of much debate. Calcium citrate may be one of the most effective types because it is more easily assimilated than other forms of calcium. Citrate is a chelating agent, which means that it binds to the calcium and enhances its absorption. In addition, citrate is more acidic than other chelating agents, which helps because you need to have adequate stomach acid in order to absorb your minerals. This makes calcium citrate a particularly good choice for older women who may have low stomach acid. Another bonus is that calcium citrate can inhibit the formation of kidney stones. (Calcium carbonate, by contrast, is very poorly absorbed, especially in older women who have low stomach acid, because it is not acidic. It may contribute to the formation of kidney stones and can be constipating.) If you have healthy digestion and adequate stomach acid (see Chapter 6), you can choose from other forms of chelated calcium, such as calcium lactate, calcium aspartate, calcium malate, or calcium succinate. For some people, these are easier on the stomach than calcium citrate.

Be aware that some calcium supplements have been found to be contaminated with lead, a toxic heavy metal.[19] A high level of lead in the body can cause anemia, hypertension, and brain and kidney damage. In children, it can result in stunted growth, increased aggressive behavior, and permanent mental impairment. I recommend that you avoid calcium supplements derived from dolomite, bone meal, or oyster shells, because they were found to have the highest levels of lead. Since an article published in the *Journal of the American Medical Association* in September 2000 reported that a substantial number of calcium products contained high levels of lead, many vitamin companies have screened for, and decreased, the amount of lead in their products.[20] I suggest that you contact the company that manufactures your calcium supplement and ask for a full disclosure of the lead content in their product, or look for the GMP (Good Manufacturing Practices) certification on the label. As we saw in Chapter 1, this certification, which is established by the National Nutritional Foods Association, indicates the supplement has been tested for quality and screened for contaminants.

Good News:
Vitamin K_2 Builds Healthy Bones!

Vitamin K_2 (menatetranone) may be one reason that Japanese women have a lower incidence of osteoporosis than women in other countries.[21] One of their traditional foods, a fermented soybean product called *natto*, has been found to contain unusually high amounts of vitamin K_2.[22] Research shows that this form of vitamin K may play a major role in bone health by preventing bone loss and reducing fracture risk.[23] In women with osteoporosis, vitamin K_2 may increase bone strength and has been found to prevent the recurrence of new fractures.[24]

Vitamin K_2 is produced in small amounts by your own intestinal bacteria, but as women get older they produce less vitamin K_2. You can obtain small amounts of vitamin

K_2 through your dietary intake of vitamin K_1, some of which is naturally converted to vitamin K_2 in the intestines. (Vitamin K_1 is found in leafy green vegetables and also plays a role in maintaining bone health.)

To make vitamin K_2 part of your bone-building plan, see if your favorite Japanese restaurant serves *natto,* or buy *natto* and try it at home. In Japan, *natto* is often eaten with chopped green onions, soy sauce, and mustard on rice. If you prefer, you can also take vitamin K_2 as a supplement; you may need to ask your naturopathic physician to order it for you.

STRONTIUM, THE NEW BONE-BUILDING MINERAL ON THE BLOCK

Strontium (not to be confused with the radioactive material known as strontium 90) is a naturally occurring mineral that was recently found to inhibit the breakdown of bone and stimulate the formation of new bone.[25] It is found in seafood, whole grains, legumes, and leafy vegetables. According to Dr. Jonathan Wright, both animal and human studies have demonstrated increases in bone density when strontium is given in fairly high doses.[26] An article published in the *New England Journal of Medicine* in January 2004 reported that two g of strontium ranelate a day decreased fracture risk and was effective in increasing bone density in postmenopausal women with osteoporosis. Bone density increases were significant; after three years of taking 2 g of strontium a day, these women's bone mineral density increased by 14.4 percent at the spine and 8.3 percent at the hip.[27] Because strontium ranelate is a semisynthetic patented form of strontium that is currently unavailable, Dr. Wright recommends using 681 mg of strontium citrate each day, which he says has been confirmed in other studies to be just as effective. For best absorption, avoid taking strontium with food or mineral supplements. See your naturopathic physician for a prescription.

HERBS FOR YOUR BONES

According to *Menopausal Years,* a delightful book by herbalist Susun Weed, drinking herbal teas high in mineral content can be beneficial to your bones. She recommends a daily infusion of horsetail, oat straw, and nettles. Horsetail is especially rich in silica, which can strengthen and regenerate connective tissue and help support your bones. Oat straw and nettles are recommended because of their calming effects on the nervous system; when you are calm, your body isn't pumping out stress hormones, which can ultimately wear down your bones. You can use these herbs on a daily basis, either separately or blended together. To vary the taste, you can add other herbs to the mixture such as peppermint, chamomile, and red raspberry.

In Chinese medicine, herbs have been used for thousands of years to support bones by building kidney Qi. Chinese herbal formulas used in the treatment of osteoarthritis can be helpful both for easing the symptoms and for addressing the underlying causes of the condition. Most herbal formulas that help with osteoarthritis are aimed at eliminating "wind," moving Qi, clearing "dampness," and dissipating cold. The herbal formula Du Huo Jisheng Wan (in English "Angelica Pubescentis and Loranthus Pill") is used to dispel "wind-cold" and dampness from the joints, strengthen Qi and Blood, and fortify kidney Qi. The dosage depends on the product, but the typical dose is nine pills twice a day. I recommend that you consult your Chinese medical practitioner for an herbal formula tailored to your specific needs.

Another method of decreasing pain associated with osteoarthritis—as well as easing joint pain due to sports injuries—is the use of Chinese herbal plasters. These plasters are like giant Band-Aids that have herbs embedded in them, which you apply to your skin and leave on for a few hours or longer. One plaster, known as Jewel and Gem Plaster, works by eliminating "wind-damp," moving Qi, and warming the meridians. (The meridians are the channels in which Qi courses through the body.) It contains a number of herbs, including camphor, wintergreen oil, and mint; when applied, it feels both hot and cold at the same time. Although you may be instructed to leave this plaster in place for a few days, I usually tell patients to remove it after twelve hours because I've seen people become allergic to the adhesive if they leave it on for too long.

Hormones and Your Bones

We saw in Chapter 7 that all your hormones work together to create health in every part of your body. The influence that your hormones have on your bones is no exception. For example, estrogen may stimulate the cells that lay down bone and inhibit the action of the cells that break down bone, while progesterone, testosterone, and DHEA are all potentially bone-building hormones. On the other hand, high levels of cortisol, the stress hormone, can decrease bone density over time. Thyroid hormones can also play an important role in your bone health.

ESTROGEN

Estrogen can help prevent bone loss, which is one of the main reasons some women have chosen to take it after menopause. Hormone levels drop after menopause, typically initiating a significant amount of bone loss that continues for at least five years. Estrogen has been one of the most commonly prescribed drugs to combat bone loss. Long-term therapy is necessary to experience the benefits, however; studies have shown that as soon as women stop taking estrogen, they begin losing bone mass at the same rate as if they'd never taken it. And not all women respond favorably to estrogen therapy. Some experience undesirable side effects such as weight gain, bloating, or headaches, and others continue to lose bone mass. And with research showing that estrogen replacement therapy can increase the risks of heart disease, stroke, breast cancer, and Alzheimer's disease, many women are reluctant to take it.

When estrogen is taken to prevent osteoporosis, lower-than-standard prescribed doses may be as effective in decreasing bone loss as higher doses. This is especially important for women who tolerate estrogen well but want to minimize its potential side effects by taking the lowest possible dose. The Women's HOPE (Health, Osteoporosis, Progestin, Estrogen) trial, sponsored by Wyeth Research in May 2002, demonstrated that early postmenopausal women were able to preserve their bone density with lower doses of hormones,[28] although the hormones used in the trial were Premarin (estrogen derived from the urine of pregnant horses) and synthetic progesterone. In another study, estriol—the weakest estrogen (and therefore considered to be the safest)—was found to increase bone density in senior women.[29]

Personally, I've witnessed with many patients over the years that low-dose natural estrogens such as Biest (80 percent estriol and 20 percent estradiol) or Triest (80 percent estriol, 10 percent estradiol, and 10 percent estrone) can have bone-preserving effects. (See Chapter 7 for more information on these estrogens.) Many of my patients take other natural hormones, such as progesterone and DHEA, that may work synergistically with estrogen to help maintain strong bones. And nearly all of the women who have come to see me with concerns about their bone health—whether they take hormones or not—are also engaged in comprehensive bone-building programs that include lifestyle and dietary factors.

PROGESTERONE

Progesterone can do many positive things for a woman's health, but one of the most controversial questions pertaining to progesterone is whether taking it in natural form can increase bone density. (Natural progesterone, as we saw in Chapter 7, is derived from soybeans or wild yams and is biologically identical to the progesterone your own body naturally produces.) In an article published in *Medical Hypotheses* in 1991, John Lee, M.D., proposed that natural progesterone, not estrogen, may be the most important hormone in helping to reverse osteoporosis.[30] He argued that women who already have osteoporosis could build bone by using progesterone on a cyclical basis that mimicked a normal menstrual cycle. Dr. Lee's theory, based on his own in-office observations of female patients who used natural progesterone, has spawned an entire industry of natural progesterone therapy with the aim of reversing osteoporosis.

For the past ten years, I have closely followed many patients with osteoporosis who have used natural progesterone, and I haven't seen the bone density increases that Dr. Lee says women will have if they follow his protocol. But I have seen that women can *decrease bone loss* by using a combination of natural estrogen and natural progesterone while practicing a bone-building diet and lifestyle. With more research on progesterone and bone health, these questions will probably be answered. In the meantime I think it's important to remember that all of your hormones work together, and that each plays a key role in maintaining your bone health—as well as the health of your entire body.

TESTOSTERONE

Testosterone is one of the most powerful bone-building hormones. One reason men are less prone than women to osteoporosis is that for most of their lives they have more of this hormone in their bodies. In women, most testosterone is released by the ovaries, and some is released by the adrenal glands. But most of the testosterone in your bloodstream is bound up with proteins, so that only one to three percent is available to act on your tissues. You can naturally increase your testosterone level by getting plenty of rest to support your adrenal glands' manufacture of testosterone, and by exercising regularly.

If you choose to take testosterone as part of your bone-building program, you should discuss your decision in detail with your health care provider. I recommend that you test your hormone level before and after beginning your treatment. If testosterone is administered in the right amount, you will be spared the symptoms of too much testosterone, such as acne, facial hair growth, and a lower voice.

DHEA

DHEA, secreted by your adrenal glands, is the most abundant steroid hormone in your body. Research has shown that DHEA plays an important role in bone health because it can stimulate the growth of new bone. It can also suppress the depletion of calcium from your bones.[31] As you age, your DHEA level drops; it has been documented that postmenopausal women have lower DHEA levels. In my practice, I've included DHEA supplementation as a part of an overall bone-building program in women who show deficient levels. For most women, a low dose of DHEA (5 to 10 mg a day) is recommended to obtain therapeutic effects.

CORTISOL

Cortisol is released by your body if you are under daily stress. When your cortisol level is chronically elevated, you are at higher risk for osteoporosis because cortisol decreases calcium absorption and contributes to bone loss. Reducing stress in your life helps keep your cortisol level under control and therefore your bones healthier. It is well known that taking strong pharmaceutical corticosteroids such as prednisone, or other drugs that are similar to your own body's cortisol, can significantly impair bone density; women who have taken these drugs for more than six months are at higher risk for osteoporosis.

THYROID HORMONES

Thyroid hormones also play an important role in bone health. Your body naturally creates certain amounts of thyroid hormones, but if your thyroid hormone levels are too high, you could lose bone faster than you can build it. Women with Graves' disease or Hashimoto's thyroiditis—hyperthyroid conditions that are associated with increased thyroid hormones—need to be extra vigilant about their bone health. Women who have taken too much thyroid hormone medication, over a long period of time, can also end up with thin, porous bones; it is essential to have your thyroid hormone levels periodically evaluated by your physician if you take thyroid medication.

Conversely, low thyroid hormone levels, or hypothyroidism, can cause poor-quality bones. According to Alan Gaby, M.D., author of *Preventing and Reversing Osteoporosis,* "Thyroid hormone is one of the triggers for the bone-remodeling cycle, which starts with bone resorption [bone breakdown] and is followed by new bone formation. If not enough thyroid hormone is present, old bone tends to accumulate—bone that is not necessarily strong or fracture-resistant."[32] Having the right levels of thyroid hormones in your body is important for your overall bone health. (See Chapter 7 for more information.)

Drugs for Your Bones?

In recent years, bone-building drugs known as biphosphonates, such as Fosamax and Actonel, have been developed for the purpose of increasing bone density. These drugs work by retaining old bone, rather than by stimulating the growth of new bone. In fact, they inhibit the action of osteoclasts (the cells that destroy old bone to make room for new bone growth). Biophosphonates are not without short-term and potential long-term consequences. Short-term side effects include ulcers in the stomach and esophagus, nausea, diarrhea, abdominal pain, back pain, and headaches. For some women, serious eye problems may be a long-term consequence of using biphosphonate drugs; there may be other long-term side effects that are not yet known because these drugs are so new.[33]

Given these concerns, do these drugs have a place in treatment for osteopenia or osteoporosis? Many women have been prescribed Fosamax and other biphosphonate drugs for this purpose, but according to Dr. Susan Love, "most experts are no longer recommending biphosphonates for women with osteopenia."[34] This is in part because we lack information about how long a woman can safely take them. According to Dr. Love, these drugs should be considered only for the treatment of osteoporosis or severe osteoporosis. The research shows that women with severe osteoporosis have a decrease in bone fractures within the first two to three years of treatment with Fosamax.[35] If you *don't* have osteoporosis, it's more prudent to approach your treatment with exercise, lifestyle and dietary changes, mineral supplementation, and if necessary, natural hormones.

Another class of relatively new drugs known as SERMs (selective estrogen receptive modulators), which includes the drug Evista, has shown promise in increasing bone density. But they too have multiple side effects, including hot flashes, leg cramps, and increased risk of blood clots. Animal studies have also raised a red flag that Evista might increase the risk of ovarian cancer.[36]

Other medications for the treatment of osteoporosis include Teriparatide, also known as Forteo. This drug, which is produced by Eli Lilly and has been approved by the FDA, is administered as a subcutaneous injection. Studies show that Forteo could increase bone density by stimulating osteoblasts (the cells that build bone). Since this is a relatively new drug, its potential long-term side effects are not yet known, but an animal study has indicated that the long-term risks may include bone cancer.[37] The researchers who conducted the animal study, which was funded by Lilly Research Laboratories, claim that it is not predictive of an increased risk of bone cancer in mature adult humans who take the drug for a limited period of time.

Interestingly, other research shows that women who take Forteo and who in the past have taken Fosamax to treat their osteoporosis have significantly less increases in bone density than women who have never taken Fosamax. The researchers conclude that previous treatment with Fosamax may lead to decreased mineralization of new bone.[38]

Regarding any of these drugs, your medical doctor will most likely prescribe what he or she thinks is best, but the decision is ultimately yours. Today we don't know what the long-term effects of taking drugs such as Fosamax, Actonel, Evista, or Forteo will be on your bones or on your health. While modern medicine continues to search for effective ways to reduce the pain and suffering associated with osteoporosis, it is important that you do everything in your power to maintain your natural bone health. With regular exercise and the Naturally Healthy Diet, you can build healthy bones every day of your life.

Preventing and Treating Osteoarthritis with Nutritional Supplements

A seasonal skier, Connie had traveled from Hawaii to Lake Tahoe every winter for many years to enjoy some deep powder. At sixty-three she was in great physical shape, and she looked forward to having more time to ski and travel after her retirement. But the osteoarthritis she had developed in her in knees was becoming increasingly painful. Her knees were stiff in the morning, and as she put it, they felt "creaky." She wondered whether skiing would only put more stress on her already irritated knees.

When Connie came to see me, she wanted to know if natural medicine could help her. I told her the good news: yes—absolutely! After a few months of taking supplements to re-build her cartilage and decrease the inflammation, along with modifying her diet, she reported that her knees felt vastly improved. That winter Connie had a great time on the slopes, and she has returned to Lake Tahoe every year since.

In Western medicine, osteoarthritis is usually treated with nonsteroidal anti-inflammatory drugs (NSAIDs). While these drugs help decrease the pain and inflammation associated with osteoarthritis, they do nothing to repair cartilage, and they may even accelerate erosion of cartilage. In addition, they have numerous side effects, including stomach ulcers, heartburn, and kidney damage. Newer NSAIDs may have less serious side effects on the stomach lining, but they can increase blood pressure in some people and may have other dire effects on the cardiovascular system, including strokes and heart attacks. (Commonly prescribed NSAIDs, including Vioxx, have come under intense scrutiny for these reasons.)

The good news is that there are a number of nutritional supplements that can help prevent or treat osteoarthritis. These include glucosamine sulfate, chondroitin sulfate, SAM-e, fish oil, and niacinamide. Some of these supplements help to rebuild cartilage, while others are natural anti-inflammatories with minimal side effects that help to increase joint mobility.

GLUCOSAMINE SULFATE AND CHONDROITIN SULFATE

These supplements are at the top of the list for women who suffer from osteoarthritis. They help to rebuild damaged cartilage by increasing the synthesis of proteoglycans in cartilage. (Proteoglycans give cartilage its strength and resiliency.) Numerous studies show that people who take glucosamine and chondroitin sulfate for osteoarthritis have reduced joint pain and tenderness, decreased swelling, and increased range of motion. There are no serious side effects associated with these compounds except for rare cases of mild digestive upset. For treating osteoarthritis, the recommended dose of glucosamine sulfate is 500 mg three times a day, and for chondroitin sulfate 400 mg three times a day. Expect to take these medicines for at least six weeks before you begin to experience the benefits.

SAM-e (S-adenosylmethionine)

SAM-e has been used in Europe for decades for the treatment of depression and more recently was found in clinical trials to decrease joint pain and inflammation. In the United States, researchers have found that SAM-e is as effective as NSAIDs in reducing pain and improving joint function in patients with osteoarthritis, without the side effects associated with those drugs.[39] SAM-e works in much the same way that glucosamine sulfate and chondroitin sulfate work—by increasing proteoglycan synthesis in cartilage.

My only hesitation in prescribing SAM-e to patients is that it is quite expensive; a therapeutic dose can cost from $2 to $4 a day. I don't prescribe it when more affordable products like glucosamine and chondroitin will do the trick. For women who have joint pain as well as depression, however, SAM-e may just be what they need to solve both problems at once. The recommended dose of SAM-e for treating osteoarthritis is 600 mg a day for two weeks, followed by 400 mg a day on a regular basis. Be sure that you purchase high-quality SAM-e; tests have found that not all products sold in the United States contain the amount of SAM-e on the label. Look for the GMP (Good Manufacturing Practices) certification.

Fish Oil

Fish oil can benefit your body in many ways, and its anti-inflammatory properties can help prevent and treat osteoarthritis. Studies show the omega 3 fats found in fish oil have a significant impact on decreasing inflammatory compounds in cartilage.[40] The recommended dose for treating osteoarthritis is 2.6 g a day of omega 3 fats. Make sure that the company you buy your fish oil from guarantees that they've removed all heavy metals and other toxins from their products. (See Appendix B for resources.)

Niacinamide

Niacinamide is a form of niacin, or vitamin B_3. More than fifty years ago niacinamide was shown in studies to have benefits in the treatment of osteoarthritis, and current research suggests that it can decrease the progression of osteoarthritis.[41] Niacinamide is much safer than niacin, which can be toxic to the liver in high amounts. But high doses of niacinamide may still cause some liver problems, so it should not be used if you have liver disease. It is recommended that you take sustained-release niacinamide because the vitamin is quickly broken down by the body. The recommended dose for treating osteoarthritis with niacinamide is 500 mg three times a day.

Building Healthy Bones for Life: Final Thoughts

As we've seen in this chapter, there are many ways to build healthy bones and support your joints, from both a Western and a Chinese medicine standpoint. If you have concerns about osteoporosis, you can use the principles of natural medicine to prevent or treat it. Many natural options are also available to you for preventing, treating, and even reversing osteoarthritis, without resorting to the use of anti-inflammatory drugs so often prescribed for the condition in Western medicine—and without worrying about their side effects.

Your bones are a powerful and dependable part of your body. Using the tools described in this chapter—including exercise, diet, natural medicine, and lifestyle choices—you can turn the fear of fragile bones and chronic joint problems into bone-building action and freedom from pain.

The Essence of Chapter 8

- Be aware that your bones are dynamic living tissues that go through many stages in your lifetime.
- Evaluate the health of your bones with DEXA testing and other methods.
- Support your bone health by nurturing your kidney Qi and kidney Essence, and by keeping your element balanced.
- Exercise on a regular basis to build your bones and keep them strong.
- Consume foods and drinks that give your body the tools it needs to maintain your bone density.
- Prevent and treat osteoarthritis with vitamin and mineral supplements, exercise, diet, and natural medicine.
- Understand the role that your hormones play in building and maintaining healthy bones.
- Remember that your bones are a powerful and resilient part of your body that can stay strong and healthy for life.

Chapter 9

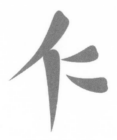

Benevolence

Creating Optimal Breast Health

"We smile knowingly; we know our breasts contain a power that is resilient,
flexible, supple, easy, and impossible to restrain. Whether the whim of
fashion says our breasts are to be large, small, pointed, or flattened, with
cleavage or without, padded or bound, accented or obscured, it matters not
to us. Our breasts fall free, untouched by current notions. The power of our
breasts is the power of life."

—SUSUN WEED, *Breast Cancer? Breast Health!*

*J*ESSICA CAME *to see me because she had a dense mass in her breast that often became*
very painful before her period. She had been dealing with this pain for years, and had
sought out the help of many health professionals who confirmed through clinical exams and
ultrasounds that her breast mass was due to fibrocystic changes. She felt that her breast
pain—which seemed to fluctuate depending on what she ate or her emotional stress level—
was her body's way of alerting her when she made unhealthy lifestyle choices.

Jessica was right; her breast pain was part of the larger picture of her overall health.
From a naturopathic perspective, it appeared that Jessica had low thyroid hormones and too
much estrogen. From a Chinese perspective, it was apparent that she suffered from stagnant

liver Qi, especially prior to her periods. After employing both medical traditions, Jessica's breast pain decreased considerably. As a result, she was inspired to become a breast massage specialist, so that she could share holistic ways to support breast health and help many other women with similar concerns. "My personal journey with breast pain," she says, "has turned into my passion for life."

✍

Your Breast Health

Your breasts are involved in many of the most intimate roles in your life. In adolescence your breasts awakened you to your changing body as it was taking on the shape of a woman. In your fertile years, your breasts may swell with each menstrual cycle or with pregnancy and, if you breast-feed, give forth life-sustaining milk. Your breasts respond to stimulation, and when aroused, your nipples harden and your areolas change color. Your breasts represent a safe haven for those you welcome into your arms, hug closely, and comfort. They lie over your heart, as if they were the guardians of your capacity for love and desire. In all these ways, your breasts are deeply connected to your femininity, compassion, and sensuality. In this chapter, we will explore how you can keep your breasts in optimal health through all the seasons of your life.

Creating a plan to optimize breast health will ultimately benefit your entire body. Problems that arise in your breasts are usually not isolated events but the result of imbalances elsewhere in your body. For instance, if you tend to develop breast cysts or have breast tenderness associated with premenstrual syndrome, you may have a hormone imbalance. If you are diagnosed with breast cancer or a precancerous condition, your whole body is involved in the process of manifesting abnormal cells. In Chinese medicine, the entire body is always taken into account when assessing health; breast cysts or breast tenderness associated with PMS are most likely to be diagnosed as an imbalance in spleen Qi and liver Qi. In all of these cases, it's important to discover the cause of the underlying imbalance and make changes that will prevent problems from recurring.

The health of your breasts can have an enormous impact on your overall health. Breast cancer is the most common type of cancer among women in the United States, and for the past two decades the incidence has been on the rise. The statistics are daunting; according to the National Cancer Institute, one in eight women who live to be eighty years of age will be diagnosed with the disease.

This chapter is especially for women who want to take measures to create optimal breast health. It will outline how the Naturally Healthy Diet and Lifestyle, along with specific nutritional and herbal supplements, can help you maintain the health of your breasts. It will delineate the ways that you can prevent and treat breast cysts and other breast conditions. You will discover tests to evaluate your estrogen levels and recommendations for breast cancer screening. And it will provide you with the tools you need to decrease the odds that you will be diagnosed with breast cancer, and map out steps you can take to help prevent a future recurrence of the disease, if applicable.

The View from the West

Your breasts are comprised of fat, arteries, veins, nerves, and lymph vessels. Each one consists of fifteen to twenty-five lobes containing milk-producing glands and milk ducts, along with connective tissue that holds everything in place. Breast size, shape, and nipple color vary considerably from woman to woman. Your nipples may be in the center of your breasts, or perhaps they point slightly to the side, which may assist with breast-feeding. Some women have nipples that protrude outward, while others have inverted nipples. Nipples can vary in color from pink to dark brown to nearly black. Your nipples may have small bumps on them, known as Montgomery's glands, or hair on or around them, both of which are perfectly natural. The images of women's breasts you see in magazines are often an artificial idealized version of how breasts should look. Your breasts are perfect in their natural state, regardless of whether they resemble the breasts on a touched-up photo of a model. Taking the time to do regular breast self-exams will allow you to become acquainted with the shape and unique qualities of your own breasts.

Your breasts respond to hormonal cues throughout your lifetime. During puberty, hormones stimulated your breast tissue to develop, and your body began to experience an ebb and flow of estrogen and progesterone that affected your breasts on a monthly basis. With every menstrual cycle, your breast size changes; right before your period your breasts may be larger and feel tender. Estrogen in particular can increase your breast size by increasing cell division in your breast tissue. While pregnant, your body begins to release the hormone prolactin in preparation for breast-feeding. Another hormone, oxytocin, is released when you start breast-feeding, which allows for the delivery of milk to the nipples. After menopause, when your hormone levels have dropped significantly, your breast size diminishes and your breast tissue becomes more flaccid.

The View from the East

"The Blood descends and becomes the menstruate;
it ascends and becomes the milk."

—HONORA LEE WOLFE AND BOB FLAWS,
Better Breast Health Naturally with Chinese Medicine

In Chinese medicine, the breasts are closely associated with the uterus, and both are related to Qi and Blood. (As we saw in Chapter 7, a healthy menstrual cycle is dependent on a steady flow of Qi and a surplus of Blood.) If you have an imbalance in the production or flow of Qi or Blood, you may have imbalances in your menstrual cycle as well as abnormalities in your breasts. Qi and Blood can determine every aspect of breast health, affecting changes in your breasts through your menstrual cycles, during breast feeding, and after menopause.

Qi and Blood, as you've discovered, are regulated by the liver and spleen. (Liver Qi is in charge of keeping Qi flowing, and spleen Qi is responsible for making Blood.) For this reason liver Qi and spleen Qi are frequently addressed when treating breast problems.

You need a surplus of Qi and Blood in order to produce milk if you are breast-feeding. If you've had a long, difficult labor resulting in profuse loss of body fluids, you are apt to have scanty breast milk, because the source of breast milk is Blood. Emotional frustration, anger, or worry can also lead to reduced milk flow because these emotions cause your liver Qi to stagnate, resulting in an obstruction of the flow of Qi to your breasts.

If you are perimenopausal, your flow of Qi and Blood is shifting upward, away from your uterus, toward your heart to nourish your spirit. Instead of moving downward toward the earth to provide for your children, your Qi and Blood now rise to feed your soul in order for you to become the wise woman of your family and community. According to Chinese medicine, breast problems associated with hormone imbalances during perimenopause will disappear when your Qi and Blood are able to make this transition smoothly. If your Qi becomes stagnant due to frustration, worry, or excessive stress, you are more likely to develop breast problems including cysts and cancer.

Tests for Breasts, and What You Need to Know About Breast Cancer

Although no one knows exactly what causes breast cancer, excessive exposure to estrogen over the course of a woman's lifetime is universally accepted as one of the contributing factors. Estrogen played a role in the development of your breasts when you were a teenager, and throughout your life it continues to stimulate estrogen-sensitive cells in your breasts to replicate themselves. Excessive estrogen exposure can contribute to cancer because when these cells are stimulated to divide, there can be "mistakes" in the translation of genetic material from one cell to another, which can lead to uncontrolled cell division, eventually resulting in tumors.

The following are some of the most important risk factors for breast cancer, according to the American Cancer Society. Some have to do with family history, because the genes you received from your parents may make your cells more susceptible to abnormal growth and cell division in your breast tissue; others pertain to dietary and lifestyle issues and to lifetime exposure to estrogen.

RISK FACTORS FOR BREAST CANCER

- A family history of relatives who have had breast cancer
- A personal history of breast cancer in one breast
- Radiation treatment to your chest earlier in life
- An abnormal breast biopsy
- Onset of menstruation before age twelve
- End of menstruation after age fifty
- No full-term pregnancies
- First full-term pregnancy after age thirty
- HRT taken for more than five consecutive years
- Current use of birth control pills (The research is still inconclusive, but it suggests a link between breast cancer and the use of birth control pills.)
- A diet high in fat, especially from red meat
- Regular consumption of alcohol
- Obesity, especially after menopause

Your Odds of Having Breast Cancer by Age Group

From age 30 to 40	*1 out of 252*
From age 40 to 50	*1 out of 68*
From age 50 to 60	*1 out of 35*
From age 60 to 70	*1 out of 27*
From age 70 to 80	*1 out of 8*
Ever	*1 out of 8*

Source: National Cancer Institute[1]

While you can't change your genetic inheritance, you may be able to prevent undesirable genes from becoming activated. On the other hand, even if you are not at all genetically predisposed to breast cancer, certain environmental and dietary factors may cause your risk to be elevated. Breast cancer is increasingly being diagnosed in women who have no family history of the disease.

Environment clearly plays a greater role in the development of breast cancer than was once generally believed. Women who have lived in countries with a low incidence of breast cancer appear to develop the same risk for breast cancer as Western women when they move to Western countries that have a high incidence of breast cancer. Research also shows that Japanese women have a low incidence of breast cancer overall, yet those who live in urban areas have a much higher rate of breast cancer than those who live in rural areas.[2]

From a naturopathic perspective, breast cancer has more risk factors than those that appear on the American Cancer Society's list. These include high exposure to environmental chemicals, the standard American diet, an inactive lifestyle, and poor breakdown and elimination of estrogen.

BREAST SELF-EXAM

One of the best tools for monitoring your breast health is literally right at your fingertips. When you do a breast self-exam (BSE), you learn the unique language of your breast tissue. The more familiar you become with your breast tissue, the more precisely you can detect subtle changes that your health care provider may not find with the same method. After all, your health care provider may see you only once every several months and may not be able to remember exactly what your normal breast tissue feels like. But by doing your own BSE at least once a month, you can reassure yourself that your breast tissue feels normal—or know that it should be further evaluated by your health care provider.

The key to a successful BSE is consistency of technique. (See the instructions on page 275.) If you are unsure how to do a BSE, first have your health care provider do one with you, and ask questions while you are examining each area of your breasts. Though women are sometimes advised to do their BSE in the shower with soap, I find that the shower itself is distracting and that this method leads to inconsistency. I recommend that you do your BSE when you are lying on your back in bed. This way you are motionless, your mind is quiet, and you can really focus on what your fingers are feeling. Using lotion or oil may help you feel changes in your breasts more easily, and you can mix in essential oils, like lavender and rose, to aid circulation or simply to create a more relaxing experience.

What are you looking for while you are doing a BSE? If your breasts feel somewhat lumpy, like a bag of grapes, this can be normal, but distinct, well-defined lumps require further attention. Lumps that are benign usually feel soft, they move some-what freely when you push them from side to side, and they can be either painless or painful. Lumps that feel hard, are fixed to the tissue around them, and are usually painless may be precancerous or cancerous. Most health care providers can show you a silicone model of a breast that can help you distinguish between a soft cyst that is typically benign and a hard lump that is more likely to be cancerous. If you find any-thing unusual or detect any changes in your breast tissue during your BSE, such as new breast lumps, nipple retraction, or breast tissue dimpling, see your health care provider right away.

Some women find that a breast self-examination pad can be a useful tool to as-sist in their BSE. The pad, which is filled with silicone and lies flat over your breast, helps you feel more clearly the underlying structures of your breast tissue. It can be purchased through your health care provider.

You can also follow up your BSE by visually examining your breasts. The best way to do this is to stand in front of a mirror and look carefully at your breasts while you are in the following four positions: with your arms relaxed at your sides, with your hands pressing firmly into your hips to contract your chest muscles, with your arms raised over your head, and bending forward so that your breasts hang straight downward. Look closely for any changes in your breasts such as bulges, dimples, swelling, flattening, or retraction of tissue or nipples. (Remember that most women's breasts are not identical; often one will be larger than the other.) In order to be able to detect any changes, you have to be familiar with the way your breasts normally look, so it's a good idea to do this visual examination often.

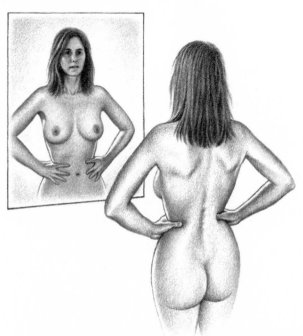

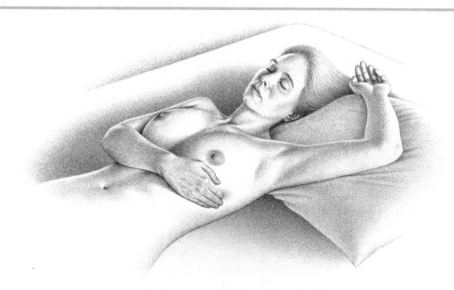

Step-by-Step Instructions for Breast Self-Exam

1. Lie down in a comfortable position with one arm over your head. To help flatten out your breast tissue, place a pillow under your shoulder on the side that you are about to examine.
2. Apply lotion or oil to your breast tissue and armpit.
3. Begin to gently feel your breast tissue with the pads of your fingers, starting near your armpit.
4. Move your fingers slowly from your underarm area toward your nipple, and then move them outward again toward the periphery of your breast, feeling for any lumps or other changes in shape or texture of your breast tissue. Next, move your fingers a quarter-inch downward, and again move your fingers toward your nipple and back out again. Repeat this pattern, circling your breast, until you've covered the entire area of your breast tissue.
5. Feel the area of your armpit and above your collarbone for any enlarged lymph nodes that feel like lumps.
6. Press straight down around the outline of your nipple, then press down on the center of your nipple; gently squeeze your nipple to see if there is any discharge.
7: Repeat these steps with your other breast.

There are many additional ways of evaluating breast health with screening tests for breast cancer. These include mammograms, ultrasound, and thermography, a relatively new type of breast screening. All these tests can be a part of your self-care; let's look at the pros and cons of each method.

MAMMOGRAPHY

Mammograms, which are detailed X-rays of breast tissue, are commonly used as a screening test for breast cancer. But according to Dr. Susan Love, author of *Dr. Susan Love's Hormone Book,* they are able to detect early breast cancer only about 30 percent of the time.[3] If you are premenopausal or take hormone replacement therapy, mammograms may be even less reliable because hormones make your breasts denser, which makes it more difficult for a mammogram to detect breast cancer in its early stages. Another problem with mammograms is that they expose women's breasts to small amounts of radiation, which over time accumulates in the body and may contribute to breast cancer.

Despite their shortcomings, mammograms can be a valuable tool. They are the standard of care, are widely available, and are covered by insurance. And even if they catch early breast cancer only 30 percent of the time, that is still much better than learning nothing 100 percent of the time without the test. According to the American Cancer Society, when breast cancer is detected and treated early, survival after treatment is 96.3 percent. Although mammograms are no guarantee that an early-stage breast cancer will be found, the American Cancer Society recommends that you begin annual mammogram screenings at age forty. If you have a strong family history of breast cancer, it's a good idea to begin screening at a younger age, and if you have any new breast lumps, you are advised to have a mammogram regardless of your age.

ULTRASOUND FOR BREASTS

An ultrasound is typically ordered if a mammogram has detected a breast lump or other abnormality, or if a patient has a palpable lump that a mammogram did not detect. In addition, some doctors are using ultrasound as a method to screen for early breast cancer in younger women whose breast tissue is so dense that mammograms are relatively inaccurate, although this has not yet become standard practice.

Ultrasound works by sending sound waves into the breast tissue to gather information about the nature of the lump. If the sound waves bounce back, the lump is likely solid (which is more indicative of cancer); if not, the lump is likely fluid-filled (which usually means it is a benign cyst).

BREAST THERMOGRAPHY

Breast thermography is a new way of evaluating breast tissue that involves taking a digital photograph of the heat patterns in a woman's breasts after her body temperature has been lowered (usually by being in a cold room for a brief period of time). Thermography relies on the fact that there is increased blood flow to tumors, and thermographic imaging picks up the heat generated by this increased blood flow. Proponents of thermography claim that increased blood flow to a woman's breasts may be a warning sign for breast cancer. But thermography simply measures levels of heat in breast tissue. Not all cancers release enough heat to show up on a thermograph; they may be too small or too deep in the chest wall to release heat. In addition, heat may be generated in a woman's breasts for reasons unrelated to cancer. For example, localized infections can create hot spots in breast tissue.

While thermography is not an extremely expensive test, usually between $175 and $250 per session, I have concerns for now about the accuracy of thermography for detecting breast cancer. If women rely solely on this method of testing, early-stage breast cancers may go undetected, with serious consequences. If you choose to use breast thermography, I recommend that you use other methods of evaluating your breast health as well.

A Hormone Test for Breasts

After having a small early-stage tumor removed from her breast, Sandra wanted to know how naturopathic medicine could help prevent a recurrence of breast cancer and enhance her overall health. She said she didn't want to take tamoxifen, a drug commonly prescribed after a woman has had estrogen-stimulated breast cancer.

Sandra was happy to learn of the existence of a test that could tell her if she was producing the kind of estrogen that could increase the potential for cancer. "I'm surprised that my medical doctor hasn't ordered this test," she said. "It seems like it should be a routine part of cancer prevention." Sandra's test results showed that her body was producing an excess of "unfriendly" pro-carcinogenic estrogen. I prescribed a diet and specific supplements to promote healthy estrogen metabolism. Three months later her follow-up test results showed that the treatment had worked. "My body was making less of the 'unfriendly' estrogen," she points out, "and more of the 'friendly' estrogen that can help prevent breast cancer."

Estrogen plays an important role in the development of most cases of breast cancer. Your naturopathic physician can order an estrogen metabolism test, which measures hormones in urine and can tell you a lot about how well you metabolize and break down estrogen. When you are healthy, estrogen is broken down in your liver in preparation for its removal from your body. At this point, it can be altered to become either "friendly" or "unfriendly." If estrogen is friendly, it acts somewhat like an antioxidant, helping to protect your tissues from damage. But unfriendly estrogen has a strong tendency to stimulate estrogen-sensitive cells, which can contribute to the development of abnormal cells. Thus high levels of unfriendly estrogen can lead to a high risk for estrogen-related cancers.

Unfriendly estrogen can form if you have nutrient deficiencies or stores of environmental toxins that alter your liver's function. Unfriendly estrogen can also convert into compounds called quinines that may attack and alter your DNA (especially that of estrogen-sensitive cells, such as those found in your breast tissue) and lead to uncontrolled cell growth. As we will see in the following section, a number of supplements can greatly enhance your liver's ability to create friendly estrogen. The estrogen metabolism test tracks the friendly and unfriendly estrogens listed in the diagram.

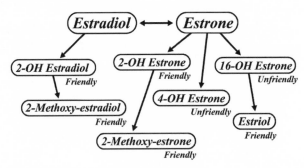

The breakdown of estrogens (Estradiol and Estrone)
into "friendly" and "unfriendly" forms

DIAGNOSING BREAST PROBLEMS FROM THE EAST

In Chinese medicine, all breast illnesses are related and part of the same continuum. As we will see throughout this chapter, most breast conditions are treated in Chinese medicine by nurturing spleen Qi and liver Qi. When your spleen Qi is abundant and your liver Qi is moving freely, you will have healthy breasts.

From the standpoint of the Five Element system, women who are Wood or Earth types may be more likely than others to manifest breast problems since they are especially prone to Qi and Blood imbalances. This is because the Wood element is associated with the liver, and liver Qi regulates the flow of Qi, and the Earth element is associated with the spleen, and spleen Qi creates Blood. At the same time, every woman is influenced by each of the elements, so imbalances in Qi and Blood can affect breast health, regardless of Element type.

Being Proactive in Creating Breast Health

There's a tremendous amount that you can do to create optimal breast health and help prevent breast cancer. Most important, you can minimize your exposure to environmental toxins, follow the Naturally Healthy Lifestyle and Diet, avoid taking hormones (including birth control pills) for any long duration, and encourage your body's breakdown and elimination of estrogen. Because Chinese medicine dictates that breast problems, including breast cancer, are the result of chronic liver Qi stagnation (due to long-term stress, emotional frustration, and toxins) and spleen Qi deficiency, treatment is focused on keeping liver Qi freely flowing through the body and strengthening spleen Qi.

YOUR ENVIRONMENT

The environment of your ancestors was very different from the one you live in today. The number of chemicals that have been dumped into the water, air, and land is staggering. All hope is not lost, however; the day-to-day choices you make can have an enormous impact on your exposure to potential cancer-causing agents. As you read on, remember that when it comes to your environment, you have the power to make healthy choices.

What exactly does the environment have to do with breast health? There has been a long-standing debate on the subject; some studies show a direct relationship between environmental chemicals and breast cancer, while others show none at all. One group of environmental chemicals, known as *hormone-disruptors,* is causing particular concern. These chemicals mimic estrogen in the body and can stimulate estrogen-sensitive cells, increasing the rate at which they multiply. The more these cells multiply, the greater the chance that an abnormal cell could multiply and grow into a cancerous tumor.

Researchers speculate that there may be more than a simple cause-and-effect relationship at work, and that the timing of exposure may be just as important as the extent of exposure.[4] For instance, women may be at increased risk of developing breast cancer later in life if they were exposed to high levels of estrogen-mimicking compounds when their bodies were rapidly maturing during their adolescent and teenage years. And a pregnant woman's exposure to estrogen-mimicking compounds may influence the risk that her unborn fetus will eventually develop breast cancer as an adult.[5]

One of the more notorious hormone-disruptors in the environment is the pesticide and insecticide DDT. Although DDT was banned in the United States in the early 1970s, it continues to be used extensively in other countries, and products imported into the United States may be contaminated with DDT. According to Charles Simone, M.D., author of *Breast Health,* the 1994 General Agreement on Tariffs and Trade allows imported produce to have significantly greater pesticide residues than American produce. Dr. Simone points out that levels of DDT much higher than U.S. standards are permitted on some fruits and vegetables sold in American markets.[6]

Other hormone-disruptors commonly found in the environment include DDE (which is formed when DDT breaks down), dioxin (from municipal and medical waste incinerators), atrazine (an herbicide frequently used on corn), the plastic by-product bisphenol-A, the plastic additive nonylphenol, and some compounds in gasoline.[7] In addition to being found in pesticides, hormone-disruptors are also found in paints, paper products, wood preservatives, lawn and pest products, and textiles. A study published in the *Journal of Occupational and Environmental Medicine* in 2003 found that women diagnosed with breast cancer had higher levels of the estrogen-mimicking, hormone-disrupting compounds DDT and HCB (hexachlorobenzene) in their blood.[8]

Hormone-disruptors are found all over the planet, from the north and south poles to your living room and bedroom, and it takes many years for most of them to break down into less toxic forms. For instance, when DDT breaks down to DDE, it takes at least thirty years for it to be eliminated from the environment.[9] Most hormone-disruptors are also fat-soluble, which means that they are stored in fat. This is very significant for breast health, because breasts are comprised of a high amount of fatty tissue. According to Dr. Simone, women are at greater risk from pesticides than men because the federal government's Allowable Daily Intake for pesticides is based on the tolerance of a 154-pound man, not a 110-pound woman with more fatty breast tissue.[10]

The good news is that you can minimize your exposure to hormone-disrupting compounds, and you can encourage their release from your fatty tissues through regular detoxification. To decrease your exposure to these chemicals, buy organic foods (you may be exposed to hormone-disruptors on a daily basis when you ingest nonorganic foods), limit your intake of foods and drinks packaged in plastic (including bottled water), minimize chemical use in your home and yard, choose all-natural cleaning agents, and use a water filter. (See Chapter 4 for more information on detoxification and removing toxins from your environment, and Chapter 3 for information on water filters.)

YOUR DIET

By choosing to follow the Naturally Healthy Diet (outlined in Chapter 1), you can keep your entire body healthy and vital. But in regard to your breasts, there's even more you can do. It has been suggested that diet may account for as much as 35 percent of all cancers,[11] and although no single food can prevent or cause breast cancer, it appears that a number of foods offer a measure of protection. I call these foods Best Breast Foods because of their unusual ability to nurture and support breasts.

For example, some foods help bind up estrogen or assist in its breakdown and elimination from the body, and others may promote breast health by blocking estrogen receptors on cells. In addition, many breast-friendly foods are loaded with nutrients and antioxidants that can help prevent cancer cells from developing into full-blown tumors. A review published by the Cancer Prevention Research Program at the Fred Hutchinson Research Center reports that at almost every stage in the development of cancer, beneficial plant chemicals known as phytochemicals have been reported to inhibit the likelihood of further development of the disease.[12]

Let's explore your Best Breast Foods, and see how each can help you optimize your breast health.

Fruits and Vegetables

Fruits and vegetables are powerhouses of nutrition, chock full of vitamins and minerals that play many roles in preventing the initiation and progression of cancer. The American Cancer Society recommends eating at least five servings of fruits and vegetables a day, and I recommend at least ten a day. (See Chapter 1.) In addition to increasing your overall health and vitality, there is little doubt that emphasizing fruits and vegetables in your diet can only optimize your breast health.

Cruciferous vegetables contain indole-3-carbinol (I3C), a potent anticancer compound that can have a profound effect on estrogen metabolism; it helps your body make the "friendly" estrogen by assisting your liver. The most commonly eaten cruciferous vegetables are broccoli, cabbage, cauliflower, kale, radishes, turnips, watercress, bitter cress, bok choy, brussels sprouts, collard greens, and horseradish. Eat plenty of these foods raw or cooked, but be aware that cooking at very high temperatures can destroy I3C.

Soy

Soy products should be a part of every woman's plan for creating optimal breast health. Among its many positive qualities, soy contains compounds that can block estrogen receptors, inhibit enzymes that can induce cancer, and act as antioxidants. For most women, consuming soy products like tofu, tempeh, and soy milk on a regular basis is a smart way to help prevent breast cancer.

A number of studies, however, have questioned whether soy is beneficial or harmful for women who have had breast cancer. Soy may slightly increase estrogen levels, resulting in increased stimulation of estrogen-sensitive cells. For women who have had the type of breast cancer that is stimulated by estrogen (known as *estrogen-receptive positive* breast cancer), ingesting a lot of soy may not be advisable. In addition, a compound found in soy known as genistein, when extracted from soy and taken in isolation, has been found in animal studies to stimulate proliferation of breast cancer cells. I recommend that my patients who are trying to prevent breast cancer eat soy three to four times a week, and those who have had estrogen-receptive positive breast cancer limit their soy intake to one serving a week. I also advise all women to avoid ingesting genistein in supplements or candy bars (although it appears that genistein, when ingested in whole soy foods, is safe).

OMEGA 3 FATS

Omega 3 fats, which are found in flax and fish oil, are important for optimizing breast health. When you ingest significant quantities of these quality fats, they become incorporated into the fat cells in your breasts, where they may help to protect you from a number of breast problems. Studies have found that omega 3 fats can stop breast cancer cell growth,[13] and that women with a lower rate of breast cancer have ingested high amounts of these fats. Animal studies have also been impressive, demonstrating that the omega 3 fats in fish oil inhibit breast tumor growth. You can use flax oil in your salad dressing or take it in capsule form. Cold-water fish, including salmon, contain high amounts of omega 3 fats, and you can also take fish oil capsules.

Greenland Eskimo women who ingest high amounts of omega 3 fats in their traditional diet have significantly lower levels of breast cancer than other women. Interestingly, they get their high levels of omega 3 fats from sea mammals that also contain high levels of "hormone-disrupting" chemicals (which are potentially cancer-causing).[14] This suggests that omega 3 fats may put the brakes on certain deleterious effects these chemicals might otherwise have.

FLAXSEEDS

Flaxseeds not only provide you with flax oil, they also contain high amounts of plant compounds called lignans. Lignans are converted by the digestive system into enterolactone and enterodiol, which protect you against breast cancer by blocking the effects of estrogen and making it less available to your cells. Studies have shown that women who have higher amounts of lignans in their diet have a reduced risk of breast cancer.[15] There are plenty of great ways to ingest these small but powerful seeds for creating optimal breast health. You can grind them up and add them to your cereal, blend them into your smoothies, or sprinkle them on your vegetables.

FIBER

Fiber is an important category of food for breast health; high-fiber diets are associated with lower estrogen levels. After your liver processes estrogen, it is eliminated through your stool. If you don't have enough fiber, you can become constipated, which results in estrogen being reabsorbed through your large intestine and returned to your circulation. To promote optimal breast health, boost your intake of fiber by increasing the fruits, vegetables, and whole grains in your diet.

GREEN TEA

Green tea contains polyphenols, which help stop free radicals in their tracks. Free radicals can damage your DNA and lead to genetic mutations and cancer. Polyphenols may also directly interfere with cancer cells themselves by attacking their energy-producing factories (mitochondria), resulting in their death. To avoid caffeine, drink decaffeinated green tea.

SEAWEED

Seaweed can contribute to optimal breast health because it contains more iodine than any other food. Intake of iodine plays an important role in maintaining healthy breast tissue because it interferes with estrogen's ability to bind to cells in breast tissue. Japanese women, who eat large amounts of seaweed, also have a low incidence of breast cancer. In laboratory tests, Japanese researchers found that wakame seaweed strongly suppressed the growth of breast cancer cells without toxic side effects.[16] There are countless ways of adding various types of seaweed to your favorite dishes. You can stir seaweed into your soups, sprinkle dulse on your food in place of salt, or make nori-rice wraps.

FOODS TO AVOID

In addition to choosing Best Breast Foods, you can also protect your breast health by knowing which foods to avoid in your diet. The standard American diet is laden with low-quality, nonorganic foods that can contribute to unhealthy breast tissue. This diet is generally too high in animal products (especially saturated animal fats), dairy products, unsaturated omega 6 fats, and refined sugar, and too low in fiber, fruits, vegetables, whole grains, quality fats, beans, and legumes. In fact, the standard American diet is deficient in many of the best food constituents—vitamins, minerals, phytochemicals, and other nutrients—that can help your body prevent diseases.

First and foremost, avoid saturated animal fats. A substantial body of research suggests that women who eat a diet high in saturated animal fats are at increased risk for breast cancer. Beef, lamb, pork, poultry, and whole-milk dairy products all contain high amounts of saturated fats. One reason saturated fats may contribute to breast cancer is that when consumed in excess they increase body fat, which can in turn increase estrogen levels. Saturated fats also contribute to insulin resistance, a hormone imbalance that results in more free estrogen in your circulation. The more estrogen you have in circulation, the more estrogen there is to stimulate estrogen receptors on your breast cells. Another reason not to eat saturated animal fats is that animals store concentrated environmental chemicals in their fatty tissues; when you eat animal fat, you may be ingesting higher levels of estrogen-mimicking chemicals.

If you do eat meat, the way you cook it can also be important for your breast health. High-heat methods of cooking meat such as barbecuing, frying, or broiling can lead to the formation of carcinogenic chemicals known as heterocyclic amines. Oven roasting, baking, boiling, stewing, or poaching meat generally produces fewer of these compounds because these methods allow you to cook at lower temperatures.

Among animal products, dairy foods are some of the worst offenders when it comes to breast health. If you consume nonorganic cream, butter, or other milk products, you are ingesting a chemical soup containing hormones, antibiotics, and environmental chemicals. In most conventional dairies in the United States, cows are injected with a substance called bovine growth hormone (BGH) in order to increase milk production. BGH increases the levels of insulinlike growth factor-1 (IGF-1) in cows, which is then passed into their milk. When humans ingest this milk, their levels of IGF-1 can also increase, potentially putting them at higher risk for cancer. According to Dr. Samuel Epstein, professor of environmental toxicology at the University of Illinois, BGH may be associated with an elevated risk for breast cancer in humans.[17] The bottom line on dairy products, as far as your breast health is concerned: steer clear of them unless they are nonfat organic.

Unsaturated omega 6 fats, which are found in safflower, corn, peanut, cottonseed, and sunflower oils, should be avoided because they have been reported to increase the risk for breast cancer when consumed in excess. The standard American diet contains an abundance of these fats[18]—they include hydrogenated fats and are found in margarines, mayonnaise, salad dressings, and many baked goods—and most Americans ingest them every day without realizing it.

To protect your breast health, I also recommend that you avoid refined sugar, which is ubiquitous in the standard American diet. Excessive sugar consumption contributes to lowered immunity, obesity, and insulin resistance—each of which elevates your risk for breast cancer. Lowered immunity increases your risk because it reduces your body's ability to destroy cancer cells; obesity can lead to more estrogen production in your fat cells and contribute to insulin resistance; insulin resistance causes more estrogen to circulate in the blood and also causes higher levels of IGF-1. The bottom line is that regular consumption of sugar is detrimental to breast health.

FOODS THAT ENHANCE BREAST HEALTH	FOODS DETRIMENTAL TO BREAST HEALTH
Fruits and vegetables	Saturated animal fats
Soy	Barbecued, fried, or broiled meats
Omega 3 fats (from flax and fish oil)	Nonorganic dairy products
Flaxseeds	Omega 6 fats (including hydrogenated fats)
Fiber	Refined sugar
Green tea	
Seaweed	

Alcohol and Breast Health

There is ample research indicating that regular consumption of alcohol increases a woman's risk for breast cancer. Alcohol is broken down in the liver to acetaldehyde, a known toxin that causes cancer in laboratory animals. Alcohol also interferes with the body's ability to utilize folic acid, an essential mineral for normal cell division. In 1997 the *New England Journal of Medicine* reported, "The mortality from breast cancer was 30 percent higher among women reporting at least one drink daily than among non-drinkers."[19] In 2004 a study published in *Cancer Epidemiology, Biomarkers and Prevention* showed that women had an elevated breast cancer risk related to their recent drinking—not to their alcohol consumption earlier in life. For postmenopausal women, this elevation in risk was 32 percent, and for perimenopausal women, 21 percent.[20]

Alcohol increases estrogen levels in women, whether they are on hormones or not. But women who take HRT need to be especially careful about avoiding alcohol. A study published in the *Journal of the American Medical Association* found that women taking estrogen and synthetic progesterone who consumed a drink containing vodka had blood levels of estrogen that were over 300 percent higher than baseline levels (levels of estrogen prior to drinking the alcohol). The levels increased within ten minutes of ingesting the alcohol and remained high for five hours.[21] Since increased estrogen puts a woman at increased risk for breast cancer, ingesting alcohol when a woman is already on HRT is extremely risky business.

Given the risks to breast health associated with alcohol use, it's troubling to see alcohol being dubiously touted in the media as an elixir for heart health. The bottom line: don't drink alcohol if you want to optimize your breast health.

YOUR DIET: THE VIEW FROM THE EAST

Most of the breast-healthy foods we've explored thus far are also considered to be breast-healthy from a Chinese medicine perspective. As we've seen, most breast problems are said to be the result of deficient spleen Qi or liver Qi stagnation. If you have breast problems, you can improve your breast health by eating foods that nourish your spleen Qi and support your liver Qi, and by avoiding foods that contribute to deficient spleen Qi and to liver Qi stagnation.

A deficiency of spleen Qi can result if you eat an excess of raw, uncooked fruits and vegetables, and especially if you eat a lot of dairy products and refined sugar. Consuming these foods in excess contributes to "dampness," which can accumulate and form lumps in your breasts. Other foods that can harm your spleen Qi and contribute to liver Qi stagnation include fatty or fried meats, refined flour products, and alcohol. Interestingly, the list of foods that can be detrimental to spleen Qi is very similar to the list of foods to avoid in the interest of optimizing breast health from a Western perspective.

To treat breast problems due to deficient spleen Qi, all foods and drinks should be eaten warm or at room temperature. If your spleen Qi is weak, it is recommended that you eat small, frequent meals; rice should be a major part of your diet because it strengthens spleen Qi and eliminates "dampness." To assist spleen Qi and help increase the movement of liver Qi, include small amounts of warming spices like cardamom, cinnamon, ginger, and nutmeg in your diet.

YOUR LIFESTYLE

All of the elements of the Naturally Healthy Lifestyle outlined in Chapter 1 will help you create optimal breast health: exercising regularly, decreasing stress, honoring your values, nurturing yourself, and getting enough sleep. Regular exercise is an especially important part of your lifestyle when it comes to the health of your breast tissue. One study found that young women who exercised vigorously at least once a day from age fourteen to age twenty-two had a 50 percent reduction in their risk for breast cancer compared with young women who did not exercise.[22] It has also been found that women who have physically strenuous jobs have a lower incidence of breast cancer than women who are sedentary at work.[23]

You can think of exercise as a way of cleansing your breast cells. Exercise increases the flow of blood to your breasts, bringing in oxygen and taking away waste products. It also acts as a pump for your lymphatic system, increasing your lymph flow dramatically and reducing the number of circulating toxins in and around your breast tissue. Exercise also increases your lean muscle mass and decreases your body fat (greater body fat means more estrogen, which increases your risk for breast cancer). In addition, exercise decreases your risk of developing insulin resistance, a condition that also elevates your risk for breast cancer. And exercise reduces your risk for other chronic diseases, makes you feel and look healthier, and gives you an excuse to have fun.

In Chinese medicine, lifestyle factors are always important for breast health. Breast problems can be due to emotional imbalances that are associated with liver Qi stagnation, such as frustration, bottled-up feelings, or anger, and regular exercise is one of the most important lifestyle recommendations for prevention or treatment. Exercise successfully counteracts liver Qi stagnation by dramatically moving Qi and Blood; it also strengthens spleen Qi and helps to eliminate "dampness" that could result in breast lumps. According to Chinese medicine, exercise is especially helpful for women who suffer from breast tenderness and swelling before their periods.

YOUR HORMONES

As we've seen, excessive hormonal stimulation of breast tissue is a potential cause of breast cancer. The July 2002 issue of the *Journal of the American Medical Association* reported that a study evaluating the long-term effects of synthetic HRT with estrogen and progesterone had to be halted because the health risks—which included a 24 percent increased risk for breast cancer—outweighed the benefits.[24] And the type of breast cancer that women developed while on HRT during the study was more aggressive, and posed a higher risk of spreading to other areas of the body, than the breast cancers of women who were not on HRT.

Many of my patients express concerns about their risks of breast cancer because of their history of using birth control pills (which contain a combination of synthetic estrogen and progesterone). Research done at the National Cancer Institute has indicated that the association between taking birth control pills and breast cancer risk is not clear, and that women in some age groups may not have increased risk whereas others might.[25] However, according to Niels Lauersen, M.D., Ph.D., and Eileen Stukane, authors of *The Complete Book of Breast Care,* "While many studies in the past have found no increased risk for breast cancer among women who were on the Pill, a growing body of medical evidence is showing that a risk exists."[26] A number of studies suggest that the younger a woman is when she starts taking the Pill, and the longer she takes it, the higher the risks that it could contribute to the development of breast cancer.

A form of birth control that many young women use is an injection of synthetic progesterone called Depo-Provera. It is also used to stop heavy menstrual bleeding in some perimenopausal women. One study showed that Depo-Provera increased the risk for breast cancer and also accelerated the growth of preexisting tumors.[27] Other studies have shown that using synthetic progesterone increases breast cancer risk.

It's not clear if natural progesterone increases or decreases your risk for breast cancer. One study indicated that natural progesterone cream applied to breast tissue for fourteen days reduced cell turnover (cell division) in breast cells and decreased estrogen's effects on breast cells.[28] This would seem to suggest that natural progesterone decreases breast cancer risk. But at this time there simply isn't enough information to know for sure if natural progesterone can help prevent breast cancer. Until we have more information, I recommend that you refrain from using natural progesterone unless you need it for specific reasons; for instance, with some women natural progesterone can make a big difference in treating heavy menstrual bleeding and insomnia associated with perimenopause. I also recommend that you avoid rubbing progesterone creams directly onto your breasts.

The bottom line on HRT and breast cancer is that you don't want to use hormones if you don't have to. If you choose to take HRT because it significantly increases the quality of your life, take the lowest possible dose for the shortest period of time needed to obtain the therapeutic effects. If you are a perimenopausal or post-menopausal woman and you are considering hormones for controlling your midlife symptoms, I highly recommend that you take only natural, bioidentical estrogen and progesterone. (See Chapter 7 for more information on HRT and hormonal health.)

Your levels of thyroid hormones may also affect your risk for breast cancer. A number of studies have suggested that hypothyroidism (low thyroid hormones) is related to an increased risk for breast cancer. According to an article published in *Medical Hypotheses,* the number of estrogen receptors on cells may increase when a woman has low thyroid hormones, which increases estrogen stimulation of breast tissue.[29] This would explain why some women with low levels of thyroid hormones tend to have exaggerated breast tenderness before their period starts or even throughout their cycles.

Your breast cancer risk could also be increased if your body's iodine levels are low, because iodine is necessary for the manufacture of thyroid hormones. Iodine is also important in the breakdown of estrogen to estriol, the "friendly" estrogen, in the liver.[30] In animal studies, iodine has been found to be necessary for normal breast tissue growth and development; without it, breast tissue showed abnormal cell growth and the development of cancer.[31]

You can be proactive in creating optimal breast health by having your thyroid hormone levels assessed (as we discussed in Chapter 7).

Breaking Down and Eliminating Estrogen to Enhance Breast Health

Estrogen is broken down in the liver and eliminated from the body in stools; poor breakdown of estrogen in the liver can lead to increased formation of unfriendly estrogen that could elevate your risk for breast cancer. Good overall detoxification is essential because it helps keep your liver and your digestive system healthy and enhances your liver's ability to break down estrogen. Detoxification also encourages the breakdown and elimination of many hormone-mimicking chemicals that are stored in your fatty tissue. Prolonged sweating in a sauna is the most effective way to remove these from your system. (See Chapter 4 for a detailed description of how to do a liver cleanse.)

Including an abundance of fiber in your diet is effective in assisting with the elimination of estrogen through stools. Another important way of eliminating estrogen is with an intestinal cleanse. (For a thorough exploration of how to do an intestinal cleanse, see Chapter 6.) Finally, the following nutritional supplements, which are special compounds derived from foods, can also play a significant role in helping your body break down estrogen.

Calcium D-glucarate. This compound contains glucaric acid, which is important in promoting breast health. It may inhibit breast cancer cell growth and help prevent other types of cancer as well. Calcium D-glucarate is naturally occurring in your body and is also found in fruits and vegetables, especially broccoli, carrots, spinach, apples, and oranges. When taken as a supplement, it can enhance the liver's ability to break down estrogen and chemical carcinogens. It also prevents bacteria in the colon from reabsorbing estrogen.

Calcium D-glucarate is especially helpful for women who have had breast cancer, or who have a high risk of developing breast cancer, and women who suffer from PMS due to too much estrogen. Many of my patients who had experienced exaggerated breast tenderness before their periods reported that calcium D-glucarate alleviated their problem. There have been no side effects reported from taking calcium D-glucarate. The recommended dose for enhancing the breakdown and elimination of estrogen is 1,500 mg a day.[32]

I3C (indole-3-carbinol). This compound, which is found in broccoli, cabbage, brussels sprouts, cauliflower, and other cruciferous vegetables, gives you another good reason to enjoy them in your diet. I3C is great for promoting breast health and preventing breast cancer because it helps your liver break estrogen down into "friendly" estrogen. One study found that women who ate lots of cruciferous vegetables had higher levels of "friendly" estrogen and were 30 percent less likely to develop breast cancer over a nineteen-year period.[33] If taken as a supplement, the recommended dose of indole-3-carbinol is 300 mg a day.

DIM (diindolylmethane). This compound, which is derived from I3C, may have even stronger effects on breast health because it can interfere with estrogen's ability to bind onto cells. I've frequently prescribed DIM to women who want extra breast health protection, or who are at high risk of developing breast cancer. DIM is especially effective in helping your body break down estrogen into "friendly" estrogen. It is safe when taken in doses of up to 300 mg a day.

MASSAGE FOR OPTIMAL BREAST HEALTH

One of the best ways of nurturing yourself and promoting your breast health is by massaging your breasts. Breast self-massage can help you create a wonderful relationship to your body and breasts. Not only does it increase the circulation of blood and lymph, which helps your breast tissue receive oxygen and takes away waste products, but it also allows you to become more familiar with this most intimate part of your body. Many women seldom touch their breasts or do so only in a clinical way. If you don't already practice breast self-massage, I invite you to explore touching and massaging your breasts in a way that is relaxing and self-nurturing.

The only reasons not to do breast self-massage are if you have an infection in your breast, or if you were recently diagnosed with breast cancer; according to some schools of thought, massage can spread the cancer into adjacent lymph nodes. But if you don't have breast cancer, or if your cancer is in remission, breast massage can be healthy. If you've had a mastectomy (surgical breast removal), I encourage you to massage your chest in a similar manner as outlined below, but with a few necessary modifications; breast self-massage can help you become more integrated with your body, which is important for your healing.

It is most comfortable to do breast self-massage while you are lying on your back in bed; you may find that it's a great way to follow up a breast self-exam. Begin by applying warm or room-temperature massage oil to your breasts with both hands. After you've spread the oil liberally over your entire chest and up into your armpits, place your left hand behind your head. Make sweeping strokes with your right hand across your left chest and breast in the direction of your left armpit, covering the entire area and including the area under your armpit on your side. By massaging toward your armpit, you enhance the circulation of lymph to the lymph nodes in your armpit. Continuing to use your right hand, massage your left breast tissue in a clockwise direction five times and in a counter-clockwise direction five times, always ending with your last stroke moving toward your armpit.

Bringing your left hand down toward your chest, use both hands to massage your left breast; with one hand under your breast and one hand on top, move your hands back and forth in opposite directions for thirty seconds to a minute. Next, direct your strokes upward from the underside of your breast toward your neck, covering the entire area of your left chest with both hands. Then place your fingertips in the cleft above your left collarbone and gently stroke inward toward the middle of your neck; this stimulates the movement of lymph. End with several long, light sweeping strokes across your left chest toward your left armpit. This completes the left side of your breast self-massage; now switch to your right side and repeat the entire process.

A number of herbs and essential oils are often blended into breast massage oils. These can help with lymph movement and circulation in your breasts, and nurture your breast tissue. A lovely breast massage oil called Breast Caress contains the herbs calendula, red clover, comfrey root, and dandelion root, along with the essential oils lavender, rose geranium, and ylang ylang. The herbs can help decongest breast tissue, and the essential oils have anti-inflammatory and tension-relieving properties. (See Appendix B for resources.)

By being proactive in creating optimal breast health, you can help prevent many problems that can affect your breasts. Your environment, diet, lifestyle, discernment in taking hormones, ability to efficiently break down and eliminate estrogen, and breast self-massage, are all important for optimizing your breast health. In the pages that follow, we will explore how to treat benign breast conditions.

Benign Breast Conditions

"Ever since I developed breasts," said Joanne, "I had experienced a great deal of pain and swelling in them with each menstrual cycle. Perimenopause, with all of its hormone fluctuations, just exacerbated the problem." She said that her hot flashes and irritability were driving her and her husband crazy. Joanne knew that taking estrogen was not an option, because it would just make her breast problem worse. But when she started taking natural progesterone, herbs, and iodine to support her thyroid, her condition changed within a few weeks. "An amazing thing happened," she said. "My breast pain improved significantly, and so did my other symptoms."

The term *benign breast conditions* refers to many different types of breast symptoms and problems that are noncancerous. As the name indicates, they are relatively harmless conditions, and although none of them are life-threatening, they can cause much discomfort for women who experience them.

Some benign breast conditions typically occur during adolescence, while others can occur at any time during a woman's life. They are often the result of imbalances in hormones, especially estrogen; too much stimulation of breast tissue by estrogen is often the culprit. If you have an excess of estrogen, it can be due to a number of causes, some of which we have already explored in this chapter: low thyroid hormone levels, high exposure to environmental estrogen, poor breakdown and elimination of estrogen, or too much estrogen compared with progesterone. According to naturopathic principles as well as Chinese medicine, if you have a benign breast lump or chronic breast pain, it is important to treat your whole body in order to heal the underlying cause. Most benign breast conditions can be successfully treated with natural medicine. I treat the following benign breast conditions most frequently in my practice.

FIBROCYSTIC CHANGES

The most common type of benign breast condition is fibrocystic changes. If you are in your menstruating years, you probably have breast tissue that feels irregular, somewhat like a bag of grapes. In most cases, this is normal and the natural result of hormones stimulating breast tissue. But if hormone imbalances occur, you can develop breast lumps of varying consistencies, sizes, and shapes. These lumps can be either hard or soft and are usually freely movable. They are often benign, but any changes that occur in your breast tissue should be evaluated by your health care provider, and further tests may be necessary. (See "Tests for Breasts" beginning on page 272.)

For years, physicians told women with lumpy or painful breasts that they had a condition called *fibrocystic breast disease*. (Many physicians now simply use the term *fibrocystic changes*.) In fact, there is no such thing as fibrocystic breast disease, and as Susan Love, M.D., points out in *Dr. Susan Love's Breast Book,* the term is "a wastebasket into which doctors throw every breast problem that isn't cancerous. The symptoms it encompasses are so varied and so unrelated to each other that the term is wholly without meaning."[34] The increased breast lumpiness or tenderness that some women feel before their periods, and that disappears after their periods, is due to changes in their hormones. As you will discover, a number of lifestyle and dietary factors can contribute to how lumpy or painful your breasts are.

BREAST PAIN

Breast pain may be your body's way of telling you that hormonal changes are taking place. One of the earliest signs of pregnancy, swollen breasts with tender nipples, is caused by hormone stimulation of breast tissue. For the same reason, many women are aware of the onset of their period due to an increase in breast size and tenderness. This is normal, but some women experience exaggerated breast tenderness or pain that can be either temporary or chronic. Their symptoms are usually benign, and Western doctors typically prescribe birth control pills or Danocrine, a drug derived from testosterone, to prevent ovulation and thus the monthly fluctuation of estrogen and progesterone. But taking a drug simply to prevent the symptoms does not address the problem. Naturopathic medicine and Chinese medicine consider it important to address exaggerated breast tenderness or pain as symptoms of an underlying imbalance; my recommendations are outlined on pages 293–295.

BREAST CYSTS

One of the most common types of benign breast lumps, cysts tend to form in the upper-outer quadrant of a breast and can range in size from a few millimeters to a few inches. They generally feel soft (they are fluid-filled) and may be tender or painful. Breast cysts are usually caused by estrogen stimulation of breast cells. Any new breast lump should be examined by your doctor; you will probably be advised to have a mammogram and an ultrasound, and your doctor may draw fluid out of the cyst to test for any cancerous cells. Once it has been confirmed that your breast cyst is benign, I recommend that you begin the natural treatments outlined on pages 293–295 to help dissolve the cyst and prevent a recurrence.

FIBROADENOMAS

Fibroadenomas are painless lumps that can be found in the breasts of women of any age, but they are more often discovered in younger women between adolescence and age twenty-five. They consist of masses of fibrous tissue that feel round, smooth, and firm with well-defined boundaries. Fibroadenomas are often found near or below the nipples, but they can be in any part of one or both breasts. It isn't known exactly what causes fibroadenomas, but one theory is that they form when there is a hormone imbalance, such as often happens during adolescence as the ovaries are "adjusting" to the onset of monthly ovulation.

One of my patients, Laura, found a small lump in her breast twenty-five years ago, when she was thirteen years old. She told her mother about it, and they went to see a doctor who said that he would have to remove her nipple in order to cut the lump out. "I was horrified at the thought of surgery," Laura told me, "but luckily, my mother insisted that we get a second opinion." They were told that the lump was a fibroadenoma, and that it didn't have to be excised. To this day, Laura says that she can still feel the lump in her breast, although it has gotten much smaller over the years.

Small fibroadenomas usually aren't surgically removed unless there are concerns that they are cancerous tissue. Fibroadenomas are not precursors to cancer, and as a rule women with fibroadenomas are not at increased risk for breast cancer. But some researchers have found that women who have a type of "complex" fibroadenoma are at higher risk for developing cancer in the future. Very large fibroadenomas may also be removed because a rare cancer, cystosarcoma phyllodes, can grow inside them. If you have a fibroadenoma and you've had it since your teenage years, my advice is to leave it alone. Regardless of your age, if you develop a breast lump, have it evaluated by your health care provider. Remember that the development of a fibroadenoma may be a sign that there is something out of balance in your body; if you have a benign fibroadenoma, have your hormone levels assessed and treat yourself with the natural methods outlined below.

TREATING BENIGN BREAST CONDITIONS NATURALLY

To treat the underlying causes of benign breast conditions, including fibrocystic changes, exaggerated breast pain, breast cysts, and fibroadenomas, it is important to follow the Naturally Healthy Diet and Lifestyle and make the other breast-healthy choices that I've outlined thus far in this chapter, including eating more Best Breast Foods. The following measures, which can all be taken simultaneously, are also important for treating benign breast conditions, and can promote optimal breast health.

AVOID CAFFEINE

Caffeine should be avoided as much as possible when you are treating (and preventing) benign breast conditions because it may cause exaggerated breast pain and lumpiness in some women. I've personally experienced more breast symptoms before my period when I drank caffeinated beverages on a regular basis, and many of my patients have described dramatic changes in their breast tissue when they drink caffeine versus when they abstain from it. For some women, eliminating caffeine from their diet can bring much relief from cyclical breast pain and result in breast tissue that feels noticeably softer.

Caffeine is a methylxanthine—a compound that is thought to interfere with enzymes in the breast, resulting in fibrocystic changes. Caffeine is found in many foods, including chocolate; some over-the-counter medications such as Excedrin and Dexatrim contain exceptionally high levels of caffeine. It does not matter if the coffee you drink is organic, you use purified water, or have the fanciest coffee machine: coffee is not breast-friendly. In Chinese medicine, coffee is considered to be a powerful Qi mover that ultimately squanders kidney Essence, leaving you more Qi-depleted than you were before you drank it. Over time this can make you more susceptible to problems in your breasts and in other areas of your body.

ASSESS FOR AND TREAT ESTROGEN DOMINANCE

In all benign breast conditions it is important to consider whether you have a condition known as *estrogen dominance*. Estrogen dominance primarily occurs if you have more estrogen than progesterone in the second half, or luteal phase, of your menstrual cycle (when you should have more progesterone); as a result, you can develop breast pain and breast lumps. There is a good chance you have estrogen dominance if you have breast pain from midcycle to the onset of your period, heavy menstrual periods, fluid retention, and depression and headaches associated with your cycles. To confirm that you have estrogen dominance, ask your health care provider to order salivary or urinary hormone tests. It's best to take the tests on day 21 of your menstrual cycle.

The best ways of treating estrogen dominance involve helping your liver break down estrogen (see the diagram on page 278) and helping your digestive system eliminate estrogen efficiently. (See Chapter 6.) You may also need to use natural progesterone to balance your estrogen level. Natural progesterone can be taken in the form of skin creams, sublingual (under the tongue) drops, or pills. For the pills, you will need a prescription. (See Chapter 7 for more information.)

EVALUATE FOR THYROID HORMONE IMBALANCES AND TAKE IODINE IF NECESSARY

Your thyroid hormones may be involved in benign breast conditions because low levels of thyroid hormones have been linked to increased estrogen stimulation of breast tissue. The more your breast tissue is stimulated by estrogen, the higher the chances that you will experience breast enlargement, have breast pain, or form breast cysts. See Chapter 7 for information on diagnosis and treatment of thyroid hormone imbalances.

Iodine, one of the key constituents of thyroid hormones, can be especially useful in the treatment of benign breast conditions. Iodine is also important for assisting with the conversion of the "unfriendly" estrogen to estriol, the "friendly" estrogen (see the diagram on page 278). There have been a number of studies on the effects of various forms of iodine supplementation on benign breast conditions. One study found that molecular iodine (also known as diatomic iodine) was much more effective than other forms of iodine in reducing fibrocystic changes.[35] This form of iodine is not found at your local health food store but can be ordered by your health care provider.

TAKE VITAMIN E AND EVENING PRIMROSE OIL

Vitamin E and evening primrose oil are two important nutritional supplements for treating benign breast conditions, especially fibrocystic changes and breast pain. One study published as far back as 1965 in the *New England Journal of Medicine* found that vitamin E can soften fibrocystic breast masses, decrease breast pain, and reduce or completely eliminate breast cysts.[36] For years I've used vitamin E with much success in my practice for treating fibrocystic changes and breast tenderness. Vitamin E is an antioxidant (which means it helps prevent free radical damage to tissues) that is stored in fatty tissue; it may protect your breast tissue from free radical damage that could be contributing to benign breast conditions. The recommended dose for most benign breast conditions is 400 to 800 i.u. of vitamin E a day. (Purchase all-natural vitamin E in the form of mixed tocopherols.)

Evening primrose oil is an omega 6 fatty acid that has a positive effect on decreasing breast pain; the recommended dosage is 1,500 mg twice a day throughout your cycle.

USE CHINESE HERBAL FORMULAS

In Chinese medicine, herbal formulas can be effective in treating benign breast conditions. In fact, as Westerners are often surprised to learn, Chinese herbal formulas have been used for thousands of years for this purpose. As we saw earlier in this chapter, Chinese medicine views all breast conditions as being related, and treating underlying Qi imbalances is essential in creating breast health. The herbs that make up an herbal formula are chosen for their ability to correct different types of Qi imbalances. You will recall that spleen Qi deficiency and liver Qi stagnation are two primary Qi imbalances associated with breast problems; the herbal formula Bupleurum Entangled Qi is one of many used for treating these imbalances.

Bupleurum Entangled Qi (a modification of the traditional Chinese formula Chai Hu Xiang Fu Tang, developed by the herbal company Health Concerns) has been used by my patients with great success in treating benign breast lumps. It contains a number of herbs that move Qi and Blood, eliminate dampness, and reduce pain, inflammation, and heat. You will need to obtain this formula from your practitioner of Chinese medicine; the typical dose is three pills three times a day for three to six months. If you don't experience relief, or if your symptoms get worse while you are using the formula, stop taking it and consult your practitioner.

Treating Breast Conditions Associated with Lactation Naturally

Many women have told me that they didn't pay much attention to their breasts until they became pregnant or started breast-feeding. During this time a woman's breasts are preparing for and performing their role of milk production. The miracle of having a baby includes the miracle of being able to feed your baby right from your own body.

One of the most important ways you can maintain milk production is simply by relaxing. When you are stressed, your milk production may decrease and you can also be more prone to breast infections. Your milk supply may be telling you that you're trying to accomplish too much and should find ways to rest and relieve stress, even with the enormous changes in your life. You can also try eating fresh fennel and drinking Mother's Milk tea (see Appendix B for resources), which contains a number of herbs, including fenugreek, coriander, and anise, that can aid in the production of breast milk.

In addition to stress, your milk supply can be decreased when you are dehydrated. According to Chinese medicine, a woman's milk supply can be reduced if she lost a great deal of fluid during her baby's delivery and she doesn't have sufficient Blood to make breast milk. In this case, get plenty of fluid and rest, and incorporate foods into your diet that are considered in Chinese medicine to be Blood-building such as seaweeds, spirulina, leafy greens, sweet rice or mochi, beans, eggs, poultry, and beef. (Red meat is generally not recommended as part of the Naturally Healthy Diet, but this is an exception; remember to eat only organic meat, and use a low-heat cooking method.) If your baby isn't properly latching on to your nipple, you can try using a breast pump and may want to see a lactation specialist.

Another common condition associated with lactation is mastitis, a local infection of the breast glands and ducts. Mastitis is caused by a blocked milk duct that causes your breast to become hard, red, and painful. If you have this condition, you may also feel like you have a flu. To treat mastitis, apply hot compresses to your breast tissue and continue to nurse or use a breast pump (the infection will not hurt your baby), drink lots of fluids, and most important of all, get some rest. This may seem out of the question with a baby to take care of, but releasing control and letting others help you may be just what your body is crying out for; like decreased milk production, mastitis can be caused by trying to do too much. For the symptoms of a hard, painful breast with fever and chills, I recommend that you take 300 mg of echinacea three times a day, 1,500 mg of vitamin C a day, and 200c of the homeopathic medicine Phytolacca. Take Phytolacca under your tongue at the onset of symptoms, and again a few hours later if needed.

There are also Chinese herbal formulas that can be used to treat mastitis. They usually contain herbs with properties that fight bacteria and yeast associated with the condition, and herbs that strengthen kidney Essence, which can be important if you are an exhausted nursing mother. You can obtain a Chinese herbal formula through a licensed acupuncturist or Chinese herbalist.

Though mastitis can often be relieved in a short period of time by using naturopathic and Chinese medicine as described above, if your condition doesn't clear up within forty-eight hours, or becomes worse, consult with your health care provider.

Natural Therapies to Support Cancer Treatment

If you've been diagnosed with breast cancer, see your oncologist for a thorough explanation of the type of cancer you have and your treatment options. Early detection and treatment of breast cancer has an excellent prognosis. While the treatment of cancer is beyond the scope of this book, the following are my general suggestions on how you can support your body, mind, and spirit through the process of healing and recovering from cancer.

The three most important things you can do to help recover from breast cancer are to support your immune system, create time for your healing, and get involved in a breast cancer support group or other therapy that allows you to express and integrate your emotions.

The information presented in Chapter 1 and Chapter 2 can help protect you from illness and keep your body balanced. Since your immune system is the foundation on which you build your health, if you've been diagnosed with breast cancer it's especially important to incorporate into your life the Naturally Healthy Lifestyle and Diet programs and immunity-enhancing techniques presented there.

Along with dietary and lifestyle support, herbal and nutritional supplements can help you boost your immune system through surgery, chemotherapy, or radiation. When you are faced with a life-threatening disease, everything can seem overwhelming; an easy way to sort through your natural treatment options is to see your naturopathic physician. If you don't have access to one, an excellent resource book is available: *How to Prevent and Treat Cancer with Natural Medicine,* written by naturo-pathic doctors Paul Reilly, Mike Murray, Joe Pizzorno, and Tim Birdsall. I recommend that you discuss your desire to use natural medicines with your oncologist to be sure that they don't conflict in any way with your cancer therapy.

Most of us live busy lives, and the thought of putting aside time every day to focus attention just on ourselves seems out of the question. But to help heal from breast cancer, I suggest that you spend at least twenty minutes each day enhancing your immune system and promoting your well-being with self-nurturing love. Many of my patients who have been diagnosed with breast cancer use this time to pray and strengthen their relationship to God, meditate, or practice healing visualizations. One woman who listened to Qi Gong meditation tapes during her chemotherapy treatments, as well as when she came in to my office for acupuncture, told me she felt that they played a powerful role in her recovery. Another patient told me that the meditation audiocassette *Health Journeys for People with Cancer* by Belleruth Naparstek was an essential part of her healing.

For most women, being diagnosed with a potentially fatal disease is understandably an ominous event that can change their self-perceptions and bring them face to face with life and death issues. A breast cancer support group or personal growth therapy can help you get through what is happening, both physically and emotionally. Many women have told me their breast cancer diagnosis changed everything in their lives overnight. In some cases, their relationships to family and close friends shifted, and they discovered that their loved ones were there for them in ways they could never have imagined. Others have described how their superficial needs seemed to disappear as they became more focused on their spiritual needs. As difficult as the experience may be, there are great gifts that can come from being diagnosed with cancer. Having a good support system can help you discover what they are, and addressing your fears while reaching out to others can be an important part of your journey toward recovery.

Creating Breast Health: Final Thoughts

Manifesting breast health is an ongoing process, and the health of your breasts depends on the health of your entire body. By being proactive and making breast-healthy choices, you can not only prevent breast problems and treat them when they arise but also continually maintain optimal breast health. Your breasts deserve special attention; they are an intimate, sensitive, beautiful, and powerful part of your body. By giving them the same kind of nurturing they were designed to give to others, you can create breast health through every stage of your life.

The Essence of Chapter 9

- Remember that your breasts change with the different stages of your life.
- Keep your liver Qi circulating and your spleen Qi abundant for healthy breast tissue.
- Know your risk factors for breast cancer, do frequent breast self-exams, and screen your breasts for cancer.
- Avoid exposure to hormone-disrupting environmental chemicals whenever possible.
- Optimize your breast health by choosing Best Breast Foods, and avoid foods that are detrimental to your breast health.
- Avoid taking hormones that can cause excessive stimulation of your breast tissue.
- Make sure that you have adequate levels of thyroid hormones.
- Improve your body's ability to break down and eliminate estrogen.
- Use natural treatments for treating benign breast conditions.
- Treat breast conditions associated with lactation with natural medicine.
- Use natural medicines to help support your treatment if you are diagnosed with breast cancer.

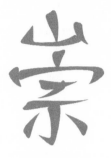

Chapter 10

Reverence

Nurturing the Cradle of Your
Intimate Self

*"Her large hips fluttered as if a bird imprisoned in her pelvis was
attempting flight."*

—MAYA ANGELOU, *The Heart of a Woman*

"My NIGHTMARE *began more than ten years ago with my first abnormal Pap test,"
Leilani said. "Over the next several years, I had numerous Pap tests that alternated
between normal and varying degrees of abnormal. It seemed like I was constantly seeing my
gynecologist."*

*About five years after her first abnormal Pap test, one of Leilani's Pap tests showed cer-
vical dysplasia, or very abnormal cells at her cervix. Her doctor recommended a surgical
procedure called cervical conization to remove the external tissue of her cervix. "I was assured that this would probably take care of the problem, so I had the procedure done," she recalls. "But five months later, another Pap test showed abnormal cells." A biopsy taken at that
time of Leilani's cervix revealed that she still had dysplasia and also had human papilloma
virus (HPV), which can cause cervical cancer. "I was told that nothing could be done to treat
the HPV, and that I would need to get a Pap test every six months for the rest of my life—or*

until I required a hysterectomy due to cervical cancer. In addition, my physician recommended another conization surgery. At that point, I decided I had to find another way. I was thirty-five years old and knew I wanted to have children."

When Leilani told me her story, I explained that merely removing tissue from her cervix was like taking away the tip of the iceberg and expecting the problem to go away. Instead of treating just her cervix, I recommended that we work with her entire body to create health. I prescribed several appropriate vitamins and minerals, a whole foods diet, and other lifestyle changes—as well as a series of treatments to her cervix twice a week for six weeks.

Leilani's treatments ended in February 1998, and since then every one of her Pap tests has come back with normal results. "The problem with my cervix woke me up to the importance of self-care," she says. "In the years since, I've continued to take good care of myself by eating a healthy diet, taking vitamins, and keeping my immune system strong. I have no doubt that my lifestyle changes have had a major impact on the continued health of my cervix—as well as my whole body."

✌

The Health of Your Pelvis

Your pelvis is the most private, mysterious area of your body. From your pelvis you can bring forth children, receive sexual pleasure, and share your most intimate self. Your pelvis is your center of gravity and creativity and the seat of your power, both physically and symbolically.

Your pelvis holds within it the potential to change the future. Your ovaries contain thousands of eggs that can develop into new life. Your uterus, cervix, vagina, and vulva are all strong, resilient, and able to expand prodigiously to allow for the growth and passage of an infant. When you are sexually excited, your pelvis releases fluids and floods with blood. Your clitoris is like a license from nature to enjoy life. It serves no physiological purpose except sexual pleasure, and it contains more nerve endings that are sensitive to touch than any other part of your body. As Natalie Angier points out in her book *Woman: An Intimate Geography,* "The clitoris is our magic cape. It tells us that joy is a serious business and that we must not take our light, our sexual brilliance, lightly."[1]

Your pelvis is something to celebrate, be in awe of, give great respect to, and honor. It is extraordinary for all of the creative roles that it plays in your life. At the same time, women can suffer from a number of pelvic problems due to infections, sexually transmitted diseases, irritants, hormonal imbalances, and other causes. And too many women disengage from this part of their body because of fear, negative sexual connotations, or cultural stigmas that have left them viewing their pelvis not as a source of power and creativity but as a place of shame. In this chapter, we will explore the cradle of your intimate self, and you will find many ways of nurturing your pelvic health and making healthy choices to keep this part of your body strong and vital.

The View from the West

"Many historians find feminine symbolism in religious architecture: two sets of doorways, inner and outer (the labia); a central hallway (the vagina) leading to an altar (the uterus). Often there are side paths (the fallopian tubes) from the altar that lead to small vestries (the ovaries)."

—Elizabeth Stewart, M.D., *The V Book*

Bounded and protected by your large, powerful pelvic bones, your remarkable female organs—your vulva, vagina, cervix, uterus, fallopian tubes, and ovaries—lie snuggled in your pelvis.

Your vulva is the external part of your genitalia that covers and protects your internal organs. It includes your mons veneris (which is Latin for "mountain of Venus"), the padded mound that lies over your pubic bone and is covered with hair; it also contains two outer labia majora, two inner labia that look like elegant wings, your delicate clitoris with its protective hood, and your vaginal and urethral openings. Your vulva is home to millions of nerve endings; at the same time, your vulva shields your delicate inner tissues from irritants. It also allows for the passage of body fluids, houses glands that provide vaginal lubrication, and plays a major role in sexual response.

Opening into your vulva, your vagina is a flexible, muscular, cylindrical-shaped organ that also leads to your cervix and your uterus. Your vagina lengthens with sexual arousal and provides access to your G-spot (Grafenberg spot), located one to two inches inside your vagina in the direction of your clitoris; when stimulated through your vagina, it can increase sexual pleasure. At the top of your vagina, the cervix forms a narrow passageway into your uterus.

In response to hormones released by your pituitary gland, every month your ovaries ripen and release an egg, along with estrogen, testosterone, and progesterone, which have far-reaching effects on your entire body. Reaching upward from your uterus toward your ovaries are the fallopian tubes. When your ovaries release a ripe egg, fernlike projections at the ends of your fallopian tubes guide it down into the tube, where (if sperm is present) it is most likely to become fertilized, and into the uterus. During your childbearing years, the uterus is stimulated by hormones to build up an inner lining called the endometrium, which allows implantation of a fertilized egg. If no egg is fertilized, the endometrium is shed every month in the menstrual flow.

The View from the East

In the West, a woman's pelvic organs and their functions have been elaborately mapped out by scientists and researchers. But research cannot explain many of the ways that a woman's emotions can affect the health of her pelvic organs. According to Chinese medicine, a number of meridians, or energetic pathways, help to direct the flow of Qi and Blood in the pelvis and play a role in sexuality, menstruation, fertility, and pregnancy. If your Qi or Blood becomes stagnant as a result of frustration or anger, or if they become deficient from too much stress, many gynecological health problems can arise. Emotions are the most common causes of disrupted Qi and Blood flow in your pelvis, along with external imbalances such as too much cold, heat, or "dampness."

In the Five Element system, keeping your dominant element balanced—whichever type you are—will help prevent gynecological problems. But if your element becomes imbalanced, you may be more susceptible, depending on your type. Women who are Earth, Wood, and Water types have the greatest tendency to develop gynecological problems. If you are an Earth type, you are particularly prone to a prolapsed uterus, fibroids, ovarian cysts, and vaginal infections. Wood types can also be vulnerable to these conditions if their Qi and Blood become stagnant. If you are a Water type, you are more apt to experience sexual difficulties—either an excessive libido or none at all—and vaginal yeast infections. Metal and Fire types are generally inclined to strong gynecological health, but if you are a Metal type, your tendency to develop skin problems may be manifested as vaginal dryness, atrophy of your vulvar tissues, and skin conditions on your vulva.

Diagnosing Pelvic Disorders

The diagnosis of pelvic disorders from the West involves an annual pelvic exam including a Pap test and bimanual exam (during which your gynecologist feels your ovaries and your uterus). If needed, other diagnostic tests such as a vaginal culture, cervical or endometrial biopsy, pelvic ultrasound, and tests for sexually transmitted diseases (STDs) may be ordered to further assess the health of your pelvic organs.

In Chinese medicine, the diagnosis of your pelvic region, as with any other area of your body, involves looking at your tongue, feeling your pulse, and evaluating the quality of your Qi; it is also based on the totality of your symptoms. The qualities of your symptoms—including some that may not seem related to your complaint—are an important part of your diagnosis. For instance, if you have a vaginal infection, your practitioner may ask you about the nature of your bowel movements, body temperature, and energy level in order to make a complete diagnosis. In this chapter, we will explore the most common Qi imbalances seen in the pelvis.

Your Vulvar Health

Your body is remarkable in its ability to provide everything you need to stay healthy, and your vulva is no exception. To keep your vulva healthy, I recommend that you do as little to it as possible. I've found that the more women try to clean, disinfect, or perfume their vulva, the more problems they have.

Your vulva is protected by glands that produce a waxy film over its tissues to shield them from urine, vaginal secretions, and bacteria. Scrubbing this film away can create an environment that makes infection and tissue irritation more likely. When my patients complain of urethral and vulvar irritation, after careful questioning I usually discover that the irritation occurred only after they used perfumed soaps or other cleansing products. I recommend that you never use perfumed soaps, cleaning lotions, or anything else directly on your vulva. Simply wash with water, separating your labia to allow the water to clean your tissues.

The exception to this recommendation is during intercourse, when lubricants can make sex more enjoyable and help prevent tissue irritation. If you use a latex barrier method of birth control (condom, diaphragm, or cervical cap), use a water-based lubricant, which you can find at your health food store; it consists primarily of water and glycerin and may also contain herbs such as chamomile, ginseng, black walnut, and calendula. If you aren't using a latex barrier method, you can use a lubricant such as coconut oil, olive oil, vitamin E oil, or almond oil. Substances to avoid include honey (I've had patients come down with raging yeast infections after using honey in their vaginas), egg whites (they become a medium for bacteria to thrive in), K-Y jelly (it contains chlorhexidine, which can cause irritation in some women, and kills sperm), and Vaseline (a petroleum product that is not the healthiest option for your tissues).

If you are menopausal or postmenopausal, you may find that even with lubrication your vaginal tissues don't feel moist enough to allow for enjoyable intercourse. The tissues of your vulva and vagina are nourished by estrogen, and when you enter menopause your estrogen level drops significantly, causing these tissues to become thin and dry, resulting in pain during intercourse as well as increased potential for urinary tract infections. If you experience vaginal dryness, you may benefit from using a very low-dose natural estrogen cream (such as estriol vaginal cream) to help rehydrate your vulvar and vaginal tissues. Estriol is a weak estrogen and the primary estrogen that supports your pelvic tissues. You can use a small dose each night for two weeks and then taper off to just two to three times a week for maintenance. See your naturopathic physician or gynecologist for a prescription.

TREATING PROBLEMS ASSOCIATED WITH VULVAR HEALTH

You can prevent many vulvar problems by keeping your entire body in peak health with the Naturally Healthy Diet and Lifestyle and by avoiding perfumed soaps and certain kinds of lubricants. But if vulvar problems arise, you can treat or alleviate them with natural approaches. Natural medicine is particularly effective in treating or alleviating two problems that many of my patients have experienced, genital herpes and vulvodynia.

GENITAL HERPES

Genital herpes is a viral infection that primarily affects the vulva, although it can occur elsewhere on the body. It is contracted through direct contact with the skin or mucous membranes of someone who is infected with the virus. There are two types of herpes virus: herpes simplex virus type 1 (HSV-1), which mainly affects the area of the mouth and lips, and herpes simplex virus type 2 (HSV-2), which primarily affects the genitals. But either type of herpes can be found at either of these locations on the body, and either can be considered genital herpes if located on the genital region. If you've contracted the herpes virus, incubation can vary from one to twenty-six days before an outbreak of the infection, although some people who have contracted the virus never experience an outbreak.

An outbreak of herpes consists of multiple small fluid-filled blisters that break open within a few days to form what appear to be small canker sores. The area around the infected site is often pink or red from irritation. The ruptured blisters can be painful and can take anywhere from one to three weeks to completely heal. During their first outbreak some women may experience other pronounced symptoms like headaches, fever, nausea, and body aches. Subsequent outbreaks may cause milder symptoms. Herpes can be diagnosed by your health care provider through a culture taken during an outbreak. A blood test can also measure antibodies to the herpes virus, but it is not as accurate as a herpes culture.

If you have sexual contact during a herpes outbreak, you risk infecting someone else with the virus. But the greatest problem associated with genital herpes may be the risk for pregnant women of transmitting the virus to a baby during delivery. Women who have an outbreak of the infection at the time of labor are often advised to have a C-section to avoid transmitting the virus, which can cause severe problems in newborns.

If you have contracted the herpes virus, an outbreak can signal that your immune system is deficient and give you an extra impetus to take extremely good care of yourself. You can think of herpes as an opportunist; when your immune system is strong, the virus remains latent, waiting in your nervous system until your guard is down. Women who have herpes often feel a tingling, burning, or painful sensation at the site of a potential outbreak before there is any visible sign of a blister. This is called the *prodrome* and can occur anywhere from a few hours to a few days before the outbreak. During this time many women have been able to prevent the infection from becoming a full-blown outbreak by intervening with immune-boosting measures. (The prodrome also allows you to prevent the spread of herpes by giving you "advance notice" that you may soon become infectious.)

As we saw in Chapter 2, there are many ways you can stimulate your immune system. If you are under a lot of stress, give your immune system some extra support by getting a massage, taking an aromatherapy bath, or practicing yoga and meditation. Nutritional supplements can also be helpful in preventing herpes outbreaks or lessening their duration and intensity, especially vitamin C, zinc, and thymus extracts. These supplements work by stimulating the immune cells into action; it's best to start taking them as soon as you feel any sensation of a prodrome, or when you know you will be under stress.

The amino acid lysine can also help prevent herpes from becoming a major outbreak, decrease the frequency of outbreaks, and reduce the severity and duration of an outbreak.[2] Lysine works by competing with arginine, another amino acid, which is required for the herpes virus to replicate. Lysine is found in high amounts in meat, dairy foods, fish, legumes, brewer's yeast, and wheat germ. Arginine is found in high amounts in chocolate, peanuts, and gelatin. By taking lysine as a supplement and eating a diet high in lysine and low in arginine, you can give your body the extra edge you need to prevent or manage herpes outbreaks. Most people consume 6 to 10 g of lysine a day in their diet. The dose of lysine recommended for preventing herpes outbreaks is 500 mg twice a day, and the dose recommended for decreasing the severity and duration of outbreaks is 1,000 mg three times a day. Lysine is best absorbed when you take it along with a calcium supplement. You should not take supplemental lysine if you have a kidney or liver disease.

An extract of the herb lemon balm (also known as *Melissa officinalis*) has been shown to have antiviral effects when applied directly to herpes lesions, and it can lessen the duration of an infection.[3] It can also decrease the symptoms of a herpes out-break and may prevent a recurrence of the infection. Melissa cream, an ointment made from lemon balm extract, can be found at most health food stores.

VULVODYNIA (VVD)

Vulvodynia is a painful, somewhat mysterious condition that affects some women with the symptoms of vulvar irritation, tenderness, burning, and painful intercourse. The patients I've seen over the years with this condition report that their vulvar pain is sometimes mild and at other times unbearable; some experience pain only when touched, while others have pain regardless of physical touch. Since we're not sure exactly what causes VVD, gynecologists are often as frustrated as their patients in trying to manage the condition, and in an effort to eradicate the symptoms of VVD they frequently prescribe topical anesthetics, antidepressants, and sometimes even surgery. Many women who suffer from the condition are often led to believe, directly or indirectly, that their pain is all in their head (which often causes them to stop seeking help). One of my patients was told by a doctor that she was fine and just needed to go out dancing and have a good time!

Since some women with VVD have found relief when they were treated for back problems by an orthopedic doctor, it has been suggested that VVD can sometimes arise from a ruptured disc in the back, resulting in pressure on the nerve that supplies the vulva. Unfortunately, the condition has in fact often proven to be much more complex and elusive. The good news is that natural treatments, including dietary changes, detoxification, homeopathic remedies, herbs, and more, have much to offer women who suffer from VVD.

Clive Solomon, Ph.D., a researcher specializing in vulvar pain, discovered that many women who suffer from VVD secrete high amounts of oxalates in their urine. Whether oxalates are a cause of VVD or simply aggravate vulvar tissue that is already irritated is not known. Oxalates are commonly found in many foods that you would ordinarily consider good for you, including leafy greens, soybeans, wheat germ, eggplant, leeks, green peppers, beets, sweet potatoes, summer squash, berries, pecans, and peanuts. But if your vulvar tissues are unhealthy, oxalates can cause irritation, histamine release, and pain. (If your tissues are healthy, oxalates do not cause these symptoms.) Dr. Solomon reported that when women stopped eating foods containing high amounts of oxalates, in most cases their symptoms improved. (For resources on low-oxalate foods, see Appendix B.)

In addition to those found in the diet, according to Dr. Solomon, oxalates can also be produced by the liver and by bacteria in the intestines. And they can be produced in higher amounts if you have leaky gut syndrome. In addition to avoiding foods high in oxalates, if you have VVD it's important to address any digestive symptom imbalances you may have, making sure that you eradicate "unfriendly" bacteria in your intestines and heal from leaky gut syndrome. It's also a good idea to find out if you have food allergies that are aggravating your condition. (For guidelines on correcting leaky gut syndrome and imbalanced intestinal flora, see Chapter 6.)

In addition to treating your digestive system, if you have VVD you will also benefit by doing a liver cleanse as outlined in Chapter 4. (Modify your cleanse to avoid high-oxalate foods.) From a naturopathic perspective, VVD is a symptom due to an underlying disorder, so it's important to treat your whole body to completely eradicate VVD. Dr. Solomon's work underscores the fact that VVD is a multidimensional problem that requires a multidimensional approach. Work with your naturopathic physician to create a plan that addresses your whole body, mind, and spirit.

Nutritional supplements that can help decrease the pain associated with VVD include calcium citrate and N-acetyl glucosamine (NAG). Taking calcium citrate reduces the effects of oxalates in your body by making it more difficult for them to irritate your tissues. The recommended dose of calcium citrate while you are following a low-oxalate diet is 200 mg three times a day. NAG helps to strengthen the connective tissues of the vulva. The Pain Project, which was directed by Dr. Solomon, reported that women who took NAG for at least four months had significant improvement in their vulvar pain. The recommended dose of NAG is 250 mg twice a day. You may also want to consult with a naturopathic physician for additional approaches to alleviate many of the symptoms associated with VVD, including the emotional chaos and frustration that may accompany it.

In Chinese medicine, the symptoms of VVD are almost always considered to be the result of "damp-heat" that has settled in the genitals. If you eat too many greasy or spicy foods, you are more prone to developing the symptoms of VVD. In addition, pent-up frustration, resentment, and repressed anger can lead to stagnation of liver Qi, which contributes to the condition. It's important to keep your dominant element balanced (refer to Chapters 2 through 6 to determine your Five Element type and learn how to keep your primary element in balance), and you may want to seek out a qualified practitioner for herbal treatments and acupuncture.

While you are treating VVD, you may continue to experience vulvar pain. I recommend the following additional steps on a daily basis to help decrease your symptoms:

- After urinating, use soft, unscented toilet paper to wipe your vulva, or rinse with water.
- Wear all-cotton underwear and use an all-natural detergent.
- Rinse your underwear two or three times after washing it and before putting it in the dryer.
- Avoid washing your bathtub with harsh chemicals.
- Refrain from using bubble bath. (You may find that even essential oils are irritating.)

- When bathing, use only water to wash your vulva. (Your body soap and shampoo should also be free of perfumes and chemicals.)
- Wear loose-fitting clothing, or go without underwear, to decrease friction against your vulva.
- During your period use soft, all-cotton tampons or pads that are not bleached with chlorine. I recommend Natracare feminine products; they are nonabrasive, perfume free, non–chlorine bleached, and 95 percent biodegradable, and the tampons are made of certified organic cotton. You can also purchase Glad-rags (reusable cotton pads), or make your own.

Your Vaginal Health

"The vagina is both path and journey, tunnel and traveler."

—Natalie Angier, *Woman: An Intimate Geography*

Your vagina is the passageway to life, the part of you that opens to receive love and give birth. When you consider the important roles your vagina can play in the life process, the significance of maintaining your vaginal health cannot be overstated.

Your vagina is healthiest when its pH is on the acidic side, which prevents "unfriendly" bacteria and yeast from thriving. A special type of "friendly" bacteria in your vagina known as lactobacillus maintains order in your vaginal tissues by producing hydrogen peroxide (which kills off unfriendly bacteria and yeast). When you have an adequate amount of friendly bacteria growing in your vagina, it is much less prone to bacterial and yeast infections, the two most common types of vaginal infections.

Your vaginal pH can be thrown off in a number of ways. Antibiotics can cause an imbalance by killing off not only unfriendly bacteria but also friendly bacteria. (This is not a healthy scenario, since your friendly bacteria help you keep the right pH balance in your vagina in the first place.) Frequent sexual intercourse can also disrupt your vaginal pH because a man's ejaculate has an alkaline pH, setting the stage for a vaginal infection.

To prevent vaginal infections from occurring while on antibiotics, take acidophilus orally (at least one capsule a day containing at least two billion organisms) and continue taking it for at least two weeks after you've stopped taking antibiotics. If you are prone to vaginal infections, insert a lactobacillus vaginal suppository into your vagina during a course of antibiotics and at least two or three times after you've finished taking them. These vaginal suppositories are available at your health food store. (See Appendix B for resources.)

Remember that yeast loves a moist environment; tight clothing that increases sweating at the vulva is also conducive to yeast overgrowth. If you swim regularly, change out of your wet bathing suit as soon as possible afterward, and if your panty-hose causes too much restriction, cut out the crotch or wear knee-highs or thigh-highs. Also avoid sugar and alcohol, which promote bacterial and yeast growth.

TREATING VAGINAL INFECTIONS

I've successfully treated many women over the years who needlessly suffered from re-current vaginal infections. With natural therapies, you can eradicate them from your life once and for all. First, determine if your infection is due to an overgrowth of un-friendly bacteria or yeast. If you have symptoms of a yellowish discharge with an un-pleasant smell, you probably have a bacterial infection; if you have symptoms of a white, curdlike discharge, it is more likely a yeast infection. You will also want to eliminate the possibility that you have chlamydia, trichomonas, or any other STD or condition that can mimic some of these symptoms, by asking your naturopathic physician or gynecologist to test for these conditions. Your partner may also need to be tested and treated, especially if you have been reinfected after intercourse.

If you've ruled out these conditions and identified a vaginal infection, the fol-lowing treatments can help eliminate the majority of vaginal infections due to un-friendly bacteria or yeast. (If the infection persists for more than a week after you begin treatment, see your naturopathic physician or gynecologist for guidance.)

Suppositories. Both goldenseal and tea tree oil vaginal suppositories are effective against bacteria and yeast. I recommend that you use one suppository twice a day for a week, then insert one lactobacillus vaginal suppository daily for a week to repopu-late friendly flora. You may need to purchase goldenseal and tea tree oil suppositories through your naturopathic physician.

Sitz Baths. I recommend sitz baths if your vulva appears red and irritated. To prepare for your bath, make a goldenseal tea: add one tablespoon of goldenseal root to four cups of boiling water, simmer covered on low heat for ten to fifteen minutes, and strain. When the tea is cool enough to bathe in, pour it into a basin large enough for you to sit in comfortably. Sit in your tea bath for at least ten minutes two to three times a day, until your redness and irritation are alleviated. It usually takes only one or two days, depending on the severity of the infection and irritation.

Douching. Many women think of douching as something old-fashioned and associ-ate it with commercials aimed at eliminating "feminine odor." But douching can be an effective way to eradicate unfriendly bacteria and yeast in the vagina. I've found that most women prefer this method over suppositories because douching doesn't cause vaginal discharge throughout the day as suppositories do. If you choose to douche, be aware that aggressive douching may drive unfriendly bacteria upward into your cervix, uterus, and fallopian tubes. I advise my patients to use very little pressure when squeezing the douche bag, and to douche either sitting upright on the toilet or standing in the shower. I also recommend against doing a *retention douche,* which involves holding the fluid in your vagina for a few minutes.

For vaginal infections due to unfriendly bacteria or yeast, you can douche with goldenseal tea. To make the tea, follow the instructions for making sitz bath tea. Or you can douche with one pint of warm water mixed with five to fifteen drops of tea tree oil. (If the oil irritates your tissues, decrease the dose.) If your tissues are red and irritated, I recommend goldenseal tea over tea tree oil. Douche twice a day for a week, then insert one lactobacillus vaginal suppository in your vagina daily for a week to repopulate friendly flora.

Frequent vaginal yeast infections are a tell-tale sign that you may have an overgrowth of yeast in your digestive tract. You would benefit from an intestinal cleanse (as outlined in Chapter 6) to prevent a recurrence.

From a Chinese medicine perspective, a chronic vaginal infection is a sign of "dampness" that has accumulated in the pelvis due to an imbalance in the liver Qi and spleen Qi; the dampness can turn into heat and create symptoms of itching. The primary causes of these imbalances are emotional problems, excessive stress, too much physical work, and consumption of too many dairy products, sweets, and greasy foods. Treatment is aimed at removing the underlying cause of the condition by making dietary and lifestyle changes and strengthening liver Qi and spleen Qi. Dietary changes include avoiding these foods, and lifestyle changes include decreasing stress and increasing enjoyable, relaxing time. To strengthen your liver Qi and spleen Qi, see Chapters 4 and 6.

Herbal treatments are also used in Chinese medicine to treat vaginal infections. A formula called Yu Dai Wan, or "Stop Leukorrhea Pills," contains herbs that can quickly clear the pelvis of heat and dampness that manifest as yellow vaginal discharge. Your Chinese medical practitioner can prescribe this herbal formula or another that suits your specific needs.

The Health of Your Cervix

The cervix is a small but powerful organ that forms the entrance to the uterus, and the opening that most of us passed through as we came into the world. Aside from playing its dramatic role in the birth process, the cervix helps create a natural lubrication during sexual intercourse and harbors sperm in the process of trying to fertilize an egg.

Yet we are probably most aware of the cervix during our annual gynecological exam, when a small sample of cells from the cervix is collected during a Pap test and sent to a laboratory to be assessed for signs of cervical cancer. Cervical cancer is the second most common cancer in women who are twenty to thirty-nine years of age,[4] but with the introduction of routine Pap tests and more advanced screening, most cases of abnormal cervical cells are found long before cancer has manifested. In recent years, however, the incidence of cervical cancer has risen due to the spread of the human papilloma virus (HPV), which is sexually transmitted and often remains latent for many years before causing abnormal cervical cell changes. Many women are unaware that most Pap tests indicating abnormal cervical cells are due to HPV.

Like my patient Leilani, whose story appears at the beginning of this chapter, many women are confronted with repeated abnormal Pap test results and a confusing array of options for treatment. If you have had a history of abnormal Pap tests, your physician will mostly likely order an HPV test to determine if you carry HPV and what strain you have. Certain strains of the virus are more virulent and potentially cancer-causing than others. If your HPV test reveals that you have a high-risk strain, it warrants more personal vigilance over your lifestyle and diet and requires regular Pap tests. Lower-risk strains rarely act as a precursor to cervical cancer but can manifest as visible warts.

If you have an abnormal Pap test, you may be advised by your health care provider to have a colposcopy if your test results indicate that you need further testing immediately. A colposcopy is a method of examining your cervix under a lighted microscope. Your doctor will be able to see areas of your cervix or vaginal wall that appear abnormal and will usually do a biopsy of the tissue, which means that a small amount of tissue will be removed and evaluated. Your doctor may also take a sample from inside your cervix where HPV infections tend to thrive.

Some women have Pap tests that show slightly abnormal cells, or *atypia*. In this case, you will be advised to have another Pap test in three months. While you wait, see your naturopathic physician to begin a program that will help you reverse your cervical cell changes. Many naturopathic physicians recommend that you take a proactive approach and use a series of vaginal suppositories that contain vitamin A and herbs including goldenseal, echinacea, and thuja. I've seen many cases of atypia effectively reversed using this method.

TREATING AND PREVENTING
ABNORMAL CERVICAL CELL CHANGES

There's no cure for HPV, but there are many ways that you can boost your immune system to prevent cervical dysplasia (abnormal cervical cell changes) and keep HPV under control. My patient Leilani made changes in her lifestyle and diet and took a number of supplements to prevent the virus from gaining a foothold in her body. If you have HPV, I recommend that you adhere to the Naturally Healthy Diet and Lifestyle to create an environment that discourages HPV from taking hold and causing abnormal cervical cell changes. In addition, refer to Chapters 2, 4, and 6 to make sure that your immune system, your liver, and your digestive system are all functioning optimally.

Certain nutritional supplements are especially important in treating and preventing HPV-related cervical cell changes. I advise my patients who have, or have had, abnormal Pap tests to eat copious amounts of cruciferous vegetables or take 300 mg a day of indole-3-carbinol (I3C). I3C helps decrease your liver's production of "unfriendly" estrogens, and there appears to be an association between the production of these unfriendly estrogens and abnormal cells in the cervix. The cells in your cervix have many estrogen receptors that, when stimulated by excessive amounts of unfriendly estrogen, can increase your risk for abnormal cell growth. (A urine test can measure which kinds of estrogens your liver is producing; see Chapter 9.) I3C is valuable for treating and preventing HPV-related cell changes because it can promote the production of the "friendly" estrogens that don't increase abnormal cell growth. Some studies show that women whose Pap tests indicate abnormal cervical cells (such as cervical dysplasia) have great improvement when they take I3C.[5]

Folic acid, a B vitamin that is important for cell replication, is an important nutrient for preventing and treating abnormal cervical cells. Some studies have confirmed that taking amounts of folic acid higher than the Recommended Daily Allowance (RDA) levels can have a positive effect on preventing abnormal cervical cell changes from progressing, especially in women who have taken birth control pills.[6] For long-term prevention, the recommended dose is 800 to 2,400 mcg a day. (Your daily multivitamin should contain 800 mcg.) Depending on whether you are treating an HPV infection or maintaining the health of your cervix, higher doses may be recommended by your naturopathic physician.

Other supplements for treating and preventing HPV-related cervical cell changes include the following antioxidants:

- Vitamin C: Take 2,000 mg a day for prevention and up to 6,000 mg a day for treatment. (Treat for at least three months.)
- Mixed carotenoids (a combination of beta-carotene, alpha-carotene, lutein,

and other carotenoids): Take 50,000 i.u. a day for prevention and 150,000 i.u. a day for treatment. (Treat for at least three months.)

- Alpha lipoic acid: Take 100 mg a day for prevention and 200 mg a day for treatment. (Treat for at least three months.)

In Chinese medicine, boosting your immune system with herbs (as outlined in Chapter 2) will help prevent and treat HPV-related cervical cell changes. In addition, a number of herbal formulas can help balance your body's Qi, which will prevent HPV from thriving. There are also herbal formulas that can dispel "damp-heat" from the vagina and help regenerate and heal cervical tissue that has abnormal cells. See your Chinese medical practitioner for an herbal prescription that is tailored to your needs.

As you've seen, my patient Leilani was successful in her treatment of cervical dysplasia with natural medicine. Because her Pap test had revealed abnormal cervical cells, I recommended that she have a series of herbal and nutritional therapies known as *escharotic treatments* to treat her cervix. Consult with your naturopathic physician to see if you are a candidate for these treatments, which have been used by naturopathic physicians for decades. In recent years, a comprehensive protocol utilizing escharotic treatments has been developed by Dr. Tori Hudson, a highly respected naturopathic physician and educator specializing in women's health care. I've had a great deal of success using her protocol to treat many women with abnormal cervical cells due to HPV and prevent their recurrence.

If you are a candidate, your naturopathic physician will probably recommend that you have one or two escharotic treatments a week for three to five weeks, depending on the severity of your condition and your HPV status. Each treatment lasts about twenty minutes and involves an application of bromelain (a digestive enzyme) to your cervix, a calendula succus wash, and an application of a solution of zinc chloride and sanguinaria to your cervix (which is left on for only one minute). To end the treatment, two vaginal suppositories are placed up against your cervix; they contain a number of compounds, including vitamin A and magnesium sulfate, which have anti-inflammatory properties and accelerate the healing of cervical tissues.

When your escharotic treatments are completed, you will be advised to use other herbal and nutritional vaginal suppositories to help heal your cervix and prevent HPV from thriving. You will also be advised to take herbal and nutritional supplements, and make lifestyle and dietary changes that support your immune system.

If you have a history of HPV or abnormal Pap tests, remember that there are myriad steps you can take to enhance your immune system and help prevent cervical cell changes that could lead to cervical cancer. I highly recommend that you work with your naturopathic physician to create a comprehensive plan that works best for you.

The Health of Your Uterus

"The uterus is related energetically to a woman's innermost sense of self and her inner world. It is symbolic of her dreams and the selves to which she would like to give birth."

—CHRISTIANE NORTHRUP, M.D.,
Women's Bodies, Women's Wisdom

The womb, the place from which we all came forth, is a wonderfully complex and creative organ. Over the course of your lifetime, your uterus sheds and regenerates its lining, known as the endometrium, many times during your menstrual cycles. Your uterus is remarkably expansive; it is capable of increasing its weight from a mere two ounces before pregnancy to as much as two pounds by the end of pregnancy. Within weeks after pregnancy, it reverts to its prepregnant size.

The health of your uterus is closely connected with your hormonal health; keeping your hormones balanced is critical to preventing many of the gynecological problems associated with the uterus. An excessive amount of estrogen in your body, along with a low level of progesterone, can increase your risk of developing abnormal cells in the uterine lining (a condition known as *endometrial hyperplasia*). To keep your hormones well balanced, see Chapter 7.

The most common symptom of endometrial hyperplasia is abnormal menstrual bleeding between periods, or bleeding in postmenopausal women. The condition, which is diagnosed with a biopsy of the endometrium, is most often seen in older women who are not menstruating. Since these women are not ovulating, they are not releasing progesterone, and they can often be successfully treated for endometrial hyperplasia with a few months' course of natural progesterone along with nutritional supplements to help their liver break down and eliminate estrogens. Although some cases of endometrial hyperplasia are resolved without any intervention, the untreated condition can lead to endometrial cancer. If you experience abnormal bleeding after menopause, seek prompt treatment.

Another way of preserving your uterine health is by preventing exposure to STDs, which can wreak havoc on a woman's gynecological system. Some STDs, such as chlamydia, can cause pelvic inflammatory disease (PID), a bacterial infection in the uterus. To treat chlamydia or PID, you will need to take antibiotics. See your naturopathic physician for immune-supportive therapies.

UTERINE FIBROIDS

One of the most common gynecological problems women experience is the growth of benign tumors known as uterine fibroids. It has been estimated that between 20 percent and 40 percent of women have them,[7] and some statistics have reported the incidence as high as 50 percent. There appears to be a genetic predisposition to fibroids, with African American women more likely to have them than Caucasian women.[8] Risk factors associated with the development of fibroids include a positive family history, obesity, and having a first period at an early age.[9] If you've had children, you are at decreased risk for developing fibroids.[10] From a Chinese medicine perspective, Earth types have the greatest likelihood to form fibroids, and Wood types may also be susceptible if their Qi becomes chronically stagnant.

A woman can have a single fibroid or many. Depending on the fibroids' size and location, some women have no symptoms associated with them while others experience heavy menstrual bleeding, pelvic pressure, and pain. (Fibroids are the most common reason women choose to have hysterectomies.) Fibroids that grow into the inner cavity of the uterus and cause heavy menstrual bleeding are known as *submucosal fibroids*. Other types of fibroids can grow large but are less likely to cause heavy bleeding and other complications. If fibroids are detected during a routine pelvic exam, a follow-up pelvic ultrasound can provide more detailed information about their size and location.

If you have uterine fibroids, your treatment depends on your symptoms and other factors. Naturopathic medicine offers you a number of tools to help stabilize fibroid growth and decrease the symptoms associated with fibroids, such as heavy bleeding and pain.

TREATING UTERINE FIBROIDS WITH NATURAL MEDICINE

Every month Diana had symptoms of severe cramping that started during her period and menstrual bleeding that lasted up to twenty-five days in a row. Her gynecologist told her that she needed to have a hysterectomy due to a small fibroid in her uterus. When Diana came to see me, she was very upset at the thought of major pelvic surgery and the effect it could have on her body. She wanted to know if natural medicine could help.

After evaluating Diana's hormone levels and assessing her condition from a naturopathic and Chinese perspective, I prescribed natural progesterone, Chinese herbs, and acupuncture treatments. After only a few months of therapy, her periods became more regular and the cramping almost nonexistent. "A year after I was told to have a hysterectomy," she now says, "my gynecologist was amazed that my fibroid had not increased in size, and had actually become slightly smaller. I continue to work out at the gym, race outrigger canoes, and enjoy life—with my uterus and ovaries!"

❧✗❧

Over the years I've treated many women with fibroids, and in many cases they were able to avoid surgery and pharmaceutical drugs by using natural therapies. But if you experience severe symptoms of excessive menstrual bleeding or pain, a surgical or pharmaceutical intervention may be warranted. In this case, natural medicine can assist you through the process while continuing to treat the underlying cause that led to the development of your fibroids.

Estrogen is the fuel that keeps uterine fibroids alive and stimulates their growth. One of the goals in treating fibroids is to reduce the rate of their growth by lowering your overall estrogen level and managing your symptoms until menopause, when your estrogen level drops naturally. After menopause fibroids often shrink and symptoms are resolved. The treatments that I use to help women with their symptoms of uterine fibroids include a combination of liver cleansing, dietary changes, natural progesterone, and Chinese herbal medicines.

Liver Cleansing. In Chapter 4 we saw that the liver cleanse includes a lipotropic formula containing herbs, amino acids, and vitamins. This formula can help your liver work better in detoxifying estrogens and other compounds. We've also seen (in Chapter 9) that women who have excessive amounts of "unfriendly" estrogen can use calcium D-glucarate and indole-3-carbinol (I3C) to help the liver deactivate and break down estrogen. These nutritional supplements can be an important part of treating the underlying causes of your fibroids. Another essential aspect of the liver cleanse is decreasing your exposure to environmental estrogens. A study published in the *Annals of New York Academy of Sciences* demonstrated that environmental estrogens, specifically organochlorine pesticides, can stimulate the growth of fibroids.[11] See Chapter 4 for detailed information on how to do a liver cleanse.

Diet. The Naturally Healthy Diet (outlined in Chapter 1) is an important part of your treatment for fibroids because, along with its many other benefits, it is a "low-estrogen" diet. By eating high-quality organic foods, consuming fewer saturated animal fats and whole-milk dairy products that can be high in estrogen-mimicking chemicals, and maintaining a healthy weight, you are essentially following a fibroid-fighting diet. In addition, the Naturally Healthy Diet also includes lots of fruits, vegetables, and whole grains—high-fiber foods that assist with the elimination of estrogens.

Progesterone. If you have fibroids, you may have a hormone imbalance, with an insufficient level of progesterone compared with estrogen. I've treated many women for fibroids by giving them natural progesterone. Most often these women had irregular or heavy menstrual bleeding or pronounced PMS, but their symptoms were resolved after they took natural progesterone for fourteen days each month, from mid-cycle until the onset of their period. For more information on natural progesterone, including guidelines on using urine or saliva tests to assess your hormone levels, see Chapter 7.

Chinese Medicine. According to Chinese medicine, fibroids are the result of stagnant Qi and Blood, which causes heat and dampness to accumulate in the pelvis; your treatment is aimed at correcting these imbalances. In Chapter 9 we discussed the Chinese herbal formula Bupleurum Entangled Qi, which is used for eliminating benign breast lumps. This formula is also used for a number of female gynecological disorders, including fibroids. To clear heat and dampness, it is often mixed with another formula called Unlocking Formula, which was developed by Dr. Bob Flaws, a specialist in Chinese medicine and female gynecology. Used together, these two herbal formulas can help treat the symptoms associated with fibroids, including heavy bleeding and pelvic pain; they can also be used to treat the underlying Qi and Blood imbalances related to the condition. You can purchase these herbal formulas through a practitioner of Chinese medicine.

The Health of Your Ovaries

"Our ovarian wisdom represents our deepest creativity, that which waits to be born from within us, that which can be born only through us, our unique creative potential."

—CHRISTIANE NORTHRUP, M.D.,
Women's Bodies, Women's Wisdom

Your ovaries are small but powerful, helping to regulate the hormones estrogen, progesterone, and testosterone, which strongly influence the health of your entire body. Your ovaries house thousands of eggs, each with the genetic potential to create a new individual. In Chinese medicine, your eggs are perceived as a direct manifestation of the kidney Essence—the Qi that is passed down from previous generations. Your ovaries bind you to your long line of ancestors and have the potential to connect you to future generations.

Keeping your ovaries healthy begins with following the Naturally Healthy Diet and Lifestyle (outlined in Chapter 1) because many of the problems that can arise in the ovaries are due to stress and nutritional deficiencies. From a Chinese medicine perspective, liver Qi imbalances due to stress and frustration, and spleen Qi imbalances due to a poor diet, play a major role in the health of the ovaries.

The ovaries typically form numerous small cysts during a normal menstrual cycle. Two of the most common types of benign ovarian cysts often go away on their own. A *follicular cyst* can form during the process of maturing an egg in the ovary. If it becomes large (greater than four centimeters) and doesn't disappear after a few months, it may require medical intervention and possibly surgery. A *luteal cyst,* which can form after an egg has been released from the ovary, is usually small and causes no symptoms, although some women experience a sharp, stabbing, cramping pain. If a luteal cyst becomes large, or if it ruptures and causes massive bleeding, medical intervention and surgery may be necessary. If your doctor feels any other type of unusual ovarian mass during your annual exam, an ultrasound is usually ordered to determine its size and location and whether it is a fluid-filled cyst or a solid mass. A solid mass may be potentially cancerous and should be further evaluated as soon as possible for early treatment.

If you consistently form follicular or luteal cysts that either cause pain at ovulation or become large enough for concern, I recommend that you have a hormone evaluation. Balancing your levels of estrogen and progesterone may be the first step in preventing future cysts. From a naturopathic perspective, ovarian cysts can also be related to poor circulation of blood and lymph in the pelvis, while according to Chinese medicine they can be caused by stagnation of liver Qi (which results in poor circulation of blood) and deficiency of spleen Qi (which leads to sluggish movement of your lymph). The goal in treating benign ovarian cysts, from both a naturopathic and a Chinese medicine perspective, is to increase the circulation of blood and lymph through the pelvis.

Many nutrients, herbs, and topical treatments can help you treat benign ovarian cysts and optimize the health of your ovaries. Eating foods containing beta-carotene and vitamin A, which are needed for healthy ovulation, taking a multivitamin, and supplementing your diet with fish and flax oils can all help prevent cysts and promote ovarian health. Herbal remedies can help decrease the formation of ovarian cysts by stimulating your circulation and assisting with the removal of waste products. The classic herbal tonic known as Turska's formula is very effective in treating ovarian cysts. It consists of a combination of herbs that have some toxicity and is not available over the counter but can be prescribed by your naturopathic physician. Chinese herbal formulas can effectively move Qi through your pelvis and clear heat and dampness; to obtain the best results, see a Chinese medical practitioner for an herbal formula prescribed according to your particular symptoms.

One of the best topical treatments for benign ovarian cysts is the application of castor oil packs, which can increase circulation and move lymph through the pelvis. To make a castor oil pack, rub a teaspoon of castor oil onto your lower abdomen, then place a piece of clean flannel or cotton (some women use an old pillowcase) on the area. Next, apply a heating pad or a hot water bottle on top of the material and allow the heat to penetrate into your tissues for at least twenty minutes. It's best to do this treatment at night before bed so that you can leave the oil on your skin until you take a shower and wash it off in the morning. If you have chronic ovarian cysts, I recommend that you do castor oil treatments three or four times a week for at least three months.

Finally, related to ovarian health is the health of the fallopian tubes, perhaps the most delicate and exquisite of all your pelvic organs. As the primary sites of fertilization, they act as conduits for a fertilized egg to enter your uterus. If your fallopian tubes become infected by chlamydia or gonorrhea, the results can include scarring and infertility. Take care to protect against STDs, and if you suspect exposure, be sure to get prompt treatment (usually requiring the use of antibiotics), and support your immune system with the nutritional and herbal supplements in Chapter 2.

Preventing and Treating Endometriosis Naturally

Endometriosis, which affects about 10 percent of women of reproductive age, is a condition that can involve any of the internal gynecological organs and surrounding tissues. It occurs when endometrial tissue, which is normally found only in the uterus, migrates to the ovaries, fallopian tubes, colon wall, or other structures. This misplaced endometrial tissue responds to estrogen stimulation as endometrial tissue in your uterus does; it proliferates and bleeds with hormonal changes associated with the menstrual cycle. There is no cure for endometriosis, which can cause chronic pelvic pain and infertility, but there are many steps you can take to prevent and treat it with natural medicine.

While we're unsure what causes endometriosis to develop, genetics may play a role, and there may be environmental factors as well as a connection to the immune system. A study published in the journal *Environmental Health Perspectives* found an association between dioxin exposure and endometriosis in monkeys.[12] A by-product of the paper mill industry, dioxin is an estrogen-mimicking chemical that is ubiquitous in the environment and can be found in trace amounts in foods that have been stored in some cardboard containers, such as milk cartons. The researchers found that dioxin adversely affected the immune system and altered the effect of estrogen on reproductive organs. The more dioxin the monkeys were exposed to, the study revealed, the higher and more severe the incidence of endometriosis.

In my practice, many women come to see me with endometriosis in varying degrees of severity, and when they use natural therapies, I often witness a dramatic reduction in their pain and improvement in the quality of their lives. My objective is initially to relieve them of their symptoms but ultimately to treat them by limiting their exposure to harmful environmental toxins, balancing hormones, enhancing the immune system, and encouraging the body's natural ability to break down and eliminate estrogens.

The Naturally Healthy Lifestyle and Diet (outlined in Chapter 1) can help minimize your exposure to estrogen-mimicking chemicals and boost your immunity. To eliminate dioxin and other chemicals that may already be in your system, support your liver function by doing a liver cleanse and practicing spa therapy as outlined in Chapter 4. If you are experiencing a great deal of discomfort with your periods due to endometriosis, see Chapter 7 to treat painful menstrual cramps and to help balance your hormones; if your pain is not influenced by your periods, see your naturopathic physician for assistance.

Choosing Birth Control

For many women, decisions about birth control are vitally important to their sexual lives, their pelvic health, and their overall health. Too often women choose a method that compromises their health in order to avoid conception. In the United States the birth control pill, which consists of synthetic hormones, has become the most common method of preventing pregnancy. The pill works by disrupting ovulation, fooling a woman's body into believing that she's pregnant. Other hormonal methods of birth control are on the rise, including hormone patches (Ortho Evra), estrogen and progestin injections (Lunelle), and progestin injections (Depo-Provera). While hormonal methods are statistically very effective at preventing pregnancy, they interfere with a woman's own natural hormone cycles and may put her at risk for a number of side effects, including irregular menstrual bleeding, weight gain, breast tenderness, nausea, headaches, and blood clots, to name a few. I often tell fertile women that the whole universe is willing them to procreate, and that if they want to block this powerful force, it's better to have sex conscientiously than to use birth control methods that can harm them.

Although there may be a time and place for hormonal methods of birth control, I don't recommend that women stay on these methods for long. Since many women want to use a reliable form of birth control for as many as thirty-five years of potential fertility, finding a method that doesn't compromise their health in any way is critical. The good news for women who want birth control is that there are many alternative methods that don't involve synthetic hormones. These methods may require diligence and some effort on the part of the woman (and often her partner as well), and at times they may interfere with spontaneity, but if used appropriately they can be extremely effective.

I recommend that my patients who are not in a monogamous relationship use a condom for every sexual encounter, even if they are on the Pill or are using another hormonal method of birth control, because hormonal methods won't protect them from STDs. If a woman is in a committed monogamous relationship and wants to prevent pregnancy, I advise a combination of methods. As you can see from the "Birth Control Methods" chart, many barrier methods (such as condoms, diaphragms, and cervical caps) have a high rate of failure. But if you use at least two of these methods, such as a condom and a diaphragm, at the same time, your chances of getting pregnant are extremely unlikely.

For couples who wish to have intercourse during part of the month without using a barrier method, I recommend reading *Taking Charge of Your Fertility* by Toni Weschler, M.P.H. This book clearly outlines the Fertility Awareness Method, which includes taking basal body temperature readings and observing changes in cervical mucus and cervical position to determine when you are ovulating and when you are not fertile. This method tells you when you need to practice abstinence, when you should use a barrier method, and when you can safely go without. According to Weschler, the method has a failure rate of 2 percent when couples abstain completely from intercourse during the fertile time of the month.[13] This method has the added benefit of making you intimately aware of your body's natural cycles, and it can also help you know exactly when to have intercourse in the event that you want to get pregnant rather than prevent pregnancy.

If you do want to conceive, in addition to the Fertility Awareness Method you can use ovulation test kits to help determine the best time to have intercourse. One innovative ovulation test kit on the market called Ovulook helps determine when you are ovulating by viewing changes in your saliva. To use the test, you gently scrape the bottom of your tongue first thing in the morning when you wake up and place a drop of saliva onto a slide. Once you are fully awake, you examine the sample (the test kit comes with a minimicroscope and light, so all you have to do is press a button and look), and you can tell by the appearance of your saliva if you are fertile. Some of my patients have used this kit to prevent pregnancy, although it is not approved by the FDA for this purpose.

Birth Control Methods

BIRTH CONTROL METHOD	PROS	CONS	FAILURE RATE*
Periodic abstinence (refraining from intercourse when you think it most likely you will get pregnant)	Easy to chart your cycle on a calendar, and convenient to *not* use any birth control during the time you think you aren't fertile	Doesn't prevent the transmission of STDs, and (because of the high failure rate) isn't the most reliable method of preventing pregnancy	20

*The failure rate is expressed as the number of pregnancies expected per 100 women per year. Failure rates are based on information from the Food and Drug Administration.[14]

BIRTH CONTROL METHOD	PROS	CONS	FAILURE RATE*
Male condom	Helps prevent the transmission of STDs; is easy to keep on hand; and may be applied with little advance preparation	Decreases sensation for both partners; latex condoms may cause an allergy in some people; and foreplay may be interrupted	11
Female condom	Helps prevent the transmission of STDs; is easy to keep on hand; and may be applied with little advance preparation	Decreases sensation for both partners; latex condoms may cause an allergy in some people; foreplay may be interrupted; and isn't a very effective method	21
Diaphragm with spermicide	Is used on an as-needed basis; can be inserted up to two hours prior to intercourse, allowing for some spontaneity	Doesn't prevent the transmission of STDs; spermicide may cause irritation; pressure from the diaphragm may contribute to urinary tract infections; and must be used correctly 100 percent of the time to be effective	17
Cervical cap with spermicide	Is used on an as-needed basis; can be inserted up to two hours prior to intercourse, allowing for some spontaneity	Doesn't prevent the transmission of STDs; spermicide may cause irritation; your partner may feel the edge of the cervical cap; and must be used correctly 100 percent of the time to be effective	17
Spermicide alone	Is easy to insert and requires no foreign object in your vagina	Doesn't prevent the transmission of STDs; not an effective method; and spermicide may cause irritation	20–50 (studies show varying failure rates)
Intrauterine device (IUD)	Allows for spontaneous intercourse; once inserted by a physician, can be left in place for up to ten years	Doesn't prevent the transmission of STDs; can increase cramps and bleeding with periods; increases risk for pelvic inflammatory disease (PID); and may cause perforation of the uterus	Fewer than 1
Birth control pills: estrogen plus progestin	Are effective and allow for spontaneous intercourse	Don't prevent the transmission of STDs; interfere with natural hormone cycles; and are associated with side effects that include depression, headaches, nausea, increased risks for stroke, high blood pressure, blood clots, and changes in mood, sexual desire, weight, and menstrual cycle	1

BIRTH CONTROL METHOD	PROS	CONS	FAILURE RATE*
Hormone patch (Ortho Evra): estrogen plus progestin	Is effective and allows for spontaneous intercourse	Doesn't prevent the transmission of STDs; interferes with natural hormone cycles; and is associated with side effects similar to those of birth control pills containing both estrogen and progestin	1
Hormone injection (Lunelle): estrogen plus progestin	Is effective and allows for spontaneous intercourse	Doesn't prevent the transmission of STDs; interferes with natural hormone cycles; and is associated with side effects similar to those of birth control pills containing both estrogen and progestin	Fewer than 1
Birth control pills: progestin only	Are effective; allow for spontaneous intercourse; can be used by women who cannot take estrogen; and may result in fewer menstrual cramps	Don't prevent the transmission of STDs; interfere with natural hormone cycles; and are associated with side effects that include irregular menstrual bleeding, depression, headaches, dizziness, breast tenderness, and weight gain	2
Hormone injection (Depo-Provera): progestin only	Is effective; allows for spontaneous intercourse for three months	Doesn't prevent the transmission of STDs; interferes with natural hormone cycles; is associated with side effects that include irregular menstrual bleeding, depression, headaches, nausea, dizziness, breast tenderness, weight gain, longer or heavier menstrual flow, nervousness, spotty darkening of the skin, hair loss, and changes in sex drive; it may take a year or more for some women to begin regular menstrual cycles after discontinuing hormone injections	Fewer than 1
Female sterilization	Is effective; allows for spontaneous intercourse without ever having to think about birth control again	Doesn't prevent the transmission of STDs; and if a woman wants to become pregnant in the future she will have to undergo additional surgery that may be ineffective	Fewer than 1

BIRTH CONTROL METHOD	PROS	CONS	FAILURE RATE*
Male sterilization	Is effective; allows for spontaneous intercourse without ever having to think about birth control again	Doesn't prevent the transmission of STDs; and if the male desires children in the future he will have to undergo additional surgery that may be ineffective	Fewer than 1

Protecting Against STDs

An important pelvic health concern for many women is the issue of sexually transmitted diseases (STDs), which can be insidious and may have long term side effects that impair fertility if not treated promptly. Most women are well aware that human immunodeficiency virus (HIV) is a silent threat that remains dormant for years before becoming active, and that the herpes virus not only is a nuisance but also can influence your decisions about giving birth. But women are often less aware that other STDs, such as human papilloma virus (HPV), can have serious consequences. If you don't know your sexual partner's history, getting screened for STDs is a self-protective act that is highly recommended. The following is a summary of the most common STDs, their screening methods, and their treatment.

STD	SYMPTOMS	TESTING METHODS	TREATMENT OPTIONS
Herpes (a virus)	Blisters on the vulva can be painful and itchy; outbreaks can also be found on the thighs, buttocks, or anywhere else on the body.	A herpes culture (blood tests are less accurate)	Naturopathic medicine treats herpes with diet, lifestyle modification, and immune support; conventional Western medicine typically employs antiviral medications, including acyclovir.
Chlamydia (a bacterium)	There may be no symptoms, but some women complain of pelvic pain, burning when they urinate, or a vaginal discharge.	A chlamydia culture or a DNA test	The antibiotics doxycycline or erythromycin
Gonorrhea (a bacterium)	There may be no symptoms, but some women complain of pelvic pain, burning when they urinate, increased urinary frequency, or a vaginal discharge.	A gonorrhea culture or a DNA test	The antibiotics doxycycline or ceftriaxone

STD	SYMPTOMS	TESTING METHODS	TREATMENT OPTIONS
Syphilis (a bacterium)	Symptoms go through stages: initially there may be a genital ulcer that heals; later a fever and a rash may develop. If untreated, there can be eventual nervous system and heart abnormalities.	A blood test	The antibiotic penicillin
Trichomonas (a parasite)	Some women experience no symptoms, while others have vaginal itching, an odorous vaginal discharge, or discomfort with intercourse.	Microscopic examination of vaginal fluids, or a trichomonas culture	The pharmaceutical drug metronidazole (also known as Flagyl)
Human papilloma virus (HPV)	Most women have no symptoms for years; HPV, which can cause cervical cancer, is usually suspected when a woman has an abnormal Pap test. With certain strains of HPV there may be warts on the vulva, vagina, or cervix.	A DNA test or a tissue biopsy	There is no cure for HPV, but natural treatments can help your immune system cope with it; conventional Western medicine often uses chemical, laser, or freezing treatments to remove visible warts.
Human immunodeficiency virus (HIV)	There may be no symptoms for many years; for some women, chronic vaginitis is the first sign of the virus. HIV attacks your immune system, making you more susceptible to infections that can be fatal.	A blood test	There is no cure for HIV; treatment with pharmaceutical drugs called protease inhibitors has been able to help keep HIV-infected individuals' immune systems functioning; natural methods can enhance the immune system's ability to cope with HIV.
Hepatitis B (a virus)	Symptoms include jaundice, fever, fatigue, and intestinal problems.	A blood test to look at antibody levels	There is no cure for hepatitis B, but it can be prevented with a series of vaccines and treated with pharmaceutical drugs and natural methods.
Hepatitis C (a virus)	There may be no symptoms, or there may be symptoms that include jaundice, fever, fatigue, and intestinal problems.	A blood test to look at antibody levels	There is no cure for hepatitis C, and no vaccine to prevent it; treatment includes antiviral drugs and natural methods.

Nurturing Your Intimate Self: Final Thoughts

There are many ways you can use gentle, effective natural medicines and treatments to promote optimal pelvic health. Most pelvic health problems don't simply appear overnight; they are the end result of imbalances elsewhere in the body. Diet, lifestyle, and emotions can all have profound effects on the health of the pelvis. Chinese medicine teaches that emotions can influence the health of the gynecological organs by affecting the flow of Qi through the pelvic region.

   You can optimize your pelvic health by keeping your whole body healthy. Your pelvis is your center of gravity and the focus of your capacity for erotic pleasure. At the same time, it is the hub of your potential for procreation, symbolizing your innermost creative powers. The value of protecting your pelvic health—honoring and nurturing the cradle of your intimate self—is immeasurable.

The Essence of Chapter 10

- Know that your pelvis is the seat of your power, both physically and symbolically, and is central to your well-being.
- Remember that in Chinese medicine emotions can influence the health of gynecological organs.
- Keep your immune system strong if you have herpes.
- Use natural medicine for relieving the symptoms of vulvodynia.
- Prevent and treat vaginal infections with natural methods.
- Boost your immune system if you have HPV, and use natural medicine if you have abnormal cervical cell changes.
- Use natural therapies to decrease the symptoms associated with uterine fibroids.
- Balance your hormones and increase the circulation of blood and lymph through your pelvis to treat ovarian cysts.
- Prevent and treat endometriosis with natural methods.
- Choose a method of birth control that doesn't compromise your health.
- Prevent STDs, and get tested for them if necessary.

Chapter 11

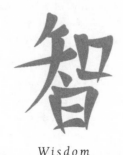

Wisdom

Tapping into the Power of Your Mind

"The brain is wider than the sky."
—EMILY DICKINSON, "The Brain"

R OSEANNE CAME *to see me after consulting a number of medical doctors about her depression. "Seeing one doctor after another," she said, "made me feel as if I'd become a collection of systems assembled into one body. Everyone was a specialist, and not one of them had taken the time to see me and my symptoms as an integrated whole."*

At first Roseanne seemed genuinely surprised that I was as interested in the state of her mind and emotions as I was in the state of her body. She had started experiencing deep depression when her husband left her in the early 1980s. "I found myself spiraling down, my feelings of humiliation alternating with despair," she told me. "It hadn't occurred to me until then that my father must have felt the same way when my mother left us during my childhood. Ever since I was a young woman I'd been battling feelings of emptiness, and now that my own kids had left home and my husband was no longer in my life, many years of suppressed emotions were surfacing. I knew that I needed professional help."

Working with Roseanne as a whole person—treating her body, mind, and emotional state with nutritional supplements, herbs, and Chinese medicine—enabled her to come up out of the dark hole that had engulfed most of her days. "My experience is that natural medicine is about so much more than just taking a pill," she says. "It made me feel truly taken care of—even with all my quirks and eccentricities!"

✍

The Power of Your Mind

The power of your mind is tremendous, and at any time you can draw on its potential to create health in your life. Your mind not only reflects the reality that you live in, it also allows you to make choices to alter that reality. Your ability to make healthy choices for your body, and in all areas of your life, is critical to your well-being.

The power of your mind touches every aspect of your life—affecting who you are, how you feel, and even what you look like—and its sphere of influence reaches far into your future. Your ability to make the healthiest choices at every moment of every day gives you the opportunity to create the life that you want—and to feel *great* while you're creating it.

In this chapter, we will discuss how to keep your brain cells as healthy as possible so that your mind can reach its fullest potential. When your brain is well nourished and functioning optimally, you are happier, you have more positive energy, and you can experience life more fully. You also have a sharper memory, greater mental and emotional clarity, and more of what is known as "presence of mind." We will explore nutritional and herbal supplements that can help you sleep, alleviate anxiety, and overcome depression, and steps you can take to decrease memory loss and reduce your risks for age-related dementia and Alzheimer's disease. You will also discover how to manifest the concept of healthy aging in your life. Knowing how to tap into the power of your mind will allow you to live each season of your life to its fullest as you gradually transform into the wise woman of your senior years.

The View from the West

Your brain is perhaps the most fascinating and complex structure in your body. Comprised of billions of nerve cells and pathways, it is the master control center for every system in your body and literally the headquarters for your entire nervous system. Your brain requires an enormous amount of fuel to do its job. Although it weighs only a few pounds, it consumes 20 percent of your body's supply of oxygen, and 25 percent of its sugar intake.[1] Your brain needs this steady supply of fuel because it is constantly active, sending trillions of messages every second of your life, even while you sleep. These messages are delivered primarily by brain chemicals (also known as neurotransmitters) such as serotonin and endorphins, which conduct signals from one nerve cell to another.

Together with certain hormones, your brain chemicals can have a major effect on your behavior, your moods, and how you feel at any given moment. For instance, having adequate levels of serotonin and endorphins can be important for your sense of well-being and happiness. And some women experience dramatic mood fluctuations due to changes in brain chemicals associated with the ebb and flow of hormones during their menstrual cycles. Many lifestyle and genetic factors can also influence the levels of these all-important compounds in the brain.

Your brain is able to defend itself from many damaging compounds with its built-in protective mechanism, known as the *blood-brain barrier,* which safeguards the brain from potentially harmful substances in the bloodstream. But your brain is susceptible to damage if it doesn't get enough oxygen and sugar or the right kind of fat from your diet, or if it is exposed to compounds that slip through the blood-brain barrier and destroy nerve cells. Protecting your brain from this kind of harm is essential to your mental and physical health.

Your brain is also vulnerable to injury if its blood supply is blocked. As we saw in Chapter 5, atherosclerosis (blocked arteries) can lead to a heart attack; it can also lead to a stroke (loss of oxygen to the brain, usually due to a blocked artery) and when severe can cause irreversible brain damage and paralysis. The Naturally Healthy Diet and Lifestyle can help prevent blocked arteries and protect your brain cells from free radical damage, toxins in the environment, and harmful chemicals in your diet. In addition, they can increase oxygen and blood flow to your brain. These powerful combined effects can keep your brain healthy and functioning optimally as you age.

Your brain is more than a physical structure; it also gives rise to your consciousness—with all of its fleeting thoughts, perceptions, memories, imaginings, and emotions. Whether your emotions arise without conscious effort or are generated by your thoughts, they can cause profound physiological changes. For example, if you are enveloped in feelings of love and support, your body feels relaxed, but if you discover that you've been slighted or betrayed, you feel anger and tension. Numerous studies have shown that laughter and positive visualizations can have a powerful impact on the mind and body. Tapping into the power of your mind, and choosing what influences you expose your mind to, can vastly enhance your health and the quality of your life.

The View from the East

In the East, the body, mind, and spirit are seen as an integrated whole. For thousands of years Chinese medicine has recognized that emotions can lead to disease, and disease can lead to disruptions in the emotions. The ancient Chinese system identifies the Seven Emotions as grief, fear, anger, excessive joy, worry, sadness, and fright. These seven emotional states can disrupt the flow of Qi and have adverse effects on certain parts of the body. Five of the seven emotions are said to correspond to the Five Elements: grief is associated with Metal, fear with Water, anger with Wood, excessive joy with Fire, and worry with Earth. By maintaining your emotional well-being, you can keep your Qi balanced and your body healthy.

When your Qi is balanced, it flows through you without interference, nourishing every tissue in your body and creating a physical, emotional, and spiritual landscape that allows you to fulfill your potential. As you move through time and have various life experiences, your Qi is continually changing and transforming. When you are in a difficult phase of your life, your Qi can become depleted or stagnant, and when you restore balance in your life, it can regenerate and flow freely again. Achieving balanced Qi is not a static process but a dynamic one that is influenced by your environment, diet, emotions, exercise, relationships, and—significantly—your mental health.

In Chinese medicine, there's a distinct connection between Qi and mental capacities. (If it helps, you can remember that *Qi* spelled backward is IQ.) In fact, the brain is intimately related to the kidney Essence, the hereditary form of Qi that you received from your parents. If your brain is nourished by sufficient kidney Essence, you are able to think clearly, your memory works well, and you have good eyesight; if your kidney Essence is insufficient, you will experience reduced concentration, forgetfulness, and poor vision. As you age, it is natural to experience a gradual depletion of your kidney Essence, but too often I see patients who have squandered their kidney Essence early in life with a high-stress lifestyle and unhealthy diet. Dementia and Alzheimer's disease are more often seen in people with prematurely depleted kidney Essence. Protecting your kidney Essence is critical to keeping your brain healthy over the course of your lifetime. Decreasing stress, getting enough sleep and exercise, and eating quality food are vital for preserving kidney Essence. See Chapter 3 for information on how you can support your kidney Essence.

In Chinese medicine, the mind and consciousness are called *shen,* a term that encompasses all mental, emotional, and spiritual characteristics. *Shen* is said to reside not in the brain but in the heart. Thus, heart Qi also has a major influence on the mind. When your heart Qi is healthy and strong, your mind and your emotions are in harmony, but if your heart Qi is not adequately nourished, problems such as depression, insomnia, and poor memory can arise. See Chapter 5 for information on nourishing your heart Qi with herbs, aromatherapy, flower essences, and other methods.

As we've seen, each of the Five Elements—Metal, Water, Wood, Fire, and Earth—is associated with distinct emotional and physical characteristics. Your unique response to your environment is affected by the ways in which the Five Elements are manifested in your life. Like every other aspect of your health, your brain, your mind, and your emotions are all influenced by which of the Five Elements dominates your personality. Keeping your dominant element well balanced will help you maintain mental and emotional health, but if your element becomes imbalanced, your brain, mind, and emotions may be compromised. (Refer to Chapters 2 through 6 for ways of balancing your element.)

If you are a Metal type, you normally have a creative and exacting mind, but when your element is out of balance, you are prone to suffer from a lack of mental clarity and emotional imbalances such as depression and grief. For Water types, the power of the mind is particularly important. If you are a Water type, you tend to be intellectual, a perpetual student of life and seeker of spiritual wisdom. As you age, you are unlikely to suffer from age-related memory loss if you've taken good care of yourself. But if you've abused your mind and body for many years, draining your kidney Essence with a stressful lifestyle, you are apt to suffer from mental deficiencies, depression, anxiety, and fear.

If you are a Wood type, your normally aggressive and disciplined mind may work against you if you've worn yourself out with too many years of hard work; you can become mentally sluggish, depressed, frustrated, angry, and lacking in ambition. If you are a Fire type, the blood vessels of your brain are healthy when your Fire element is well nourished; if your Fire element is imbalanced, you are prone to poor memory, anxiety, strokes, and what is described as an excess of joy. (In Chinese medicine, joy is a wonderful emotion, but too much joy, or excessive excitement, can injure heart Qi.) If you are an Earth type, you are both compassionate and mentally alert, but if your health is out of balance, you can become mentally scattered, chronically worried, and unable to stay focused, especially as you enter your later years.

Evaluating Mental Health

In the West, mental health is assessed by a qualified psychologist or psychiatrist through a description of mental and emotional symptoms. (Some conditions, such as Alzheimer's disease, are best diagnosed by a neurologist.) Unfortunately, no blood test can tell you if you are depressed, and neurotransmitters such as serotonin, which in low levels is associated with depression, are not easily measured. Researchers can measure levels of serotonin only through invasive means (for instance, by evaluating a sample of a person's cerebrospinal fluid) that are not appropriate for general use.

In the East, mental and emotional health is evaluated by assessing the flow and quality of Qi. Because the heart houses the mind, mental problems are typically perceived as heart Qi imbalances. Your heart Qi is particularly affected if you suffer from depression. The primary emotion of the heart is joy, but when heart Qi becomes imbalanced, a lack of joy (depression), or symptoms such as insomnia and anxiety, can occur. See Chapter 5 for more information on common heart Qi imbalances and how to evaluate your heart from a Chinese perspective.

Mental health can also be diagnosed in Chinese medicine through the Five Elements. As you've seen, each element is uniquely connected to states of mind and is associated with emotional tendencies that can affect mental health. Once you discover your dominant element, you will have a greater understanding of any emotional and mental imbalances you may have.

How to Tap into the Power of Your Mind

When it comes to creating health, my patients often ask me which comes first, the body or the mind. Do a healthy diet and lifestyle positively influence your mind, or do you have to first alter your consciousness in order to make healthier choices for your body? The answer, it seems, is both. All of the essential aspects of the Naturally Healthy Lifestyle that you've discovered in this book—including diet, exercise, detoxification, and balanced Qi—are also important for your brain performance and the stability of your mental and emotional health. Your mind, in turn, affects every cell in your body in countless ways. In this chapter, we'll look at the key ways that you can tap into the relationship between your body and mind to achieve optimal physical and mental health.

YOUR BODY INFLUENCES YOUR MIND

The Naturally Healthy Diet can have a very beneficial effect on your brain chemistry, emotions, memory, moods, and thoughts. It is loaded with brain-boosting carbohydrates, protein, and fats; at the same time it provides you with plenty of brain-friendly fruits and vegetables—and keeps many potentially brain-damaging food additives out of your body. Along with the Naturally Healthy Diet, you can support your brain health with nutritional supplements, exercise, and the removal of harmful substances from your environment. Let's explore each of these important ways the health of your body can influence your mind.

CARBOHYDRATES

Carbohydrates are an important source of fuel for the brain, but too much of the wrong kind of carbohydrates can negatively impact brain cells and cause erratic changes in brain chemicals that leave you feeling depressed, tired, and anxious. As we saw in Chapter 1, not all carbohydrates are the same. Eating complex carbohydrates that are digested slowly, like beans and whole-grain breads, results in a gradual increase in blood sugar. Ingesting simple carbohydrates with a high glycemic index, such as candy, causes a sudden increase in blood sugar levels, followed by a crash. Some people are particularly sensitive to these sudden drops in blood sugar, which can lower levels of brain chemicals (serotonin and endorphins), resulting in mood and behavioral changes. The symptoms of low blood sugar levels include fatigue, confusion, irritability, difficulty with sleep, impulsive behavior, low pain and stress tolerance, sugar cravings, and feelings of hopelessness. The Naturally Healthy Diet can help ensure that your blood sugar is balanced and your serotonin and endorphin levels remain optimal; you will have steady energy throughout the day, your mind will be clear and focused, and you will feel emotionally stable, optimistic, creative, and relaxed.

In addition to the undesirable effects that simple carbohydrates can have on your blood sugar level, a diet consistently high in simple carbohydrates can also increase the formation of compounds known as advanced glycosylation end products (AGEs), which accelerate aging. AGEs are damaging to brain cells because they create free radicals and can clog blood vessels, increasing the risk of atherosclerosis and stroke.

Finally, the way high-carbohydrate foods are cooked may affect brain health, whether they are simple or complex carbohydrates. When some carbohydrates, such as potatoes, are baked or fried at high temperatures, they form compounds called acrylamides, which are not only toxic to brain and nerve cells but have been classified as a "probable" cancer-causing agent by the Environmental Protection Agency.[2] Acrylamides are found in especially high amounts in french fries. When you cook potatoes and other high-carbohydrate foods at lower temperatures, such as by boiling, steaming, or toasting, you will eat fewer of these toxins.

PROTEIN

Protein is brain friendly for a number of reasons. Eating some high-quality protein at each meal stabilizes your blood sugar, which can influence your mood, behavior, and mental clarity. Protein in the diet also provides you with amino acids, which your body uses to produce brain chemicals that govern your brain cell functions. For instance, turkey is high in the amino acid tryptophan, which your body can convert to the brain chemical serotonin. The amino acid tyrosine, found in almonds, pumpkin seeds, sesame seeds, and dairy products, can benefit your brain by acting as a precursor to brain chemicals that regulate your mood and energy. There are many other important amino acids that support brain health; by eating a diet with adequate protein, you gain the building blocks for balanced brain chemistry.

> ### Why Eat Eggs for Your Brain?
>
> Eggs are good brain food because the yolks are full of lecithin, which contains choline. An important brain nutrient, choline played a significant role in your developing brain when you were an infant, and it continues to be important for your brain function throughout your life. Choline is incorporated into brain cells and plays a role in cell-to-cell communication. The memory neurotransmitter acetylcholine is made from choline, and some evidence indicates that an abundance of choline can enhance memory. Other foods high in choline include whole grains, legumes, and vegetables.

FATS

The brain contains a high level of fats, which comprise the membranes that wrap around the brain's nerve cells like insulation. This is, in part, why the fats in your diet can have a major influence on your intelligence, memory, moods, and overall brain health. The "friendly" omega 3 fats found in fish, which as you know are good for your heart, are great for your brain as well. Studies show that dietary consumption of one of these fats, DHA (your nerve cells are comprised of 30 percent DHA), is especially important for healthy brain development during infancy and childhood,[3] and animal studies suggest that high levels of DHA in the brain can improve the ability to learn.[4] These friendly fats make brain cells "smarter" by increasing the production of a compound in the brain, phosphatidylserine, that can affect the number and quality of nerve cell connections[5] and improve communication among brain cells.

The unfriendly fats—saturated fats and the excess of omega 6 fats typically found in the standard American diet—that are bad for your heart are also bad for your brain. These fats can contribute to clogging of your blood vessels, which can lead to atherosclerosis and strokes. They also add to the formation of eicosanoids, hormone-like substances that increase inflammation and free radicals, which can damage brain cells. DHA helps to protect brain cells by making them more resistant to inflammation and by blocking free radical damage.

The fats you eat can also affect your mood. One study showed that low levels of omega 3 fats and high levels of "unfriendly" omega 6 fats contributed to depression.[6] Fish oils in particular may affect levels of mood-altering brain chemicals such as serotonin,[7] which is important for preventing and treating depression. To support your brain health, I recommend that you eat low-mercury seafood and take a fish oil supplement containing at least 300 mg of DHA once a day.

FRUITS AND VEGETABLES

Fruits and vegetables are a major part of the Naturally Healthy Diet because they are packed with antioxidants that protect the brain. The blood vessels in your brain are just as vulnerable to atherosclerotic plaque as your heart. By helping to keep your brain's blood vessels free of debris, the antioxidants in fruits and vegetables can assist you in preventing strokes. In addition, antioxidants protect your brain cells from the destruction caused by free radicals. The cell membranes in your brain are rich in fats, making them especially susceptible to free radical damage. The fruits and vegetables that contain the highest amounts of brain-protective antioxidants include blueberries, blackberries, strawberries, raspberries, prunes, raisins, tomatoes, kale, and spinach.

FOOD ADDITIVES

The standard American diet contains numerous food additives that can be harmful to your brain. In the landmark book *Excitotoxins: The Taste That Kills,* neurosurgeon Russell Blaylock, M.D., reveals that the food additives aspartame and monosodium glutamate (MSG) are excitotoxins, which can cause excessive stimulation of nerve and brain cells, resulting in their death. Although the FDA considers these food additives safe, Dr. Blaylock points out that their potential dangers are greatest in the developing brains of infants and children—and that with chronic use they also affect adults and may contribute to the development of age-related dementia, Alzheimer's disease, and other degenerative diseases of the brain.

Diet soft drinks are one of the major sources of aspartame, but it is also found in many processed, low-calorie foods. Aspartame consists of methanol and two amino acids, aspartic acid and phenylalanine. According to Dr. Blaylock, both methanol and aspartic acid are powerful neurotoxins (toxins to nerve cells), and phenylalanine, when in high concentrations in the brain, can also be a neurotoxin. He says that although aspartic acid and phenylalanine are naturally found in some foods, they're not safe when taken as individual amino acids and in the amounts found in aspartame. You can easily avoid ingesting processed foods containing aspartame by checking their ingredient lists. Its common names include NutraSweet, Equal, Spoonful, and Natrataste.

MSG is most commonly found in processed foods, especially in Asian cuisine. In addition to avoiding this obvious source of MSG, you can minimize the MSG in your diet by avoiding other food products that may contain hidden amounts of MSG. These include malt extract, malt flavoring, bouillon cubes, hydrolyzed vegetable protein, hydrolyzed plant protein, yeast extract, sodium caseinate, calcium caseinate, textured protein, hydrolyzed oat flour, autolyzed yeast, and plant protein extract. Incredibly, MSG may also be found in some products that list "natural flavoring" or "seasoning" in their ingredients, so if you want to further eliminate MSG from your diet, adhere to the Naturally Healthy Diet and eat unprocessed, whole foods as often as possible.

If you are exposed to aspartame or MSG in your diet, Dr. Blaylock suggests that taking magnesium can help protect your brain cells from injury. (Be sure you are getting at least the amount of magnesium recommended in Chapter 2 as part of your multivitamin.) Making sure that your brain cells regularly receive optimal nutrition and steady levels of blood sugar can also help.

Vitamin Supplements

If you want additional brain-health insurance, you can take extra antioxidants. The fats in the brain are vulnerable to free radical damage, but antioxidants can squelch free radicals before they are able to cause destruction. The most important antioxidants are vitamin C, coenzyme Q10, and those that work in fatty tissues, such as vitamin E and alpha lipoic acid. Antioxidants work both alone and together to stop free radicals in their tracks. Alpha lipoic acid is uniquely helpful because it has the capacity to regenerate itself and other antioxidants so that they can all continue to protect brain cells. To enhance your antioxidant status, make sure that your multivitamin contains at least 1,000 mg of vitamin C and 400 i.u. of vitamin E in the form of mixed tocopherols; in addition, take 100 mg of alpha lipoic acid, and 50 mg of coenzyme Q10.

B vitamins can also give you an extra layer of brain-health insurance by helping to manufacture brain chemicals and other compounds that your brain needs to make energy and function optimally. You get plenty of B vitamins in the Naturally Healthy Diet, although additional supplementation may be necessary if you don't assimilate the nutrients well due to advanced age or other factors. Taking a good multivitamin (as outlined in Chapter 2) will provide you with the B vitamins you need for healthy brain function.

One type of vitamin B_{12}, methylcobalamin, may be especially important for healthy brain function. Your body naturally makes this type of B_{12}, but as you get older you may have lower levels because of poor B_{12} absorption. Methylcobalamin can help protect your brain cells from injury by a variety of toxins, including acrylamide, heavy metals such as mercury, and excitotoxins like MSG.[8] It may also play a role in regenerating nerve cells that have been damaged by nerve toxins. As a supplement, take 1,500 mcg of methylcobalamin a day in addition to your multivitamin.

Exercise

One of your greatest tools for a healthier mind is regular exercise. Exercise boosts your level of endorphins, brain chemicals that make you feel more alive, confident, and optimistic. Evidence suggests that exercise can also increase your level of serotonin, your "happy" brain chemical, which can elevate your sense of well-being. If you have dramatic mood changes when you eat sugar, exercise can help you keep sugar cravings in check.

Regular exercise can also enhance your memory.[9] According to Jean Carper, author of *Your Miracle Brain,* exercise induces your brain cells to create new networks of cell-to-cell communication.[10] Exercise is especially important as you get older; having more memory power can compensate for the normal brain changes that are associated with aging. One study reported that regular physical activity was a potent protective factor for preventing the onset of dementia and Alzheimer's disease.[11] Exercise can also improve your clarity of mind by increasing the amount of oxygen that reaches your brain cells. For all these reasons, I highly recommend that you exercise for at least thirty minutes five to six times a week to boost your brain power.

A HEALTHY ENVIRONMENT

It's well known that many commonly used environmental chemicals and heavy metals are toxins that can damage the brain and nervous system. The class of chemicals known as solvents—found in gasoline, kerosene, paint, paint thinners, and some cleaning fluids—can harm your brain cells with excessive exposure. Protect yourself by wearing a mask if you work with these substances.

Heavy metals can have injurious effects on many systems in the body and the brain in particular. You regularly ingest the heavy metal mercury when you eat fish and other forms of seafood, and you are also exposed to mercury if you have silver dental fillings. Mercury can accumulate in your brain, as well as in your nervous system, liver, and kidneys. Studies have found that animals exposed to mercury develop brain lesions that resemble the lesions found in people with Alzheimer's disease.[12] Chronic accumulation of mercury can also lead to symptoms of depression, poor memory, and emotional instability.[13] You can limit your exposure to mercury by eating only low-mercury seafood (see Chapter 1) and requesting nonmercury dental fillings. If you already have mercury fillings, consider having them replaced with porcelain or palladium-free gold fillings.

Aluminum, another heavy metal, has been implicated in Alzheimer's disease. It also directly contributes to memory loss because it inhibits the enzymes responsible for producing the brain chemical acetylcholine, which is important in memory functions.[14] To minimize your exposure to aluminum, be aware of its hidden sources in baking powders, nondairy creamers, underarm deodorants, and antacids. Avoid using aluminum pots and pans, or wrapping your food in aluminum foil.

Because your brain is especially sensitive to free radical damage, it's important not only to minimize your exposure to these kinds of toxic substances but also to take antioxidants. Detoxifying your body from solvents, mercury, aluminum, and other heavy metals is another important part of keeping your brain healthy; your brain and nervous system work best when environmental chemicals and other harmful substances are effectively neutralized and removed from your system. For a general plan to help your body cope with and detoxify environmental chemicals, see Chapter 4. Consult with your naturopathic physician for a comprehensive heavy metal detoxification plan.

YOUR MIND INFLUENCES YOUR BODY

Western science has only just begun to "discover" what some cultures have known for centuries: that the mind can influence every system in the body and cause profound physiological changes. Positive and peaceful thoughts can stimulate your immune cells, influence your hormones, decrease pain, and create an environment for spontaneous healing. When you tap into the power of your mind with guided visualizations, affirmations, prayer, or meditation, you can create changes in your brain waves, resulting in deep relaxation and a sense that your body, mind, and spirit are one. From this quiet place, many women create a feeling of peace and gain the strength to heal themselves.

Just as healthy choices about what you eat make you physically healthier, healthy choices about what you expose your mind to make you mentally healthier. On a daily basis, you have the ability to make conscious decisions about what you "ingest" mentally. For instance, you can choose to listen to music that makes you feel depressed or music that nourishes your soul; you can choose to read books that make you feel discouraged about your body and your health, or books that encourage you to be as healthy as you can possibly be; and you can choose to watch sad or violent movies, or you can watch movies that are hopeful and uplifting.

You can also tap into your mind's power through positive thinking. Most people have a kind of inner voice or monologue that they "hear" when they are going about their daily activities. Often this voice is either self-affirming or self-negating. Positive thinking boosts your energy and helps you bring about your greatest dreams and desires, but negative thinking pulls your energy down and often manifests your worst fears.

If you find that you are sabotaging yourself with thoughts like "I can't do this" or "I'm not good enough," focus on reversing the direction of your thoughts to "I can do this" and "I am more than good enough." Know that it's never too late to alter your thoughts; you can always change your mind, literally, and doing so can help manifest what you want in life. Ultimately, you can choose to have an inner voice that is as loving and caring toward yourself as it is toward the most cherished person in your life.

Practicing positive thinking can do wonders for the quality of your life. It can be as simple as a shift in thoughts, or it may involve a much more complex, long-term process. For some people, it may mean seeing a therapist who specializes in cognitive therapy or another means of countering negative thought patterns and creating more productive, life-affirming thoughts.

In the Five Element system of Chinese medicine, you can use affirmations to help keep your mind healthy and your element well-balanced. Depending on your type, you display certain characteristic emotional tendencies when you are not in balance: Metal types tend to have low self-esteem and difficulty letting go of the past; Water types are apt to feel afraid and lack self-confidence; Wood types are prone to anger, a lack of purpose, and feelings of helplessness; Fire types tend to feel emotionally unstable, anxious, and depressed; and Earth types are inclined to worry obsessively and feel abandoned. The following are examples of affirmations that you can repeat to yourself during times of distress to help you regain your emotional footing. Affirmations are a powerful tool that you can use at any time; throughout the day, they can help lift your spirits, bring you peace, and remind you that you are a positive, upbeat, happy person.

If you are a Metal type:
"I am strong and capable; I am able to let go of the old and let in the new."

If you are a Water type:
"I am secure and confident that I can achieve anything I put my mind to."

If you are a Wood type:
"I have purpose and direction in my life; I am at ease with my environment, and I am capable of change."

If you are a Fire type:
"I am happy and joyful; I feel love for everything in my world."

If you are an Earth type:
"I am at peace within myself; I feel deeply connected to the important people in my life."

Many women tap into their emotional lives through counseling and therapy. A good therapist can be a potent catalyst for emotional growth and change. If you find that something seems to block you from caring deeply for yourself, or that dysfunctional relationships keep emerging, I recommend that you participate in some type of personal growth therapy. Discovering the emotional and psychological patterns that keep you stuck and prevent you from defining and realizing your goals is the first step toward making change.

Change is not always easy and doesn't always happen overnight. It's important to understand that most real change is a gradual process rather than an immediate shift; it may take time before real mental and physical transformation occurs. Many of the women whose stories you've read in this book needed to change their lives in fundamental ways in order to reach their health goals. They had to make long-term changes in lifestyle and diet and often in the ways they perceived themselves.

In most cases, the first step toward change in your life is to become conscious of exactly what has to happen to make the change possible. As I told one of my patients who wanted to permanently change her eating habits, your mind must first become aware of precisely what your obstacles are, and form a specific plan to overcome those obstacles, in order to reach your goal. The second step is to take whatever action is necessary to follow the plan and make the change happen; for this patient, it meant identifying particular foods that she had been eating, becoming aware of why she was eating them, and consciously making healthier choices at certain times. The third step is to make the change a conscious and an unconscious part of who you are; ultimately, my patient began making healthy diet and lifestyle choices on a daily basis without even realizing it.

Natural Solutions for Sleeping Disorders, Anxiety, and Depression

Natural medicines provide you with many ways of resolving some of the most common health issues that can affect your brain and the quality of your mental life, including problems with sleep, anxiety, and depression. Herbs, aromatherapy, and nutritional supplements, when combined with one of the first tenets of naturopathic medicine—"remove the obstacles to cure"—can help your brain function better while nourishing and restoring your body, mind, and spirit.

SWEET DREAMS

Sleep is one of your greatest healers, regenerating your brain along with every other part of your body. When you are awake, the electrical activity of your brain, measured by brain waves, is highly active; during sleep your brain waves become slow, interspersed with periods of activity associated with dreaming. When you are asleep, your blood pressure drops, you breathe more slowly, and your body's metabolism slows down. All of these changes are essential for the health of your brain and body.

To get regular sleep, create a plan for it. Make sure that you're in bed by a certain time every night, even if you aren't tired, because your brain and body need regularity. If you don't fall asleep easily, or you have trouble staying asleep, you aren't alone: millions of people suffer from bouts of insomnia. The most common reasons that women have insomnia include stress, caffeine, poor blood sugar regulation, and hormonal changes. Let's look at the simple steps you can take to address each of these problems.

STRESS

Stress causes your adrenal glands to release hormones that make you feel alert and ready for action. Unfortunately, these hormones can also prevent your body from slipping into a restorative sleep state. If you have stress-induced insomnia, try melting away the tension of the day with gentle stretching exercises, meditation, a candle-lit bath, or a good book (but not an action-packed suspense novel), or by listening to soothing music. By giving yourself time to wind down, relax, and take the pressure off your brain and nervous system, you will be much more likely to sleep restfully.

CAFFEINE

Caffeine can prevent sleep because it blocks the action of the brain chemical adenosine, which tells your brain to go to sleep. In addition to preventing sleep, caffeine can also cause feelings of agitation. If you have insomnia and you regularly drink caffeinated beverages or eat a lot of chocolate, stop ingesting these substances before you try other means of improving your sleep.

POOR BLOOD SUGAR REGULATION

Blood sugar can contribute to insomnia because, when it is low, the body compensates by releasing hormones that make you feel more agitated. If you have problems with regulating your blood sugar, eating a balanced dinner can make all the difference in whether you get a good night's sleep. Many common protein sources, including chicken, turkey, tofu, salmon, and kidney beans, contain an amino acid called tryptophan that can increase your serotonin level and help you sleep. But since tryptophan has to be escorted into your brain by insulin to be effective, eating these foods alone may not be enough. Eating a complex carbohydrate with dinner will increase your insulin and serotonin levels and enhance the quality of your sleep.

HORMONAL CHANGES

Hormonal changes can also cause insomnia; when women have low levels of estrogen, progesterone, or both, they can experience disruptions in their sleep patterns. Correcting these hormonal imbalances can make a huge difference in their ability to sleep. (See Chapter 7 for more information.)

If you've addressed the most common reasons that may cause you to have insomnia and you still aren't getting a good night's sleep, the following natural medicines can help you get the rest and the sweet dreams you need for your brain and body. It's best to try one of these at a time and see what works for you. (I don't recommend using all of them simultaneously.)

VALERIAN ROOT

Valerian root calms and restores your nervous system; it is recommended for insomnia associated with nervousness and anxiety and is especially helpful if you can't get to sleep because your mind is racing. The herb contains compounds that bind to receptors in the brain called GABA receptors, exerting a relaxing effect. According to Chinese medicine, valerian root calms the spirit and helps you get a good night's sleep because it nourishes heart Qi. For insomnia, take 300 to 500 mg of valerian root about an hour before bedtime. Valerian root should not be taken with alcohol.

MELATONIN

Melatonin is a potent sleep hormone that helps to regulate sleep cycles and also has antioxidant effects. It has been popularized for its ability to reset sleeping and waking patterns disrupted by jet lag. Melatonin is safe to use in low doses when needed, but if you take it when you don't need it, you may feel drowsy the next morning. If you take melatonin for chronic insomnia, you will need to take it for at least two weeks to determine if it is effective. For jet lag, I recommend that you take melatonin after you reach your destination and before you go to bed; avoid taking it in the middle of the day if you want to nap, and take it for three consecutive nights to reestablish your sleep cycle. The daily dose for treating insomnia and jet lag is 1 to 3 mg taken right before bedtime. The best way to take melatonin is under your tongue, for immediate absorption.

5-HYDROXYTRYPTOPHAN (5-HTP)

5-HTP, which is derived from the amino acid tryptophan, can help you sleep if your insomnia is due to a low level of the brain chemical serotonin. 5-HTP not only increases the level of serotonin in your brain and nervous system, it can also increase your levels of melatonin, endorphins, and other brain chemicals. For insomnia, take 100 to 300 mg of 5-HTP once a day, before bedtime for best results. Do not use 5-HTP if you are taking an antidepressant medication that is classified as a selective serotonin reuptake inhibitor (SSRI), such as Prozac, Zoloft, Wellbutrin or Paxil. (If you're on antidepressant medication, check with your doctor if you aren't sure if it's an SSRI.)

NATURAL PROGESTERONE

Natural progesterone can help some women who experience insomnia prior to their period. Women who start to have insomnia when they are going through their midlife hormonal transition may also benefit from natural progesterone. Natural progesterone can influence the GABA receptors in your brain, resulting in a calming effect. It's best to test your progesterone level before taking natural progesterone. (See Chapter 7 for information on how to test your progesterone level.) If your level is low, take 25 to 50 mg before bedtime to help you sleep. Side effects of taking natural progesterone, including nausea, headaches, vertigo, and diarrhea, will most likely occur if you take more than your body needs. You will need a prescription if you are taking progesterone in pill form, but not if you are using progesterone creams or sublingual (absorbed under your tongue) progesterone.

AROMATHERAPY

Aromatherapy can calm your mind, relieve tension, and soothe your nervous system. For peaceful sleep, use a combination of lavender, melissa, and clary sage; apply these essential oils to your skin, or add them to your bath. You can also dilute them with water, put them in a spritzer bottle, and spray the mixture on your chest and neck before you go to bed.

FLOWER ESSENCES

Flower essences can help to quiet your mind and induce sleep. Chaparral is recommended if you have disturbing dreams and agitated sleep, and white chestnut if your sleep is blocked by obsessive, repetitious thoughts; the flower essence St. John's wort is used if fear and emotional stress are getting in the way of sleep. Put a few drops under your tongue and slip into a deep, comforting sleep.

FINDING CALM

If you find yourself frequently feeling uneasy, nervous, or panicky for no apparent reason, you may suffer from anxiety. Women who have anxiety can experience symptoms that include a faster heart rate, agitation, and an urge to immediately flee their environment. Anxiety can develop for many reasons, including low blood sugar, stress, and hormonal and brain chemical imbalances.

There are a number of natural solutions for treating anxiety. In most cases, anxiety can be relieved by maintaining balanced blood sugar levels, eating regular meals, avoiding caffeine, getting enough sleep, and keeping your body healthy with the Naturally Healthy Lifestyle and Diet. According to Chinese medicine, you can prevent and treat anxiety by keeping your heart Qi well nourished. There are also many herbs that can help you reduce anxiety and calm your mind.

Hormones can play a significant role in the genesis of anxiety. When your level of the stress hormone cortisol is high, you are more apt to feel agitated, nervous, and anxious. Phosphatidylserine (PS), which can be taken as a soy-based supplement, is an effective compound for decreasing your cortisol level. The recommended dose for reducing anxiety is 90 mg of PS taken two to three times a day (best taken with meals).

A low level of progesterone can also induce anxiety in some women. Progesterone affects receptors in the brain that induce a calming state. Women who experience anxiety only before their periods, or whose symptoms of anxiety begin when they are in perimenopause, often have a deficiency of progesterone. If you suspect you have low progesterone, test your hormone levels on day 21 of your menstrual cycle. (See Chapter 7 for information on how to test your progesterone level.) If you find that your progesterone level is low, consider using natural progesterone from midcycle until the onset of your period each month; for treating anxiety, take 25 to 50 mg of progesterone each night before going to bed. If you are postmenopausal, progesterone may also help with anxiety; take this amount in three-week cycles with a week between each (three weeks on, one week off). You can purchase most natural progesterone products over the counter.

Anxiety can also be caused by brain chemical imbalances, which are often treated with pharmaceutical drugs that increase serotonin levels. These medicines have their place, but they may have side effects and should not be used until natural solutions have been fully explored. I've seen many women successfully treat their anxiety with L-theanine, an amino acid derived from the leaves of green tea. L-theanine increases your level of another amino acid, gamma-aminobutyric acid (GABA), which makes you feel more calm and centered by binding to the GABA receptors in your brain. L-theanine may also increase your tryptophan level, which could in turn increase your serotonin level. And L-theanine doesn't cause drowsiness or interfere with your mental clarity. In fact, it may even increase your ability to concentrate. The recommended dose of L-theanine is 200 mg, with or without food, once or twice daily. You should feel the calming affects of L-theanine within thirty minutes of taking it.

Many herbs that help you sleep can also be taken in smaller amounts to reduce anxiety. For instance, valerian root, which is recommended for insomnia, can also help with anxiety because it affects GABA receptors in the brain, slowing down your overactive nerve cells. The following herbs, called nervines, gently nourish the nervous system, creating an overall calming effect.

Wood betony. An excellent herb for anxiety associated with nervous exhaustion, wood betony, with its relaxing and restoring effects, can help you think clearly and feel more grounded.

Chamomile. Chamomile can decrease physical restlessness and an agitated mind with its calming, relaxing effects. It can help calm an irritated digestive system and can also ease an irritated nervous system.

Passionflower. A gentle sedative that can be used for anxiety, especially with insomnia, this herb is often recommended for women who have anxiety while going through their midlife hormonal transition.

Blue vervain. Blue vervain nourishes and supports the nervous system, while acting as a mild sedative. It can be especially helpful if you have an overactive nervous system or headaches due to anxiety.

One of the best ways to use these herbal nervines is to blend them together as tea: mix all four dried herbs in equal parts and steep one teaspoon of the blend in one cup of boiling water for five minutes; strain, and drink either hot or cold. You can do this on a daily basis, or make a larger quantity of the tea and keep it covered in the refrigerator until ready to drink; most herbal teas will keep up to three days. To enhance your herbal nervine blend, add equal parts of lemon balm (melissa) and lavender, which can calm the spirit, relieve tension, and nourish heart Qi.

Treating Depression

Nan came to my office after years of self-medicating her depression with alcohol. "I started experiencing depression in my early teens but wasn't officially diagnosed with the condition until my thirties," she told me. "Now I can see that over the years I became an alcoholic as a way of coping with pain. In my forties I started taking antidepressants, which at first seemed like a quick-fix miracle. But after a few years their effectiveness slowly decreased and I became mired once again in despair."

In addition to starting treatment with naturopathic and Chinese medicine, Nan joined Alcoholics Anonymous and began seeing a psychotherapist. The results of the changes she has made in her life since are profound and inspiring. "Now I'm drug free and living a life that's full of joy and hope," she says. "I'm experiencing more clarity of mind, and I've developed a strong spiritual life. Today I feel that I'm supporting my health and well-being rather than treating a disease—an empowering difference. I've moved from surviving to thriving."

The darkness of depression affects almost twice as many women as it does men.[15] Some estimate that as many as 33 percent of American women will suffer from a major episode of depression in their lifetime.[16] The causes are manifold, but among the most common reasons women suffer from depression are stressful life events and imbalances in their brain chemicals—especially serotonin—along with hormonal changes associated with menstrual cycles, pregnancy, or menopause.

The level of serotonin in your brain has a major influence on your moods. When your serotonin level is normal, you are optimistic and have a sense of well-being, but if your serotonin level is low, you can experience symptoms of depression, including changes in appetite, fatigue, excessive sleeping, insomnia, feelings of hopelessness, or low self-esteem. Usually a diagnosis of depression is made when symptoms have been present for a significant period of time.

Many natural solutions for treating depression involve encouraging the body's ability to manufacture serotonin. Regular exercise, a balanced diet, and nutritional supplementation can all help increase your serotonin levels. The amino acid 5-HTP, which can help you sleep, can also boost serotonin levels. For depression, the recommended dose of 5-HTP is 50 mg three times a day.

The herb St. John's wort can help treat mild cases of depression by increasing your serotonin level; the recommended dosage is 900 mg a day of 0.3 percent hypericin (the herb's active constituent). I recommend that you avoid taking St. John's wort if you are taking 5-HTP, and avoid using both if you are taking any drug classified as a selective serotonin reuptake inhibitor (SSRI), or if you are on a monoamine oxidase (MAO) inhibitor. Some studies have found that the herb can also have negative interactions with birth control pills and chemotherapeutic agents. But if you are not currently taking prescription drugs, this herb can be of value in helping you overcome depression.

Depression can occur if you have fluctuations in hormones, because a drop in estrogen can lead to a drop in serotonin levels in the brain. In some women these changes are felt acutely and result in changes in mood. Many women are able to affect their response to changes in their estrogen level by taking one of the serotonin boosters mentioned above or by balancing their hormones. If you suspect that you are depressed due to hormonal changes, see Chapter 7 for information on how to balance your hormones.

Your thyroid and your adrenal glands can play a role in the genesis of depression as well. If your thyroid hormones are deficient or you have exhausted adrenal glands from too much stress, symptoms of depression can arise. Low thyroid function may be one of the hidden causes of depression; many women who are diagnosed with low thyroid function have had symptoms of thyroid deficiency for quite a long time before low thyroid levels show up on standard blood tests. See Chapter 7 to find out ways to determine if you have "subclinical" hypothyroidism or if your adrenal glands are compromised.

Brain chemical imbalances often play an important role in depression, but many aspects of depression remain mysterious to Western science. For reasons that are not fully understood, aromatherapy can be a powerful tool to help move from the darkness of depression toward the light. Aromatherapy, which has a direct effect on the limbic system—the emotional center of your brain—seems to be able to stimulate shifts in moods in unique ways. It can help calm your spirit, lift your mood, and create a sense of inner peace and harmony. The effects of the essential oils used in aromatherapy can be especially penetrating when combined with the principles of ancient Chinese medicine.

According to Chinese medicine, depression can occur when your Qi is deficient and your primary element (your type in the Five Element system) is out of balance due to excessive stress or physical and emotional exhaustion. When you have abundant Qi and your element is balanced, you are happy and calm and you have the vitality you need to fulfill your goals. But if your element is out of balance and you become depressed, your depression will affect you in unique ways, depending on your type. Metal types are prone to chronic anxiety associated with emotional numbness when they are depressed; Water types tend to feel a sense of total hopelessness along with depression; Wood types tend to burn out their Qi, resulting in depression mixed with anger; Fire types typically become completely exhausted when they are depressed, experiencing anxiety along with a lack of joy; and Earth types are apt to have low self-esteem, feel abandoned, and be extremely lethargic when depressed.

Aromatherapy oils have different effects on each of the Five Element types; when you are treating depression, aromatherapy is most effective if you use the essential oil that best balances your type. You can use your essential oil as often as you like: place a few drops in your bath or wear it as you would a perfume. The following aromatherapy oils are most beneficial for relieving depression, according to your type:

> **If you are a Metal type:** Use clary sage oil for its emotionally elevating effects.
> **If you are a Water type:** Use ginger oil for its ability to uplift and stimulate your mind.
> **If you are a Wood type:** Use orange oil to encourage a carefree, playful state of mind.
> **If you are a Fire type:** Use rose oil to rekindle your natural sense of inner joy.
> **If you are an Earth type:** Use marjoram oil for its ability to comfort and soothe your spirit and promote self-nurturing.

Flower essences can have a strong effect on the mind and emotions and provide you with another way of lifting yourself out of depression. Using flower essences along with the Naturally Healthy Lifestyle and Diet can help you overcome feelings of anguish, apathy, and unhappiness that perpetuate depression. The following flower essences can help you break the cycle of depression and lift up your energy.

Wild Rose. Wild Rose is recommended if you feel drained of your enthusiasm for life, unhappy, and apathetic. Use this remedy if you feel "stuck" in your present circumstances and lack the energy to change them.

Milkweed. This remedy is recommended if you have a tendency to escape from the realities of life, either by using recreational drugs to alter your consciousness or by losing yourself in addiction; milkweed can also be used if you are in a deeply depressed state and unable to cope with your daily affairs.

Sweet Chestnut. Use sweet chestnut if you are overwhelmed by a sense of despair and hopelessness. This remedy is for severe depression or anguish; it is recommended if you've reached the limits of your ability to cope, and you feel utterly alone and abandoned.

You can combine wild rose, milkweed, and sweet chestnut to create a synergistic effect. To use flower essences, place four drops or pellets under your tongue four times a day, or more frequently if you need to strengthen the effects of a remedy. Flower essences can also be mixed into your drinking water, applied to your skin, or added to your bath.

CHINESE HERBAL MEDICINES FOR INSOMNIA, ANXIETY, AND DEPRESSION

Chinese medicine has a long history of using "*shen* tonics" for the treatment of insomnia, anxiety, and depression; these three conditions are often treated simultaneously, because they are considered to have a common cause. *Shen* includes all of your mental, emotional, and spiritual characteristics, which are said to reside within your heart. Many of the herbs that nourish heart Qi are considered to be *shen* tonics because they also help nourish the mind, emotions, and spirit. When your *shen* is not securely rooted in your heart, you can experience insomnia, anxiety, nervousness, sadness, and grief. The following popular *shen* tonics are often found in Chinese herbal formulas.

Zizyphus seed. Used to treat insomnia caused by "excessive thinking," zizyphus seed is traditionally known as "Calm the Heart Seed" because it can calm the spirit and nourish the heart. It is also used for disturbed dreams and nightmares.

Biota. Biota is also known for its ability to nourish the heart and calm the spirit. It is particularly useful for treating anxiety, insomnia, and irritability.

Asparagus root. Used by Chinese herbalists for centuries as a strong mood elevator and to "open the heart," asparagus root can help bring about feelings of love, warmth, and kindness.

Margarita. Margarita (also known as pearl) is an effective mood stabilizer, considered to be especially useful if the heart and spirit are not at peace. Margarita can help relieve anxiety and tension and promote peaceful sleep.

Polygala root. Polygala root can relax the mind, yet it also has the ability to strengthen the will. It "smooths" the flow of Qi through your heart and calms the spirit. It is used to treat insomnia, anxiety, and restlessness and is recommended if you feel mentally disoriented.

I have not included dosages for these herbs because in Chinese medicine they are traditionally blended into herbal formulas. A Chinese herbal formula that contains a number of these *shen* tonics is the product Calm Spirit (also known by its Chinese name, Ding Xin Wan) made by the herbal company Health Concerns. The recommended dose is three pills three times a day; see your Chinese medical practitioner to obtain this formula.

Healthy Aging

"I would work very hard to figure out my responsibilities at forty, only to realize that I was now fifty, and suddenly sixty. What does it mean to be an elder in this culture? What are my new responsibilities? What has to be let go to make room for the transformations of energy that are ready to pour through the body-soul? . . . As life asks new things of me, I feel I must pause, go inward, and ask, 'What is my weight now? What are my new values? . . . Do I have the courage to live with this evolving me?'"

—MARIAN WOODMAN, *Bone*

For many women in Western culture, the idea of growing older is associated with loss and is met with nervous jokes about being "over the hill." The subject fills some women with anxiety—about losing their mental faculties, their physical health, or even their value in society. In my practice I see many women struggling with the aging process, desperately searching for the latest elixir of youth as soon as they begin to have wrinkles or gray hair. I often tell my patients to think of aging in terms of gaining rather than losing. (After all, we say that we are "getting" older.) Living a full life, and becoming the wise woman of your later years, is your crowning glory.

In May 2000, when the "anti-aging" medicine movement was in full swing, I presented a public lecture on the topic of aging in Honolulu. It occurred to me that the term *anti-aging* reinforces the misguided notion that aging is something we should be opposed to. I named my lecture "Healthy Aging" because I've always felt that we shouldn't be taking a stance against aging but rather embracing the process and doing it in the healthiest way possible.

Healthy aging is about taking care of your body, every step of the way, as you change from the woman that you are to the woman that you will become. Healthy aging also means taking care of your mind—not only because keeping your mind sharp will enable you to make the most of your age, but because your mind determines how you feel about yourself and your world, and how you perceive the aging process itself. When your mind is healthy, you can be tuned in to who you are as you move through each of the seasons of your life. The power of your mind enables you to choose the life you want and how you define yourself. You can honor and celebrate your changing self, and you can fully experience the incredible changes that take place in your body, mind, and spirit on your journey through the cycle of life.

In Chinese medicine, the cycle of life is understood in terms of the Five Elements; each element is associated with a season of the year and also with a phase of life, from birth to old age. By becoming conscious of the role that each of the elements plays in the different phases of your life, you can shift your self-perceptions as you move through the seasons of time.

The Wood element, which influences new growth, provides you with the energy for the rapid physical, emotional, and mental changes that occur between birth and childhood; Fire, the element of passion, rules the dramatic transformations you experience during adolescence and young womanhood—when your energy is directed outward, and you are exploring the world. The Earth element guides the time of adulthood when you seek out a home, put down roots, and take on responsibilities. During this phase of your life you become grounded and centered, and you have a strong sense of stability and purpose. Many women in this phase are either raising children or actively involved in their careers.

The Metal element is in full force between late middle age and your senior years, the season of fall when your energy is turning inward and slowing down in preparation for winter. For many women, this is the time when their children have left home and they find themselves having extra time for spiritual or creative pursuits; the Metal time in your life offers you the freedom to give to yourself. Finally, the Water element influences the last phase of your life, when you contemplate a return to the primordial water that you came from. At this stage you have the opportunity to quietly reflect on all of the preceding seasons of your life.

In our culture, moving through time in a healthy way may mean letting go of society's limited definitions of aging and using the power of your mind to be present with your evolving self. You may hear a message from our culture that people are "over the hill" at a certain age, but it's not a message you ever have to listen to. Though our society may not respect the wisdom of its elders as much as some other cultures do, that doesn't prevent you from attaining that wisdom. Healthy aging is knowing that the age you are now, the ages you have been, and the ages you will become are all part of your journey through life.

PRESERVING THE POWER OF YOUR MIND

When you are in your seventies, eighties, or nineties, you'll want your mind to be strong, agile, and as sharp as possible. The future power of your mind depends, to a great extent, on the choices you make *now*. By making brain-healthy choices, you are helping to preserve the power of your mind and avoiding some of the pitfalls of the aging process. As women grow older, they are three times more likely to suffer from a loss of intellectual function than men.[17]

Alzheimer's disease (AD), one of the causes of dementia, affects twice as many women as men.[18] For years, women were told that hormone replacement therapy could prevent AD. Then in May 2003 the *Journal of the American Medical Association* published the news that postmenopausal women who were prescribed synthetic hormone replacement therapy (Premarin and Provera) had twice the risk of developing AD compared with women who didn't take it.[19] Now women want to know more than ever what they can do to reduce their chances of having AD.

Alzheimer's disease is a debilitating condition that can result in severe memory loss and changes in mood, personality, and behavior. The symptoms, which usually don't occur until after sixty-five, include a decreased ability to learn or recall new information. AD is a progressive disease, which means it gets worse over time. People with AD have increased brain cell loss, and scans of their brains reveal neurofibrillary tangles and other structural changes that result in abnormal memory and behavior. AD is also characterized by a deficiency of the brain chemical acetylcholine. Some of the medications used to treat AD are aimed at increasing the level of acetylcholine, a natural brain chemical that allows brain cells to communicate with one another.

The causes of AD are unknown, but risk factors include depression, head trauma, thyroid disease, and exposure to solvents or aluminum.[20] There is also a strong genetic link; if you have a family member who has or has had AD, you are at higher risk for the disease. But it is important to remember that your risk factors and your genes aren't the only determinants of your destiny. Your choices, over the course of your life, can have a major influence on the health of every cell in your body, including the cells of your brain.

There is no cure for AD, but Western doctors typically recommend that women with AD take anti-inflammatory medications. While these drugs may play a role in preventing the progression of the disease, their long-term side effects can include gastritis, stomach ulcers, and cardiovascular problems. The good news is that there's a tremendous amount that you can do to help prevent memory loss, dementia, and AD with natural medicine.

The first step to keeping your brain as healthy as possible is to follow the Naturally Healthy Diet and Lifestyle. The second step is to enhance your brain function with specific lifestyle and nutritional interventions, especially if you are experiencing memory loss or you are at high risk for AD. You can keep your memory intact for years to come with plenty of physical exercise, mental exercise, and memory- and brain-supportive supplements.

Regular physical exercise increases the amount of oxygen flowing to your brain, allowing it to work more efficiently, and can help prevent memory loss, dementia, and

AD in the elderly.[21] With regular mental exercise, your brain can continue to function optimally as you age. It has been found that when people regularly use their brain, no matter what their age, their brain cells respond by forming more connections among cells. As neurologist Russell Blaylock, M.D., points out, "The brain, in this way, is much like a muscle; the more you exercise it the more powerful it becomes. Thinking is the exercise of the mind."[22] At any age, learning new skills, or practicing old ones, will stimulate your brain and increase its capacity. Your brain needs a workout like the rest of your body, so use it regularly!

Certain supplements can also boost your brain function. According to a study in the journal *Neurology,* the soy-based supplement phosphatidylserine (PS) is a promising candidate for treating memory loss associated with age,[23] while other studies have found that it may help people who suffer from dementia and AD. In addition to its uses for decreasing anxiety, this superstar supplement can help keep your brain cells healthy and functioning well into your senior years. PS enhances cell-to-cell communication and plays a role in increasing your acetylcholine level. When you are young, your brain cells are rich in PS, which is produced naturally in your brain when you have adequate levels of vitamins B_{12}, folic acid, and the "friendly" fats found in fish and flax oils. As you increase in age, your body produces less PS. Taken as a supplement, PS becomes incorporated into your brain cell membranes and revitalizes them. If you are concerned about your memory, take 100 mg three times a day with meals. For dementia or AD, 500 mg of PS a day is recommended. PS is very safe; there are no known side effects.

A high level of homocysteine, an amino acid that is made in the body, can increase your risk for AD and contribute to memory loss, depression, and stroke. Homocysteine can also cause damage to blood vessel walls, setting the stage for clogged arteries, and may affect the synthesis of certain brain chemicals. In addition, it may directly kill brain cells by acting as a toxin to nerve cells. Vitamins B_{12}, B_6, and folic acid, which are found in your basic multivitamin, break down homocysteine so that it doesn't wreak havoc on your brain and blood vessels.

Free radical damage in the brain can also contribute to the progression of dementia and AD. High doses of the antioxidant vitamin E can help prevent AD, and a study published in the *New England Journal of Medicine* found that a high dose of vitamin E—2,000 i.u. a day—slowed the progression of AD.[24] Vitamin E is the perfect brain-friendly antioxidant because it is stored in the fatty portion of brain cell membranes, providing your brain with "on-site" protection from free radical damage.

Enhancing Your Memory with Chinese Medicine

Chinese herbal medicines have been used to increase memory for centuries, their secrets passed down over many generations. Only in modern times has Western science been able to isolate their active constituents, but it's fascinating how frequently Western analysis backs up the medicinal properties that have long been recognized in China. The following three herbs have been used traditionally in Chinese medicine to help increase memory as people age.

GINKGO BILOBA

Ginkgo biloba increases blood flow to the brain, bringing oxygen and other nutrients to brain cells. The herb also acts as a powerful antioxidant and may increase the ability of acetylcholine to work in the brain. For prevention of memory loss in the elderly, the recommended dose is 40 mg of a standardized extract of ginkgo biloba containing 24 percent ginkgoflavonglycosides three times a day; for the treatment of dementia or AD, the recommended dose is 80 mg three times a day. Refrain from taking ginkgo biloba if you are on blood-thinning medications. Side effects are rare, but some people have reported headaches or stomach discomfort.

HUPERZINE A

Huperzine A is a compound derived from *Huperzia serrata,* also known as the herb club moss, that is used to enhance memory in seniors. It is a promising candidate for preventing the progression of AD because it is a potent inhibitor of the enzyme that breaks down acetylcholine, the brain chemical that is severely depleted in the brain cells of people with AD. Huperzine A may also help prevent brain cell death from toxins and could play a role in reducing injury from strokes.[25] The recommended dose of huperzine A is 200 mcg twice a day.

SCHIZANDRE

Schizandre is used to enhance memory and tone up the nervous system when you feel mentally and physically exhausted. It is known for its ability to increase alertness, intellectual functioning, and concentration without increasing anxiety. In fact, it is also used to *decrease* agitation and calm the spirit. Schizandre is a unique herb in Chinese medicine because it strengthens the Three Treasures (kidney Essence, spirit, and overall Qi), enters all of the meridians, and has a broad range of effects on the body. It is typically found in herbal formulas that nourish kidney and heart Qi. Taken as an individual herb, the recommended dose is one 400 mg capsule two to three times a day. You can also get the benefits of this herb in schizandre berries, though they are quite sour and are best eaten with cereal or with other fruit.

Tapping into the Power of Your Mind: Final Thoughts

Your mind is central to your capacity to create health. At any moment you can influence your health through conscious awareness and the choices that you make. In this chapter, we've seen many ways of nourishing the brain and nervous system with diet, exercise, detoxification, natural medicines, balancing Qi, and more. All of these methods can help you keep your brain cells healthy, enhance your memory and moods, and boost your mental and emotional clarity. The more healthy, self-esteeming choices become a part of your Naturally Healthy Lifestyle, the better you will feel and the easier it will be to continue making choices that will optimize the health of your body and mind.

The Essence of Chapter 11

- Remember that the power of your mind is vast and right at your fingertips.
- Keep your kidney Essence abundant to maintain your brain health, and nurture your heart Qi to keep your mind and spirit healthy.
- Nourish the power of your mind by eating "friendly" fats, steering clear of certain food additives, and taking antioxidants.
- Exercise to keep your brain healthy.
- Minimize your exposure to toxic chemicals.
- Tap into the power of your mind with guided visualizations, affirmations, prayer, and meditation.
- Take natural medicines if you have insomnia, anxiety, or depression.
- Use the power of your mind to honor, celebrate, and fully experience who you are at every season in the cycle of your life.
- Preserve the power of your mind, and prevent dementia and Alzheimer's disease, with your lifestyle, diet, and natural medicines.

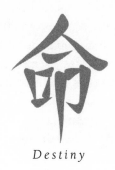

Destiny

Manifesting Your Naturally Healthy Lifestyle

"The journey is the reward."
—CHINESE PROVERB

WHEN WE began this journey toward optimal health, we started with the question: what is health? In the chapters that followed, we've explored many answers to that question. We've seen how to use natural, nontoxic means—food, exercise, nutritional supplements, herbs, Chinese medicine, and much more—to create the highest vision of your health.

Health is freedom from illness, but it is much more than that; it is a dynamic state of mind, body, and spirit. When you are in peak health, your immune system is a force-field of pure wellness that enables you to achieve the fullest possible expression of your genetic potential. Great health allows you to create the life you want and fulfill your dreams and your destiny.

Health is a choice, and the choice is yours. Choosing health means taking the time to care for yourself, honor yourself, and commit to making your health your first priority. Every day you make choices about your health that affect who you are and who you will become. Healthy choices are self-perpetuating; the healthier your choices, the better you feel and the more you want to continue making beneficial choices. Your health is comprised, to a great extent, of all the healthy choices you make over the course of your lifetime.

Your health is like a beautiful, intricately crafted puzzle, with all of your body's systems fitting precisely together as a unified whole. The chapters of this book have outlined ten key areas of health, each essential to your well-being. In each chapter, you've encountered many ways that you can create radiant health. By incorporating the basic principles I've outlined in each chapter, you can profoundly improve your health at each stage of your life. Maintaining a Naturally Healthy Lifestyle will provide you with a strong foundation that allows you to make the best possible choices every step of the way.

This book has given you the tools you need to make great health a reality. As you put these tools to use, keep in mind that taking good care of yourself is not a full-time job or an overwhelming task. At the same time, remember that creating optimal health doesn't happen overnight; some changes occur slowly, in small increments. Be kind and loving to yourself as you continue on your journey into greater health, and allow yourself the time it may take to arrive at your destination.

One of the things I love most about natural medicine is that it gives *you* the opportunity to nurture and heal yourself; after all, only you have the power to create great health in your own life. My hope is that this book can serve as your guide as you treat yourself to a lifetime of optimal health.

Appendix A

KEY ELEMENTS OF NATURE'S PHARMACY

Herbal Medicines

Herbal medicines are generally available at health food stores as dried herbs, tinctures, capsules, or tablets. Depending on the circumstances and the age of the patient, any of these forms can be used effectively. Dried herbs can be purchased as tea bags or in bulk form (often referred to as "single" herbs). Herbal tinctures are usually made by extracting properties from herbs and preserving them in an alcohol or glycerin solution. If you use herbs in capsule or tablet form, I recommend you purchase products that are standardized to contain the principal active constituents of the herb.

Nutritional Supplements

Nutritional supplements include vitamins, minerals, amino acids, and compounds derived from plants and foods. I highly recommend that you avoid using synthetic supplements that have colors and fillers in them. The supplements you take should be made from a natural source. If you have digestive problems, it's best to buy your supplements in the form of powders, liquids, or capsules; your body can break down and absorb these more easily than tablets.

When you buy nutritional supplements, choose the highest-quality products you can find at your health food store. Look for the GMP (Good Manufacturing Practices) certification on the label; this certification is established by the National Nutritional Foods Association and indicates that a nutritional supplement has been screened for contaminants and quality-tested.

Homeopathic Medicines

You can safely self-prescribe, for a short period of time, low-dose homeopathic medicines. These medicines can treat a variety of acute ailments, and low-dose remedies (with potencies of 3x, 6x, 12x, 30x, 6c, 12c, and 30c) are found in most health food stores and in some pharmacies. You may also find homeopathic preparations for specific ailments that contain multiple low-dose remedies in combination.

The dose of a homeopathic remedy reflects the strength of the remedy: it may seem counterintuitive, but the more diluted a remedy is, the greater its potency (a notion that is not yet explainable in Western scientific terms). The "x" series of remedies is based on the decimal scale; for example, if one-tenth of a compound is added to nine-tenths of alcohol and shaken vigorously, the result is a remedy with a "1x" potency. The "c" series of remedies, which is more diluted and stronger than the "x" series, is based on the centesimal scale; for example, if one-hundredth of a compound is diluted with ninety-nine hundredths of alcohol and shaken vigorously, this renders the remedy a "1c" potency. The number of a remedy represents the number of times this process is repeated. For instance, a "3x" remedy has been diluted and shaken three times in succession, and a "6c" remedy has been rediluted and shaken six times. High-dose homeopathic prescriptions (doses of 200c and above) require the consultation of a naturopathic physician or other practitioner who has extensive training in homeopathic medicine.

Homeopathic medicines are prepared (diluted and shaken) by homeopathic pharmacies and sold as liquids or pellets. The two preparations are equally effective, but it is generally easier to administer pellets to children. To take a homeopathic medicine, dissolve the remedy under your tongue at least fifteen minutes away from eating or drinking anything. A remedy can be taken three to four times a day until symptoms resolve, or for a maximum of three days, unless otherwise directed. You should avoid ingesting coffee or mint on the days you are taking a remedy, because they can antidote the remedy. Also refrain from using essential oils such as peppermint and eucalyptus, because they will render the remedy less effective.

To know which homeopathic remedy to use, it's important to read what it is recommended for before taking it; for a precise prescription, consult your naturopathic physician. Side effects can occur if the wrong remedy is used, too high a dose is taken, or a remedy is taken for too long a period of time. If side effects occur, the remedy can be antidoted by drinking coffee, ingesting mint, or applying essential oils to your skin.

A p p e n d i x B

SUPPLEMENT COMPANIES, SUPPLIERS, AND OTHER RESOURCES

Supplement Companies

Products from the following supplement companies can be purchased either over the counter or online. Some companies sell only certain products to consumers who are not licensed health care providers.

Eclectic Institute

36350 Southeast Industrial Way
Sandy, OR 97055
(800) 332-4372
www.ecleticherb.com
For over-the-counter nutritional and herbal supplements; they carry an excellent multivitamin and lipotropic formula.

Emerita

621 Southwest Alder, Suite 900
Portland, OR 97205-3627
www.emerita.com
For over-the-counter progesterone cream, vaginal lubricants, and other women's health products

Enzymatic Therapy

www.enzy.com
For over-the-counter nutritional supplements, including Heartburn Free

Health Concerns

8001 Capwell Drive
Oakland, CA 94621
www.healthconcerns.com
A source of Chinese herbal medicines. They offer a number of products for the general public. You can purchase them online.

Herb Pharm

www.herb-pharm.com
For herbal tinctures and salves. Search their website for a store that carries their products near you.

Metagenics

www.metagenics.com
Produces UltraClear Sustain, a rice-based protein powder designed to support patients with conditions associated with gastrointestinal problems, including IBS and leaky gut syndrome. The company only sells directly to licensed physicians, but many other companies sell the product online.

Natren

www.natren.com
For oral and vaginal acidophilus

Nordic Naturals

www.nordicnaturals.com
For over-the-counter fish oil supplements

Ron Teeguarden's Herb Garden

P.O. Box 42030
Los Angeles, CA 90049
(310) 471-0404
www.dragonherbs.com
A source of Chinese herbal medicines

Standard and Hyland Homeopathic Remedies

www.arrowroot.com
For low-potency homeopathic medicines

Vitanica
www.vitanica.com
For women's herbal products. Search their website for a store that carries their products near you.

Suppliers

Alexandra Avery
4747 Southeast Belmont Street
Portland, OR 97215
www.alexandraavery.com
For aromatherapy and all-natural skin care products

Gaiam Living Arts
www.gaiam.com
For exercise, yoga, Pilates, Qi Gong, and meditation resources, and for aromatherapy diffusers and other personal and household items that promote health

Ho'ano Botanicals and Women's Holistic Health Services
www.hoano.com
For Breast Caress Massage and Body Oil

Natracare Feminine Products
www.natracare.com
The products are also often found at your health food store.

Saffron Rouge Cosmetics
www.saffronrouge.com
For all-natural organic cosmetics

Snowlotus Aromatherapy
www.snowlotus.org
For aromatherapy oils

Other Resources

Bach Flower Essences
www.bachcentre.com
To locate a retailer carrying Bach flower essences near you

Progest-E (Sublingual Progesterone)
Progest-E was developed by Dr. Ray Peat and can be purchased at a health food store or online. (Many supplement companies sell it.) Each drop of Progest-E contains 3 mg of progesterone.

Traditional Medicinals Herbal Tea
You can find these herbal teas, including Mother's Milk tea, at most health food stores.

Compounding Pharmacy
Key Pharmacy
23422 Pacific Highway South
Kent, WA 98032
(800) 878-1322
www.keynutritionrx.com
For natural and bioidentical hormones

Super-Blenders
www.vitamix.com
High-powered blenders for home use

Exercise and Weight Lifting Video
Strong Women Stay Young video and other supplies for creating an exercise program at home can be purchased at www.aswechange.com.

Ovulook
www.ovulook.com
For ovulation test kits

For Testing Wood for Arsenic
Environmental Working Group
www.ewg.org

Information on Quality of Dietary Supplements
www.consumerlab.com
www.nnfa.org

Information on Fluoride
Fluoride Action Network
www.fluoridealert.org

Chinese Herbal Medicines
Free and Easy Wanderer (also known as Xiao Yao Wan) is sold in most Chinese herbal stores. But in my practice I use only herbs that have been processed in the United States, due to reports that some prepared herbal medicines from China have been contaminated with heavy metals and pharmaceutical drugs. A number of herbal companies (see "Supplement Companies") sell high-quality Free and Easy Wanderer.

Information on Gluten-free Foods
www.glutenfree.com

Information on Purchasing Alkaline-Forming Salt
www.realsalt.com
www.celtic-seasalt.com

Information on Assessing Breast Cancer Risk
www.halls.md/breast/risk.htm

Information on Low-Oxalate Foods
www.vulvarpainfoundation.org
A low-oxalate cookbook is available.

A p p e n d i x   C

LABORATORIES

To have tests done through the following laboratories, you will need to work with your naturopathic physician or holistically oriented medical doctor.

AAL Reference Laboratories
1715 East Wilshire #715
Santa Ana, CA 92705
(800) 522-2611
Offers comprehensive hormone testing, including estrogen metabolism tests

Accu-Chem Laboratories
990 North Bowser Road, Suite 800–880
Richardson, TX 75081
(800) 451-0116
Offers comprehensive environmental toxin testing through blood, urine, and tissue biopsy

Diagnos-techs Laboratory
6620 South 192nd Place, Bldg. J
Kent, WA 98032
tel. (800) 878-3787
fax (425) 251-0636
www.diagnostechs.com
Offers stool and salivary tests, including the Adrenal Stress Index (ASI) and female hormone panels

Elisa/Act Biotechnologies
14 Pidgeon Hill #300
Sterling, VA 22181
tel. (800) 533-5472
fax (703) 450-2981
Offers comprehensive food and chemical allergy testing

Great Smokies Diagnostic Laboratory
63 Zillicoa Street
Asheville, NC 28801-1074
(800) 522-4762
www.gsdl.com
Offers comprehensive tests including complete digestive stool analysis, hormone testing, heavy metal testing, liver detoxification tests, and more

A p p e n d i x   D

HOW TO CHOOSE A PHYSICIAN TRAINED IN NATURAL MEDICINE

This book is designed to serve as a guide for optimizing your health. But if you also need professional guidance, knowing how to choose a personal physician who is well trained in natural medicine can be one of the most health-protecting lifestyle choices you ever make.

When you look at your health care options, you may feel as if you've entered a confusing maze. The success of natural medicine has led to a surge of popularity, giving rise to many clinics offering various combinations of conventional and unconventional medicine. For example, an "integrated" clinic may provide the services of a medical doctor trained in conventional pharmaceutical-based therapies as well as the services of practitioners trained in acupuncture or nutrition.

The most important question you can ask yourself is no longer "How can I find a doctor who offers natural medicine?" but "What, exactly, is the *training* of a doctor who offers natural medicine?" As a consumer, you may have no way of telling at first glance if a physician is adequately trained to provide natural medicine. Anyone licensed to practice medicine can legally offer "natural medicine" to the public with no credentials from an accredited school of natural medicine and with little or no background whatsoever in natural medicine. Doctors may have the best of intentions but simply not be trained to provide you with the wealth of natural options that are available. It takes many years of training to assimilate the complex understanding required to practice the science and art of natural medicine. There is much, much more to it than attending a few seminars and prescribing a token selection of the natural remedies and therapies popularized by the media.

To guarantee that your doctor is trained in natural medicine, I strongly recommend you find a graduate of an accredited naturopathic medical school. These schools stand in a category all their own: they are currently the only medical schools in the United States that *require* students to become highly trained in the full range of natural and alternative therapies.[1, 2] They offer by far the most thorough, rigorous, in-depth education of its kind available anywhere—in short, the world's best training in natural medicine.

I urge you to compare the course requirements of accredited naturopathic medical schools with those of any other medical programs. According to the Association of American Medical Colleges, in 2000–2001 no conventional medical school in the United States required a single separate course in alternative and complementary medicine. (At some schools, these topics were taught only as a part of a required course, or offered as an elective).[3] By contrast, accredited naturopathic medical programs require more than seven hundred hours of therapeutic nutrition and naturopathic therapeutics.

In addition, according to the American Association of Naturopathic Physicians, the naturopathic medical school curriculum includes a comparable number of hours of basic biological sciences as conventional medical schools such as Yale and Stanford.[4] As a result, many believe that graduates of the naturopathic medical programs are the only doctors whose *training* is truly "integrated," making them uniquely qualified to balance conventional and unconventional medical approaches. Their training places them squarely between the two worlds, in the truest sense of the word able to "integrate" the best of each.

You can find graduates of accredited naturopathic medical schools throughout this country. One note of caution: naturopathic physicians are not yet licensed in some states, so *be sure that your naturopathic physician is a graduate of one of the accredited schools*. As a rule, anyone else using the term *naturopath* is doing so without adequate training. You can do a quick check to be sure you are putting your care in the hands of a legitimate graduate of one of the accredited schools: contact the American Association of Naturopathic Physicians. (See the following list for contact information.)

Organizations

American Association of Naturopathic Physicians
3201 New Mexico Avenue, NW, #350
Washington, DC 20016
tel. (866) 538-2267; (202) 895-1392
fax (202) 274-1992
www.naturopathic.org

National Certification Commission for Acupuncture and Oriental Medicine
11 Canal Center Plaza, Suite 300
Alexandria, VA 22314
tel. (703) 548-9004
fax (703) 548-9079
www.nccaom.org

Naturopathic Medical Schools

Bastyr University
14500 Juanita Drive Northeast
Kenmore, WA 98028-4966
tel. (425) 823-1300
fax (425) 823-6222
www.bastyr.edu

Boucher Institute of Naturopathic Medicine
200–668 Carnarvon Street
New Westminster, BC V3M 5Y6
(604) 777-9981
www.binm.org

Bridgeport University
126 Park Avenue
Bridgeport, CT 06601
(203) 576-4552
www.bridgeport.edu

Canadian College of Naturopathic Medicine
2300 Yonge Street
Toronto, ONT M4P 1E4
(416) 486-8584
www.ccnm.edu

National College of Naturopathic Medicine
049 Southwest Porter Street
Portland, OR 97201
(503) 499-4343
www.ncnm.edu

Southwest College of Naturopathic Medicine and Health Sciences
2140 East Broadway
Tempe, AZ 85282
(602) 990-7424
www.scnm.edu

Additional Information on Naturopathic Medicine

www.schools.naturalhealers.com/bastyr
www.drlauriesteelsmith.com

Appendix E

RECOMMENDED READING

Chapter 1
To Create Overall Health

Pizzorno, Joseph, N.D. *Total Wellness.* (Rocklin, Calif.: Prima Publishing, 1998).

Reichstein, Gail. *Wood Becomes Water: Chinese Medicine in Everyday Life* (New York: Kodansha America, 1998).

Chapter 2
To Support Your Immune System

Elias, Jason, L.Ac., and Katherine Ketcham. *Chinese Medicine for Maximum Immunity: Understanding the Five Elemental Types for Health and Well-Being* (New York: Three Rivers Press, 1998).

Murray, Michael, N.D. *Dr. Murray's Total Body Tune-Up* (New York: Bantam Books, 2000).

Teeguarden, Ron. *The Ancient Wisdom of the Chinese Tonic Herbs* (New York: Warner Books, 2000).

Chapter 3
To Support Your Kidneys
and Urinary System

Gillespie, Larrian, M.D. *You Don't Have to Live with Cystitis* (New York: Avon Books, 1996).

Hulme, Janet A., M.A., P.T. *Beyond Kegels* (Missoula, Mont.: Phoenix Pub., 2002).

Rodman, John, M.D., Cynthia Seidman, M.S., R.D., and Rory Jones. *No More Kidney Stones* (New York: John Wiley & Sons, 1996).

Rovner, Eric, M.D., Alan Wein, M.D., and Donna Caruso. *A Woman's Guide to Regaining Bladder Control: Everything You Need to Know for the Diagnosis and Cure of Incontinence* (New York: M. Evans and Company, 2002).

Chapter 4
To Support Your Liver
Health

Bennett, Peter, N.D., and Stephen Barrie, N.D., with Sara Faye. *7-Day Detox Miracle* (New York: Prima Publishing, 2001).

Steinman, David, and Samuel Epstein, M.D. *The Safe Shopper's Bible: A Consumer's Guide to Nontoxic Household Products, Cosmetics, and Food* (New York: Hungry Minds, 1995).

Chapter 5
To Support Your Heart Health

Pashkow, Fredric, M.D., and Charlotte Libov. *The Women's Heart Book: The Complete Guide to Keeping Your Heart Healthy* (New York: Hyperion, 2001).

Sinatra, Stephen, M.D., Jan Sinatra, R.N., M.S.N., and Roberta Jo Lieberman. *Heart Sense for Women: Your Plan for Natural Prevention and Treatment* (New York: Penguin Putnam, 2001).

Rippe, James M., M.D. *The Healthy Heart for Dummies* (Foster City, Calif.: IDG Books Worldwide, 2000).

Chapter 6
To Support Your Digestive System

Buillory, Gerard, M.D. *IBS: A Doctor's Plan for Chronic Digestive Troubles* (Vancouver, B.C.: Hartley & Marks Publishers, 2001).

Lipski, Elizabeth, M.S., C.C.N. *Digestive Wellness* (Lincolnwood, Ill.: Keats Publishing, 2000).

Semon, Bruce, M.D., Ph.D., and Lori Kornblum. *Feast Without Yeast* (Milwaukee, Wis.: Wisconsin Institute of Nutrition, 1999).

Chapter 7
To Support Your Hormonal System

Laux, Marcus, N.D., and Christine Conrad. *Natural Woman, Natural Menopause* (New York: HarperCollins Publishers, 1997).

Love, Susan, M.D. *Dr. Susan Love's Menopause and Hormone Book* (New York, Three Rivers Press, 2003).

Northrup, Christiane, M.D. *The Wisdom of Menopause* (New York: Bantam Books, 2001).

Northrup, Christiane, M.D. *Women's Bodies, Women's Wisdom* (New York: Bantam Books, 1994).

Shames, Richard, M.D., and Karilee Halo Shames, R.N., Ph.D. *Thyroid Power: 10 Steps to Total Health* (New York: HarperCollins Publishers, 2002).

Sichel, Deborah, M.D., and Jeanne Watson Driscoll, M.S., R.N., C.S. *Women's Moods: What Every Woman Must Know About Hormones, the Brain, and Emotional Health* (New York: HarperCollins Publishers, 1999).

Rako, Susan, M.D. *The Hormone of Desire: The Truth About Testosterone, Sexuality, and Menopause* (New York: Three Rivers Press, 1996).

Chapter 8
To Support Your Bone Health

Colbin, Annemarie. *Food and Our Bones* (New York: Penguin Putnam, 1998).

Gaby, Alan, M.D. *Preventing and Reversing Osteoporosis* (Rocklin, Calif.: Prima Publishing, 1994).

Nelson, Miriam, Ph.D. *Strong Women, Strong Bones* (New York: Penguin Putnam, 2001).

Sanson, Gill. *The Osteoporosis Epidemic: Well Women and the Marketing of Fear* (Auckland, New Zealand: Penguin Books, 2001).

Chapter 9
To Support Your Breast Health

Curties, Debra, R.M.T. *Breast Massage* (Toronto, Ontario: Curties-Overzet Publications, 1999).

Lauersen, Neils, M.D., and Eileen Stukane. *The Complete Book of Breast Care* (New York: Ballantine Books, 1996).

Love, Susan, M.D., and Karen Lindsey. *Dr. Susan Love's Breast Book* (Cambridge, Mass.: Perseus Publishing, 2000).

Wolfe, Honora Lee, and Bob Flaws. *Better Breast Health Naturally with Chinese Medicine* (Boulder, Colo.: Blue Poppy Press, 1998).

Chapter 10
To Support Your Pelvic Health

Henderson, Gregory, M.D., Ph.D., and Batya Swift Yasgur, M.A., MSW. *Women at Risk: The HPV Epidemic and Your Cervical Health* (New York: Avery Publishing, 2002).

Hudson, Tori, N.D. *Women's Encyclopedia of Natural Medicine: Alternative Therapies and Integrated Medicine* (Lincolnwood, Ill.: Keats Publishing, 1999).

Stewart, Elizabeth, M.D., and Paula Spencer. *The V Book: A Doctor's Guide to Complete Vulvovaginal Health* (New York: Bantam Books, 2002).

Weschler, Toni, MPH. *Taking Charge of Your Fertility: The Definitive Guide to Natural Birth Control, Pregnancy Achievement, and Reproductive Health* (New York: Quill/ HarperCollins Publishers, 2002).

Chapter 11
To Support Your Mental Health

Blaylock, Russell L., M.D. *Excitotoxins: The Taste That Kills* (Sante Fe, N.M.: Health Press, 1997).

Carper, Jean. *Your Miracle Brain* (New York: HarperCollins Publishers, 2000).

A p p e n d i x   F

A CHECKLIST FOR GETTING STARTED
ON YOUR NATURALLY HEALTHY LIFESTYLE

- Locate a natural foods store where you can purchase organic foods.
- Buy olive oil for cooking and flax oil to mix into your favorite salad dressings. Take one tablespoon of flax oil each day.
- Decrease your exposure to environmental chemicals by purchasing all-natural shampoo, body soap, toothpaste, cosmetics, and other personal care items. Also buy nontoxic cleaning agents for use in your home.
- Purchase a multivitamin derived from natural sources and void of synthetic chemicals. Make sure that it provides the amounts outlined in Chapter 2. For high-quality supplements, look for the GMP certification on the label.
- Begin a regular exercise program: purchase comfortable workout clothes, sneakers, light weights, and an exercise tape, and consider investing in a gym membership.
- Buy a reverse osmosis water filter if you live in an area that adds fluoride to the water. If your water is not fluoridated, use a good carbon filter. Consider a water filter for your showerhead or for your entire household.
- Avoid dry cleaning as much as possible. If you need to dry-clean, use a perc-free dry cleaner exclusively. If you cannot find a perc-free dry cleaner, hang your clothes in a well-ventilated area before you wear them.
- Find a licensed naturopathic physician and acupuncturist who can be a part of your health plan.
- Create time to nurture yourself each day.

Notes

Chapter 1. Creating Health

1. E. Koop, *1988 U.S. Surgeon General's Report on Health,* online at Profiles in Science website, http://profiles.nlm.nih.gov/NN/B/C/Q/G/(accessed Jul. 2, 2003).

2. J. S. Bland, *Genetic Nutritioneering* (New York: McGraw-Hill/Contemporary Books, 1999), 7.

3. A. Sanchez et al., "Role of sugars in human neutrophilic phagocytosis," *American Journal of Clinical Nutrition* 26, no. 11 (1973), 1180–84.

4. E. Guallar et al., "Mercury, fish oils, and the risk of myocardial infarction," *New England Journal of Medicine* 347, no. 22 (Nov. 28, 2002), 1747–54.

5. "FDA Announces Advisory on Methyl Mercury in Fish," FDA Talk Paper, online at U.S. Food and Drug Administration website, www.fda.gov/bbs/topics/ANSWERS/2001/ANS 01065.html (accessed May 3, 2003).

6. "Illegal Pesticides in Produce," online at Environmental Working Group website, www.ewg.org/reports/fruit/chapter2.html (accessed Aug. 1, 2004).

7. T. Colborn et al., *Our Stolen Future* (New York: Penguin Books, 1997), 183.

8. D. K. Asami, Y. Hong, and D. M. Barrett, "Comparison of the total phenolic and ascorbic acid content of freeze-dried and air-dried marionberry, strawberry, and corn grown using conventional, organic, and sustainable agricultural practices," *Journal of Agricultural and Food Chemistry* 51 (2003), 1237–41.

Chapter 2. Your Protective Shield

1. S. E. Taylor, L. Cousino Klein, and B. P. Lewis, "Biobehavioral responses to stress in females: Tend-and-befriend, not fight-or-flight," *Psychological Review* 107, no. 3 (2000), 411–29.

2. B. T. Gaffney, H. M. Hugel, and P. A. Rich, "The effects of *Eleutherococcus senticosus* and *Panax ginseng* on steroidal hormone indices of stress and lymphocyte subset numbers in endurance athletes." *Life Sciences* 70, no. 4 (Dec. 14, 2001), 431–42.

3. E. Rogala et al., "The influence of *Eleutherococcus senticosus* on cellular and humoral immunological response of mice," *Polish Journal of Veterinary Sciences* 6 (3rd supp.) (2003), 37–39; B. Bohn, C. T. Nebe, and C. Birr, "Flow-cytometric studies of *Eleutherococcus senticosus* extract as an immunomodulatory agent," *Arzneimittel-Forschung* 37, no. 10 (Oct. 1987), 1193–96.

4. A. Szolomicki et al., "The influence of active components of *Eleutherococcus senticosus* on cellular defense and physical fitness in man," *Phytotherapy Research* 14, no. 1 (Feb. 2000), 30–35.

5. Ibid.

6. R. Teeguarden, *The Ancient Wisdom of the Chinese Tonic Herbs* (New York: Warner Books, 1998), 113.

7. M. Williams, "Immuno-protection against herpes simplex type II infection by *Eleutherococcus* root extract," *International Journal of Alternative and Complementary Medicine* 13, no. 7 (Jul. 1995), 9–12.

8. M. Davydov and A. D. Krikorian, "*Eleutherococcus senticosus* as an adaptogen: A closer look," *Journal of Ethnopharmacology* 72, no. 3 (Oct. 1, 2000), 345–93.

9. Anonymous, "Astragalus Monograph," *Alternative Medicine Review* 8, no. 1 (Feb. 2003), 72–77.

10. Ibid.

11. R. Teeguarden, *The Ancient Wisdom of the Chinese Tonic Herbs* (New York: Warner Books, 1998), 121.

12. M. J. Hsu et al., "Signaling mechanisms of enhanced neutrophil phagocytosis and chemotaxis by the polysaccharide purified from *Ganoderma lucidum,*" *British Journal of Pharmacology* 139, no. 2 (May 2003), 289–98; L. Z. Cao and Z. B. Lin, "Regulation on maturation and function of dendritic cells by *Ganoderma lucidum* polysaccharides," *Immunology Letters* 83, no. 3 (Oct. 1, 2002), 163–69.

13. Teeguarden, *The Ancient Wisdom,* 88.

14. Ibid.

15. S. Wachtel-Galor, B. Tomlinson, and I. F. Benzie, "*Ganoderma lucidum* ('Lingzhi'), a Chinese medicinal mushroom: Biomarker responses in a controlled human supplementation study," *British Journal of Nutrition* 91, no. 2 (Feb. 2004), 263–69.

16. Y. Gao, S. Shou, and W. Jiang, "Effects of ganopoly (a *Ganoderma lucidum* polysaccharide extract) on the immune function in advanced-stage cancer patients," *Immunological Investigations* 32, no. 3 (Aug. 2003), 201–15; H. Hu et al., "*Ganoderma lucidum* extract induces cell cycle arrest and apoptosis in MCF-7 human breast cancer cell," *International Journal of Cancer* 102, no. 3 (Nov. 20, 2002), 250–53; D. Silva, "*Ganoderma lucidum* (Reishi) in cancer treatment," *Integrative Cancer Therapies* 2, no. 4 (Dec. 2003), 358–64.

17. Teeguarden, *The Ancient Wisdom,* 88.

18. D. Cui, Z. Moldoveanu, and C. B. Stephensen, "High-level dietary vitamin A enhances T-helper type 2 cytokine production and secretory immunoglobulin A response to influenza A virus infection in BALB/c mice," *Journal of Nutrition* 130, no. 5 (May 2000), 1132–39.

19. D. O. Freier, K. Wright, and K. Klein, "Enhancement of the humoral immune response by *Echinacea purpurea* in female Swiss mice,"

Immunopharmacology and Immunotoxicology 25, no. 4 (Nov. 2003), 551–60; X. H. Gan et al., "Mechanism of activation of human peripheral blood NK cells at the single cell level by Echinacea water soluble extracts: Recruitment of lymphocyte-target conjugates and killer cells and activation of programming for lysis," *International Immunopharmacology* 3, no. 6 (Jun. 2003), 811–24.

Chapter 3. Flowing Water

1. Centers for Disease Control, Division of Bacterial and Mycotic Diseases, *Disease Information: Urinary Tract Infections,* online at www.cdc.gov/ncidod/dbmd/diseaseinfo/urinary tractinfections_t.htm (accessed Sept. 8, 2003).

2. E. Rovner, A. Wein, and D. Caruso, *A Woman's Guide to Regaining Bladder Control* (New York: M. Evans & Co., 2002), 3.

3. G. Reichstein, *Wood Becomes Water* (New York: Kodansha America, 1998), 174.

4. R. M. Jaffe, *Host Defenses,* part 2, *Evoking the Human Healing Response,* part 2: *Dysbiosis* (1992–93), 5–62.

5. Medline Plus Health Information, *Sodium in Diet,* online at www.nlm.nih.gov/medlineplus/ency/article/002415.htm (accessed Dec. 25, 2002).

6. M. Murray, *Encyclopedia of Nutritional Supplements* (Rocklin, Calif.: Prima Publishing, 1996), 179.

7. P. Pitchford, *Healing with Whole Foods* (Richmond, Calif.: North Atlantic Books, 1993), 158.

8. E. N. Whitney and E. M. N. Hamilton, *Understanding Nutrition,* 2nd ed. (St. Paul, Minn.: West Publishing Co., 1981), 497.

9. Environmental Working Group, "Weed Killers by the Glass," online at www.ewg.org/pub/home/reports/weed_killer/weed3.html (accessed Dec. 25, 2002).

10. Environmental Working Group, *Consider the Source: Farm Runoff, Chlorination Byproducts, and Human Health*, online at www.ewg.org/reports/ConderTheSource/es.html (accessed Dec. 2002).

11. H. Limeback, "Guest Editorial: Fluoride," *International Society of Fluoride Research* 34, no. 1 (2001), 3.

12. Ibid, 3.

13. Fluoride Action Network, online at http://fluoridealert.org/govt-statements.htm (accessed Jan. 2, 2002).

14. A. M. Colbin, *Food and Healing* (New York: Ballantine Books, 1986), 297.

15. J. X. Li, Y. Hong, and K. M. Chan, "Tai Chi: Physiological characteristics and beneficial effects on health," *British Journal of Sports Medicine* 35, vol. 3 (Jun. 2001), 148–56; L. Qin et al., "Regular Tai Chi Chuan exercise may retard bone loss in postmenopausal women: A case-control study," *Archives of Physical Medicine and Rehabilitation* 83, no. 10 (Oct. 2002), 1355–59.

16. G. Mojay, *Aromatherapy for Healing the Spirit* (Rochester, Vt.: Healing Arts Press, 1997), 59.

17. National Kidney and Urological Disease Information Clearinghouse, "Urinary tract infections in adults," online at www.niddk.nih.gov/health/urolog/pubs/utiadult/utiadult.htm (accessed Jan. 12, 2003).

18. L. Gillespie, *You Don't Have to Live with Cystitis* (New York: Avon Books, 1996), 194–95.

CHAPTER 4. NEW SHOOTS

1. L. Clorfene-Casten, *Breast Cancer: Poisons, Profits, and Prevention* (Monroe, Me.: Common Courage Press, 1996), 54.

2. D. Steinman and S. Epstein, *The Safe Shopper's Bible: A Consumer's Guide to Nontoxic Household Products, Cosmetics, and Food* (New York: Hungry Minds, 1995), 17.

3. C. M. Ardies and C. Dees, "Xenoestrogens significantly enhance risk for breast cancer during growth and adolescence," *Medical Hypotheses* 50, no. 6 (Jun. 1998), 457–64.

4. T. Colborn, D. Dumanoski, and J. P. Myers, *Our Stolen Future* (New York: Plume Books, 1997), 182–83.

5. F. Falck Jr. et al., "Pesticides and polychlorinated biphenyl residues in human breast lipids and their relation to breast cancer," *Archives of Environmental Health* 47, no. 2 (Mar.–Apr. 1992), 143–46.

6. R. Abel, *The Eye Care Revolution* (New York: Kensington Books, 1999), 339.

7. J. Houlihan, C. Brody, and B. Schwan, "Not too pretty: Phthalates, beauty products and the FDA," *New York Times,* Jul. 8, 2002.

8. J. Pizzorno and M. Murray, *The Textbook of Natural Medicine* (London, Eng.: Churchill Livingstone, 2000), 443.

9. Ibid., 442.

10. Ibid., 443.

11. Ibid.

12. Ibid.

13. B. Flaws, *The Tao of Healthy Eating* (Boulder, Colo.: Blue Poppy Press, 1998), 106.

14. Ibid., 60–63.

15. Pizzorno and Murray, *Textbook of Natural Medicine,* 447.

CHAPTER 5. A FIRE WITHIN

1. A. Clark, A. Seidler, and M. Miller, "Inverse association between sense of humor and coronary artery disease," *International Journal of Cardiology* 80, no. 1 (Aug. 2001), 87–88.

2. National Heart, Lung, and Blood Institute, *Facts About Heart Disease and Women: Are You At Risk?,* online at www.nhlbi.nih.gov/health/public/heart/other/wmn_risk.htm (accessed Nov. 2001).

3. J. P. Strong et al., "Early lesions of atherosclerosis in childhood and youth: Natural history

and risk factors," *Journal of the American College of Nutrition* 11 (1991), 51S–54S.

4. Clark, Seidler, and Miller, "Inverse association," 87–88.

5. R. Williams et al., "The impact of emotions on cardiovascular health," *Journal of Gender Specific Medicine* 2, no. 5 (Sept.–Oct. 1999), 52–58.

6. R. Ballou, *The Viking Portable Library World Bible* (New York: Viking Press, 1967), 572.

7. *Third Report of the Expert Panel on Detection, Evaluation, and Treatment of High Blood Cholesterol in Adults* (Adult Treatment Panel III), National Cholesterol Education Program, online at www.nhbi.nih.gov/guidelines/cholesterol/atglance.htm (accessed Dec. 2001).

8. *Seventh Report of the Joint National Committee on Prevention, Detection, Evaluation, and Treatment of High Blood Pressure*, National Institutes of Health, National Heart, Lung, and Blood Institute, online at www.nhlbi.nih.gov/guidelines/hypertension/jncintro.htm (accessed Sept. 2003).

9. J. Pizzorno and M. Murray, *The Encyclopedia of Natural Medicine* (Rocklin, Calif.: Prima Publishing, 1998), 88.

10. B. Christensen et al., "Abstention from filtered coffee reduces the concentrations of plasma homocysteine and serum cholesterol—a randomized controlled trial," *American Journal of Clinical Nutrition* 74 (2001), 302–7.

11. J. P. Wang et al., "Antihemostatic and antithrombotic effects of capsaicin in comparison with aspirin and indomethacin," *Thrombosis Research* 37, no. 6 (Mar. 1985), 669–79.

12. M. C. Ramirez-Tortosa et al., "Oral administration of a turmeric extract inhibits LDL oxidation and has hypocholesterolemic effects in rabbits with experimental atherosclerosis," *Atherosclerosis* 147, no. 2 (Dec. 1999), 371–78.

13. Y. Wan et al., "Effects of cocoa powder and dark chocolate on LDL oxidative susceptibility and prostaglandin concentration in humans," *American Journal of Clinical Nutrition* 74 (2001), 596–602.

14. E. Rimm, "Alcohol and cardiovascular disease," *Current Atherosclerosis Reports* 2, no. 6 (Nov. 2000), 529–35.

15. K. A. Meister, E. M. Whelan, and R. Kave, "The health effects of moderate alcohol intake in humans: An epidemiologic review," *Critical Reviews in Clinical Laboratory Sciences* 37, no. 3 (Jun. 2000), 261–96.

16. A. Klatsky, "Should patients with heart disease drink alcohol?" *Journal of the American Medical Association* 385, no. 15 (Apr. 18, 2001), 2004–6.

17. Meister, Whelan, and Kave, "Health effects of moderate alcohol intake," 261–96.

18. U.S. Department of Health and Human Services, Office of Applied Studies, *National Household Survey on Drug Abuse, Main Findings* (1997), 106, 110–11.

19. M. P. Longnecker, "Alcohol consumption and risk of cancer in humans: An overview," *Alcohol* 12, no. 2 (Mar.–Apr. 1995), 87–96.

20. N. Lu, *A Woman's Guide to a Trouble-Free Menopause* (New York: HarperCollins, 2000), 103.

21. P. Boffetta et al., "Mortality from cardiovascular diseases and exposure to inorganic mercury," *Occupational and Environmental Medicine* 58, no. 7 (Jul. 1, 2001), 461–66.

22. J. Wright, "Chlorinated water," *Dr. Jonathan V. Wright's Nutrition and Healing with Alan R. Gaby, M.D.* 4r, no. 8 (August, 1997), 10.

23. M. Imamura et al., "Repeated thermal therapy improves impaired vascular endothelial function in patients with coronary risk factors," *Journal of the American College of Cardiology* 38 (2001), 1083–88.

24. J. A. Simon and E. S. Hudes, "Relation of serum ascorbic acid to serum lipids and lipoproteins in U.S. adults," *Journal of the American*

College of Nutrition 17, no. 3 (Jun. 1998), 250–55.

25. "The role of vitamin E in the prevention of heart disease," *Archives of Family Medicine* 8, no. 6 (Nov.–Dec. 1999), 537–42.

26. A. A. Qureshi et al., "Lowering of serum cholesterol in hypercholesterolemic humans by tocotrienols," *American Journal of Clinicial Nutrition* 53, no. 4 (supp.) (Apr. 1991), 1021S–1026S.

27. A. Miller and G. Kelly, "Homocysteine metabolism: Nutritional modulations and impact on health and disease," *Alternative Medicine Review* 2, no. 4 (July 1997), 244.

28. S. Sinatra, *Heart Sense for Women* (New York: Penguin/Putnam, 2001), 116.

29. G. Castano et al., "Effects of policosanol on postmenopausal women with type II hypercholesterolemia," *Gynecological Endocrinology* 14, no. 3 (Jun. 2000), 187–95.

30. D. Brown and S. Austin, "Hyperlipidemia and prevention of coronary heart disease," *Quarterly Review of Natural Medicine* (Spring 1997), 61–76.

31. S. Panda and A. Kar, "Gugulu (*Commiphora mukul*) induces triiodothyronine production: possible involvement of lipid peroxidation," *Life Sciences* 65, no. 12 (1999), PL 137–41.

32. Brown and Austin, "Hyperlipidemia and prevention of coronary heart disease," 61–76.

33. Qureshi et al., "Lowering of serum cholesterol," 1021S–1026S.

34. A. Gaby, "Commentary: Chelation therapy," *Dr. Jonathan V. Wright's Nutrition and Healing with Alan R. Gaby, M.D.* 4, no. 7 (Jul. 1997), 11.

35. J. Kleijnen and P. Knipschild, "Ginkgo biloba for cerebral insufficiency," *French Journal of Clinical Pharmacology* 34 (1992), 352–58.

36. N. Kohashi and R. Katori, "Decrease of urinary taurine in essential hypertension," *Japanese Heart Journal* 24, no. 1 (Jan. 1983), 91–102.

37. M. A. Creager et al., "L-arginine improves endothelim-dependent vasodilation in hypercholesterolemic humans," *Journal of Clinical Investigation* 90, no. 4 (Oct. 1992), 1248–53.

CHAPTER 6. GIFTS OF THE EARTH

1. P. Pietinen et al., "Intake of dietary fiber and risk of coronary artery disease in cohort of Finnish men," *Circulation* 94, no. 11 (1996), 2696–98.

2. M. Soler et al., "Fiber intake and risk of oral, pharyngeal and esophageal cancer," *International Journal of Cancer* 91, no. 3 (2001), 283–87.

3. C. D. Cocky, "Diagnosing irritable bowel syndrome," *AWHONN Lifelines* 3, no. 6 (Dec./Jan.1999–2000), 11.

4. N. Plummer, "Unseen epidemic," *Townsend Letter for Doctors and Patients* 252 (Jul. 2004), 91.

5. D. Brown, *Herbal Prescriptions for Better Health* (Rocklin, Calif.: Prima Publishing, 1996), 97–109; J. Stiles et al., "The inhibition of *Candida albicans* by oregano," *Journal of Applied Nutrition* 47, no. 4 (1995), 96–102; T. Birdsall and G. Kelly, "Berberine: Therapeutic potential of an alkaloid found in several medicinal plants," *Alternative Medicine Review* 2, no. 2 (Mar. 1997), 94–103; P. M. Furneri et al., "In vitro antimycoplasmal activity of oleuropein," *International Journal of Antimicrobial Agents* 20, no. 4 (Oct. 2002), 293–96; G. Bisignano et al., "On the invitro activity of oleuropein and hydrozytyrosol," *Journal of Pharmacy and Pharmacology* 51, no. 8 (Aug. 1999), 971–74.

6. J. A. Cantanzaro and L. Green, "Microbial ecology and probiotics in human medicine (part II)," *Alternative Medicine Review* 2, no. 4 (Jul. 1997), 296–305.

7. Ibid., 302.

CHAPTER 7. ORCHESTRATING YOUR HORMONAL DANCE

1. C. Northrup, *Women's Bodies, Women's Wisdom* (New York: Bantam Books, 1994), 95.

2. Ibid., 101.

3. Ibid., 99.

4. G. Maciocia, *Obstetrics and Gynecology in Chinese Medicine* (London, Eng.: Churchill Livingstone Books, 1998), 11.

5. R. Trickey, *Women, Hormones and the Menstrual Cycle* (St. Leonards, NSW, Australia: Allen and Unwin, 1998), 107.

6. D. Sichel and J. W. Driscoll, *Women's Moods* (New York: Quill Books, 1999), 83.

7. S. Love, *Dr. Susan Love's Hormone Book* (New York: Random House, 1998), 2.

8. B. Flaws, *My Sister the Moon* (Boulder, Colo.: Blue Poppy Press, 1992), 315.

9. J. E. Rossouw et al., "Risks and benefits of estrogen plus progestin in healthy postmenopausal women: Principal results from the Women's Health Initiative randomized controlled trial," *Journal of the American Medical Association* 167, no. 4 (Aug. 20, 2002), 377–78.

10. Dr. Susan Hendrix, a gynecologist, on the government decision to require labels on drugs containing estrogen, "Quote of the day," *New York Times,* Jan. 9, 2003.

11. S. R. Rapp et al., "Effect of estrogen plus progestin on global cognitive function in postmenopausal women," *Journal of the American Medical Association* 289 (2003), 2663–72.

12. T. Hudson, "Hormone Replacement Therapy: Benefits, Risks, and Options," *Integrative Medicine* 2, no. 1 (Feb.–Mar. 2003), 22.

13. M. F. McCarty, "Androgenic progestins amplify the breast cancer risk associated with hormone replacement therapy by boosting IGF-1 activity," *Medical Hypothesis* 56, no. 2 (Feb. 2001), 213–16.

14. R. Shames and K. H. Shames, *Thyroid Power* (New York: Quill Books, 2002), 16–17.

15. R. Bunevicius et al., "Effects of thyroxine as compared with thyroxine plus triiodothyronine in patients with hypothyroidism," *New England Journal of Medicine* 340, vol. 6 (Feb. 11, 1999), 424–29.

16. J. A. Bralley and R. Lord, *Evaluations in Molecular Medicine* (Norcross, Ga.: Institute for Advances in Molecular Medicine, 2001), 296.

17. Shames and Shames, *Thyroid Power,* 169.

18. W. Crinnion, "Environmental Medicine, Part 1: The Human Burden of Environmental Toxins and Their Common Health Effects," *Alternative Medicine Review* 5, no. 1 (Feb. 2000), 52–63.

19. Bralley and Lord, *Evaluations in Molecular Medicine,* 307.

20. T. Hertoghe, *The Hormone Solution: Stay Younger Longer* (New York: Harmony Books, 2002), 63–64.

21. American Association of Clinical Endocrinologists, online at www.aace.com/pub/BMI/findings.php (accessed Mar. 3, 2003).

22. Bralley and Lord, *Evaluations in Molecular Medicine,* 307.

23. A. S. Rayn et al., "Hormone replacement therapy, insulin sensitivity and abdominal obesity in postmenopausal women," *Diabetes Care* 25, no. 1 (Jan. 2002), 127–33.

24. J. M. Holly, D. J. Gunnell, and G. Davey Smith, "Growth hormone, IFG-1 and cancer. Less intervention to avoid cancer? More intervention to prevent cancer?" *Journal of Endocrinology* 162 (1999), 321–30.

CHAPTER 8. BUILDING HEALTHY BONES FOR LIFE

1. National Institutes of Health, *Fast Facts on Osteoporosis,* online at www.osteo.org/newfile.asp?doc=fast&doctitle=Fast+Facts+on+Osteoporosis&docty (accessed Apr. 12, 2003).

2. National Institute of Arthritis and Musculoskeletal and Skin Diseases, online at www.niams.nih.gov/hi/topics/arthritis/oahandout.htm (accessed Apr. 12, 2003).

3. J. A. Kanis and C. Gluer, "An Update on the Diagnosis and Assessment of Osteoporosis with Densitometry," *Osteoporosis International* 11 (2000), 192.

4. National Institute of Arthritis and Musculoskeletal and Skin Diseases, online at www.niams.nih.gov/hi/topics/arthritis/oahandout.htm (accessed Apr. 12, 2003); A. Gaby, "Natural treatments for osteoarthritis," *Alternative Medicine Review* 4, no. 5 (1999), 330–41.

5. A. I. Ahmed, G. M. Blake, and J. M. Rymer, "Screening for osteopenia and osteoporosis: Do the acceptable normal ranges lead to overdiagnosis?" *Osteoporosis International* 7, no. 5 (1997), 432–38.

6. S. Love, *Dr. Susan Love's Menopause and Hormone Book* (New York: Three Rivers Press, 2003), 98.

7. Ibid., 95.

8. "Vitamin D deficiency, the silent epidemic," interview with Michael F. Holick, *Nutrition Action Newsletter* (Oct. 1997), 1–6.

9. M. Nelson and S. Wernick, *Strong Women, Strong Bones* (New York: Penguin Putnam, 2000), 30.

10. M. T. Hannan, "Dietary protein and effects upon bone health in elderly men and women," *Nutritional Aspects of Osteoporosis* (San Diego, Calif.: Academic Press, 2001), 246.

11. Y. Takada et al., "Whey protein stimulated the proliferation and differentiation of osteoblastic MC3T3-E1 cells," *Biochemical and Biophysical Research Communications* 223, no. 2 (Jun. 14, 1996), 455–59.

12. D. Barclay, "Calcium bioavailability from foods," *Nutritional Aspects of Osteoporosis* (San Diego, Calif.: Academic Press, 2001), 91.

13. S. A. New et al., "Dietary influences on bone mass and bone metabolism: Further evidence of a positive link between fruit and vegetable consumption and bone health?" *American Journal of Clinical Nutrition* 71, no. 1 (Jan. 2000), 142–51.

14. K. L. Tucker et al., "Potassium, magnesium and fruit and vegetable intakes are associated with greater bone mineral density in elderly men and women," *American Journal of Clinical Nutrition* 69, no. 4 (Apr. 1999), 727–36.

15. C. M. Weaver, L. A. Spence, and E. R. Lipscomb, "Phytoestrogens and bone health," *Nutritional Aspects of Osteoporosis* (San Diego, Calif.: Academic Press, 2001), 322.

16. N. Morabito et al., "Effects of genistein and hormone-replacement therapy on bone loss in early postmenopausal women: A randomized double-blind placebo-controlled study," *Journal of Bone and Mineral Research* 17 (2002), 1904–12.

17. T. Hudson, "Women's Health Update: Essential Fatty Acids and Osteoporosis," *Townsend Letter for Doctors and Patients* (Aug.–Sept. 2001), 186–87.

18. N. F. Childers and M. S. Margoles, "An apparent relation of nightshades (solanaceae) to arthritis," *Journal of Neurological and Orthopedic Medical Surgery* 12 (1993), 227–31.

19. R. P. Heaney, "Lead in calcium supplements: Cause for alarm or celebration?" *Journal of the American Medical Association* 284, no. 11 (Sept. 20, 2000), 1432–33.

20. E. A. Ross, "Lead content of calcium supplements," *Journal of the American Medical Association* 284, no. 11 (Sept. 20, 2000), 1425–29.

21. M. Kaneki et al., "Japanese fermented soybean food as the major determinant of the large geographic difference in circulating levels of vitamin K_2: Possible implications for hip-fracture risk," *Nutrition* 17, no. 4 (Apr. 2001), 315–21.

22. H. Katsuyama et al., "Usual dietary intake of fermented soybeans (Nato) is associated with bone mineral density in premenopausal women," *Journal of Nutritional Science and Vitaminology* 48, no. 3 (Jun. 2002), 207–15.

23. A. Zitterman, "Effects of vitamin K on calcium and bone metabolism," *Current Opinion in Clinical Nutrition and Metabolic Care* 4, no. 6 (Nov. 2001), 483–87.

24. M. Shiraki et al., "Vitamin K$_2$ effectively prevents fractures and sustains lumbar bone mineral density in osteoporosis," *Journal of Bone and Mineral Research* 15, no. 3 (Mar. 2000), 515–21.

25. O. Lamy, C. Mischler, and M. A. Krieg, "Treatment of osteoporosis (with the exception of hormone replacement and its derivates)," *Revue Medicale de la Suisse Romande* 122, no. 8 (Aug. 2002), 389–93.

26. J. V. Wright, "Fight—even prevent—osteoporosis with the hidden secrets of this bone-building miracle mineral," *Nutrition and Healing Newsletter* 10, no. 2 (Feb. 2003).

27. P. J. Meunier et al., "The effects of strontium ranelate on the risk of vertebral fracture in women with postmenopausal osteoporosis," *New England Journal of Medicine* 350, no. 5. (Jan. 2004), 459–68.

28. R. Lindsay et al., "Effect of lower doses of conjugated equine estrogens with and without medroxyprogesterone acetate on bone in early postmenopausal women," *Journal of the American Medical Association* 287, no. 20 (May 2002), 2668–76.

29. T. Hayashi et al., "Estriol (E$_3$) replacement improves enodethialia function and bone mineral density in very elderly women," *Journals of Gerontology Series A—Biological Sciences and Medical Sciences* 55, no. 4 (Apr. 2000), B183–90; discussion B191–93.

30. J. R. Lee, "Is natural progesterone the missing link in osteoporosis prevention and treatment?" *Medical Hypotheses* 35, no. 4 (Aug. 1991), 316–18.

31. C. M. Gordon, J. Glowacki, and M. S. LeBoff, "DHEA and the skeleton (through the ages)," *Endocrine* 11, no. 1 (Aug. 1999), 1–11.

32. A. Gaby, *Preventing and Reversing Osteoporosis* (Rocklin, Calif.: Prima Publishing, 1993), 231.

33. F. W. Fraunfelder and F. T. Fraunfelder, "Bisphosphonates and ocular inflammation," *New England Journal of Medicine* 348, no. 12 (Mar. 20, 2003), 1187–88.

34. S. Love, *Dr. Susan Love's Menopause and Hormone Book* (New York: Three Rivers Press, 2003), 277.

35. A. Cranney et al., "Meta-analyses of therapies for postmenopausal osteoporosis II. Meta-analysis of alendronate for the treatment of postmenopausal women," *Endocrine Reviews* 23, no. 4 (Aug. 23, 2002), 508–16.

36. Anonymous, "Raloxifene: Not better than estrogen," *Canadian Family Physician* 46 (Aug. 2000), 1592–96, 1599–603; G. G. Long, I. R. Cohen, and C. L. Gried, "Proliferative lesions of ovarian granulosa cells and reversible hormonal changes induced in rats by selective estrogen receptor modulator," *Toxicologic Pathology* 29, no. 6 (Nov.–Dec. 2001), 719–26.

37. J. L. Vahle et al., "Skeletal changes in rats given daily subcutaneous injections of recombinant human parathyroid hormone for 2 years and relevance to human safety," *Toxicologic Pathology* 30, no. 3 (May–Jun. 2002), 312–21.

38. M. L. Zoler, "Teriparatide may build bone best when used alone," Center for Clinical Age Management, online at www.natural-hrt.com/artman/publish/printer_118.shtml (accessed Apr. 17, 2003).

39. K. L. Soeken et al., "Safety and efficacy of S-adenosylmethionine (SAM-e) for osteoarthritis: A meta-analysis," *Journal of Family Practice* 51, no. 5 (May 2002), 425–30.

40. C. I. Curtis et al., "Pathologic indicators of degradation and inflammation in human osteoarthritic cartilage are abrogated by exposure to n-3 fatty acids," *Arthritis and Rheumatism* 46, no. 6 (Jun. 2002), 1544–53; L. G. Darlington and T. W. Stone, "Antioxidants and fatty acids in

the amelioration of rheumatoid arthritis and related disorders," *British Journal of Nutrition* 85, no. 3 (Mar. 2001), 251–69.

41. A. Gaby, "Natural treatments for osteoarthritis," *Alternative Medicine Review* 4, no. 5 (1999), 331–32.

CHAPTER 9. CREATING OPTIMAL BREAST HEALTH

1. National Cancer Institute, "Lifetime probability of breast cancer in American women," online at *http://cis.nci.nih.gov/fact/5_6.htm* (accessed Sept. 7, 2003).

2. S. Tominaga and T. Kuroishi, "Epidemiology of breast cancer in Japan," *Cancer Letters* 90, no. 1 (Mar. 1995), 75–79.

3. S. Love and K. Lindsey, *Dr. Susan Love's Hormone Book* (New York: Times Books, 1998), 125.

4. L. H. Kuller, "The etiology of breast cancer from epidemiology to prevention," *Public Heath Reviews* 23, no. 2 (1995), 157–213.

5. M. S. Wolff et al., "Breast cancer and environmental risk factors; epidemiological and experimental findings," *Annual Review of Pharmacology and Toxicology* 36 (1996), 573–96.

6. C. Simone, *Breast Health* (New York: Avery Publishing Group, 1995), 124.

7. E. Ness, "Masquerading as hormones," *MAMM: Women, Cancer and Community,* Jul.–Aug. 2000, 34–54; S. H. Safe and T. Zacharewski, "Organochlorine exposure and risk for breast cancer," *Progress in Clinical Biological Research* 396 (1997), 133–45.

8. C. Charlier, A. Albert, and P. Herman, "Breast cancer and serum organochlorine residues," *Occupational and Environmental Medicine* 60, no. 5 (May 2003), 348–51.

9. L. C. Casten, *Breast Cancer, Poisons, Profits and Prevention* (Monroe, Me.: Common Courage Press, 1996), 30.

10. Simone, *Breast Health,* 124.

11. G. Ramaswamy and L. Krishnamoorthy, "Antioxidant vitamins and cancer," *American Journal of Medicine* 97, no. 3A (Sept. 26, 1994), 2S–4S; discussion 22S–28S.

12. J. D. Potter and K. Steinmetz, "Vegetables, fruit and phytoestrogens as preventive agents," *IARC Scientific Publications* 139 (1996), 61–90.

13. V. Chajes et al., "Influence of n-3 fatty acids on the growth of human breast cancer cells in vitro: Relationship to peroxides and vitamin E," *Breast Cancer Research and Treatment* 34, no. 3 (Jun. 1995), 199–212.

14. P. Ayotte et al., "PCBs and dioxin-like compounds in plasma of adult Inuit living in Nunavik (Arctic Quebec)," *Chemosphere* 34, nos. 5–7 (Mar.–Apr. 1997), 1459–68.

15. S. E. McCann et al., "The risk of breast cancer associated with dietary lignans differs by CYP17 genotype in women," *Journal of Nutrition* 132, no. 10 (Oct. 2002), 3036–41.

16. H. Funahashi et al., "Seaweed prevents breast cancer?" *Japanese Journal of Cancer Research* 92, no. 5 (May 2001), 483–87.

17. J. Kohen, *The Truth about Breast Cancer* (Larkspur, Calif.: Parissound Publishing, 1999), 42.

18. A. Wolk et al., "A prospective study of association of monounsaturated fat and other types of fat with risk of breast cancer," *Archives of Internal Medicine* 158, no. 1 (Jan. 12, 1998), 41–45.

19. M. J. Thun et al., "Alcohol consumption and mortality among middle-aged and elderly U.S. adults," *New England Journal of Medicine* 337, no. 24 (Dec. 11, 1997), 1705–14.

20. P. L. Horn-Ross et al., "Patterns of alcohol consumption and breast cancer risk in the California Teachers Study cohort," *Cancer Epidemiology, Biomarker and Prevention* 13, no. 3 (Mar. 2004), 405–11.

21. E. S. Ginsburg et al., "Effects of alcohol ingestion on estrogen in postmenopausal women,"

Journal of the American Medical Association 276, no. 21 (Dec. 1996), 1747–51.

22. R. Mittendorf et al., "Strenuous physical activity in young adulthood and risk of breast cancer," *Cancer Causes and Control* 6, no. 4 (Jul. 1995), 347–53.

23. P. F. Coogan, P. A. Newcomb, and R. W. Clapp, "Physical activity in usual occupation and risk of breast cancer," *Cancer Causes and Control* 8, no. 4 (Jul. 1997), 626–31.

24. J. E. Rossouw et al., "Risks and benefits of estrogen plus progestin in healthy postmenopausal women: Prinicpal results from the Women's Health Initiative Randomized Trial," *Journal of the American Medical Association* 288, no. 3 (Jul. 17, 2002), 321–33.

25. M. Althuis and L. A. Brinton, "Oral contraceptives and the risk of breast cancer," *New England Journal of Medicine* 347, no. 18 (Oct. 31, 2002), 1448–49.

26. N. Lauersen and E. Stukane, *The Complete Book of Breast Care* (New York: Ballantine Books, 1996), 135.

27. D. C. Skegg et al., "Depot medroxyprogesterone acetate and breast cancer: A pooled analysis of the World Health Organization and New Zealand studies," *Journal of the American Medical Association* 273, no. 10 (Mar. 8, 1995), 799–804.

28. J. M. Foidart et al., "Estradiol and progesterone regulate the proliferation of human breast epithelial cells," *Fertility and Sterility* 69, no. 5 (May 1998), 963–69.

29. A. Clur, "Di-iodothyronine as part of the oestradiol and catechol estrogen receptor—the role of iodine, thyroid hormones and melatonin in the etiology of breast cancer," *Medical Hypotheses* 27, no. 4 (Dec. 1988), 303–11.

30. B. V. Stadel, "Dietary iodine and risk of breast, endometrial, and ovarian cancer," *Lancet* 1, no. 7965 (Apr. 24, 1976), 890–91.

31. B. A. Eskin, "Iodine and mammary cancer," *Advances in Experimental Medicine and Biology* 91 (1977), 293–304.

32. Monographs, *Alternative Medicine Review* 7, no. 4 (2002), 336–39.

33. M. S. Brignall, "Prevention and treatment of cancer with indole-3-carbinol," *Alternative Medicine Review* 6, no. 6 (Dec. 2001), 583.

34. S. Love and K. Lindsey, *Dr. Susan Love's Breast Book* (Cambridge, Mass.: Perseus Publishing, 2000), 83.

35. W. R. Ghent et al., "Iodine replacement in fibrocystic disease of the breast," *Canadian Journal of Surgery* 36, no. 5 (Oct. 1993), 453–60.

36. A. A. Abrams, "Use of vitamin E in chronic cystic mastitis," *New England Journal of Medicine* 272 (1965), 1080–81.

CHAPTER 10. NURTURING THE CRADLE OF YOUR INTIMATE SELF

1. N. Angier, *Woman: An Intimate Geography* (New York: Anchor Books, 1999), 78.

2. F. Tomblin and K. Lucas, "Lysine for management of herpes labialis," *American Journal of Health-System Pharmacy* 58, no. 4 (Feb. 15, 2001), 298, 300, 304.

3. M. Murray and J. Pizzorno, "Herpes simplex," *Textbook of Natural Medicine* vol. 2 (London, Eng.: Churchill Livingstone, Harcourt Publishers, 2000), 1273–76.

4. K. Marshall, "Cervical dysplasia, early intervention," *Alternative Medicine Review* 8, no. 2 (May 2003), 156–70.

5. Ibid.

6. C. Butterworth et al., "Improvement in cervical dysplasia associated with folic acid therapy in users of oral contraceptives," *American Journal of Clinical Nutrition* 35 (1982), 73–82.

7. Interviews by Jodi Godfrey Meisler, M.S., R.D., "Toward Optimal Health: The Experts

Respond to Fibroids," *Journal of Women's Health and Gender Based Medicine* 8, no. 7 (1999), 879.

8. Ibid.

9. C. L. Walker, "Role of hormonal and reproductive factors in the etiology and treatment of uterine leiomyoma," *Recent Progress in Hormone Research* 57 (2002), 277–94.

10. Ibid.

11. L. C. Hodges et al., "An in vivo/in vitro model to assess endocrine disrupting activity of xenoestrogens in uterine leiomyoma," *Annals of the New York Academy of Science* 948 (Dec. 2001), 100–11.

12. S. Rier et al., "Immunoresponsiveness in endometriosis: implication of estrogenic toxicants," *Environmental Health Perspectives* 103, supp. 7 (1995), 151–56.

13. T. Weschler, *Taking Charge of Your Fertility* (New York: Quill Books, 2002), 355.

14. U.S. Food and Drug Administration, "Consumer Friendly Birth Control Information," online at www.fda.gov/fdac/features/19997/conceptbl.html (accessed Jun. 26, 2003).

Chapter 11. Tapping into the Power of Your Mind

1. R. Blaylock, *Excitotoxins: The Taste That Kills* (New Mexico: Health Press, 1997), 15.

2. U.S. Environmental Protection Agency, Technology Transfer Network Air Toxics, "Acrylamide," online at www.epa.gov. (accessed Oct. 1, 2003).

3. D. A. Clayman et al., "Life Extension," *Disease Prevention and Treatment,* 4th ed. (Hollywood, Fla.: Life Extension Media, 2003), 62.

4. T. Moriguchi et al., "Behavioral deficits associated with dietary induction of decreased brain docosahexaenoic acid concentration," *Journal of Neurochemistry* 75, no. 6 (Dec. 2000), 2563–73.

5. N. Salem Jr. et al., "Mechanisms of action of docosahexaenoic acid in the nervous system," *Lipids* 36, no. 9 (Sept. 2001), 945–59.

6. H. Tiemeier, H. R. van Tuijl, and A. Hofman, "Plasma fatty acid composition and depression are associated in the elderly: The Rotterdam study," *American Journal of Clinical Nutrition* 78, no. 1 (Jul. 2003), 40–46.

7. J. R. Hibbeln et al., "Essential fatty acids predict metabolites of serotonin and dopamine in cerebrospinal fluid among healthy control subjects, and early-and-late-onset alcoholics," *Biological Psychiatry* 44, no. 4 (Aug. 15, 1998), 235–42; H. Li, D. Liu, and E. Shang, "Effect of fish oil supplementation on fatty acid composition and neurotransmitters of growing rats," *Journal of Hygiene Research* 29, no. 1 (Jan. 30, 2000), 47–49.

8. A. Akaike, Y. Tamura, and Y. Sato, "Protective effects of a vitamin B_{12} analog, methylcobalamin, against glutamate cytotoxicity in cultured cortical neurons," *European Journal of Pharmacology* 241, no. 1 (Sept. 7, 1993), 1–6; M. Kasuya, "The effect of methylcobalamin on the toxicity of methylmercury and mercuric chloride on nervous tissue in culture," *Toxicology Letters* 7, no. 1 (Nov. 1980), 87–93.

9. M. Richards, R. Hardy, and M. E. Wadsworth, "Does active leisure protect cognition? Evidence from a national birth cohort," *Social Science and Medicine* 56, no. 3 (Feb. 2003), 785–92.

10. J. Carper, *Your Miracle Brain* (New York: HarperCollins, 2000), 35.

11. D. Laurin et al., "Physical activity and risk of cognitive impairment and dementia in elderly persons," *Archives of Neurology* 58, no. 3 (Mar. 2001), 498–504.

12. D. Quig, "Cysteine metabolism and metal toxicity," *Alternative Medicine Review* 3, no. 4 (Aug. 1998), 266.

13. Ibid.

14. Blaylock, *Excitotoxins,* 180.

15. J. Endicott, M. M. Weissman, and K. A. Yonkers, "What's unique about depression in women?" *Contemporary Ob/Gyn,* Jun. 1997, 51–71.

16. C. Landau and F. Milan, "Assessment and treatment of depression during the menopause: A preliminary report," *Menopause: The Journal of the American Menopause Society* 3, no. 4 (1996), 201–7.

17. R. Diaz Brinton, "Estrogen replacement therapy and Alzheimer's disease," *Menopausal Medicine* 5, no. 1 (Spring 1997), 5.

18. A. Paganini-Hill, "Alzheimer's disease, women, and estrogen replacement therapy," *Contemporary Ob/Gyn,* May 1999, 110–27.

19. S. A. Shumaker et al., "Estrogen plus progestin and the incidence of dementia and mild cognitive impairment in postmenopausal women: The Women's Health Initiative Memory Study," *Journal of the American Medical Association* 289, no. 20 (May 2003), 2717–19.

20. Paganini-Hill, "Alzheimer's disease," 110–27.

21. Laurin et al., "Physcial activity and risk of cognitive impairment," 498–504.

22. Blaylock, *Excitotoxins,* 137.

23. T. H. Crook et al., "Effects of phosphatidylserine in age-associated memory impairment," *Neurology* 41, no. 5 (May 1991), 644–49.

24. M. Sano, C. Ernesto, and R. G. Thomas, "A controlled trial of selegiline, alpha-tocopherol, or both as treatment for Alzheimer's disease," *New England Journal of Medicine* 336, no. 17 (Apr. 24, 1997), 1216–22.

25. A. Skolnick, "Old Chinese herbal medicine used for fever yields possible new Alzheimer's disease therapy," *Journal of the American Medical Association* 277, no. 10 (Mar. 12, 1997), 776.

APPENDIX D.
HOW TO CHOOSE
A PHYSICIAN TRAINED
IN NATURAL MEDICINE

1. Academic Programs; Graduate Program: Naturopathic Medicine 2002–2003 Bastyr University website. Available at http://www.bastyr.edu/academic/profiles/naturopath/curriculum. Accessed July 1, 2003.

2. The Association of American Medical Colleges Curriculum Directory. Association of American Medical Colleges website. Available at http://www.aamc.org. Accessed July 1, 2003.

3. The Association of American Medical Colleges Curriculum Directory; *Hot Topics in Medical Education.* Number of U.S. Medical Schools teaching selected topics. From the Liaison Committee on Medical Education Part II Annual Medical School Questionnaire for 2000–2001, compiled by the AAMC Institutional Profile System. Association of American Medical Colleges website. Available at http://services.aamc.org/currdir/section2/LCMEHotTopics.pdf. Accessed July 1, 2003.

4. Naturopathic Medical Education Comparative Curricula: Comparing Naturopathic Med Schools with Conventional Med Schools. The American Association of Naturopathic Physicians website. Available at http://www.naturopathic.org/education. Accessed Juy 1, 2003.

Acknowledgments

As the quotation at the beginning of this book says, "A long journey begins with a single step." This book had its first steps deep in the past when I was discovering my life purpose and choosing to become a naturopathic physician and practitioner of Chinese medicine. Numerous people along my path have profoundly influenced me; this book is the result of many years of benefiting from their accumulated wisdom.

In recent years, a number of people have played key roles in helping with the creation of this book. I especially wish to acknowledge the following.

Thank you, Sara Levins, for encouraging me to write, for dreaming big dreams, and for helping me to launch this project. Without your assistance in taking the first steps, this book would not exist. It is rare for two people to work so well together for so many years, and your dedication to my business has made my life richer and my work more joyful.

Alex Steelsmith, how do I thank you when you have contributed so much to this book? You have brought to my life many gifts and supported me through every life challenge for so many years. This book, our latest challenge, is what it is largely because of your precise mind, high IQ (and abundant Qi!), creative rewriting of the text, and invaluable perseverance with meaning and clarity. Your coauthorship and your artwork in these pages are priceless. I love you more than life itself.

Deirdre Mullane, thank you for being so much more than an agent. You have helped shape this book since its conception and brought to it so much of your creative energy. It continues to be an honor to work with you.

Jennifer Kasius, I am uniquely grateful to you for seeing the potential of this project in its earliest phase nearly four years ago, for putting your faith in it, and for sharing your vision of what it could become.

Shana Drehs, editor extraordinaire, I feel very fortunate that you have brought to this project your keen eye for organization and your many wonderful insights. I am so impressed with and appreciative of all that you have done for this book, despite taking on the project after it was under way. Thank you, Shana, for bringing this book to life! (I'm grateful to the powers that be at Crown Publishers for their improvements to this book, as well.)

So many others have helped me in numerous ways on this journey. Dr. Laura Louie, thank you for your brilliant mind and for being my colleague and one of my dearest friends. All the postgraduate training we have done together has helped make this book what it is. Dr. Leah McNeill, thank you for our special friendship and the countless hours we've spent on the phone discussing women's health issues; our dialogue has been an integral part of this book. Dr. Eric Jones, thank you for being my teacher, believing in me, and spending many hours carefully reading and editing the manuscript. Your feedback has been invaluable. Dr. Mark Nolting, I am honored to have been one of your students and I thank you for giving such close attention to the manuscript on such short notice. Catherine Yi-Ling Low, I am most grateful for your excellent instruction in Chinese herbal medicine, and for your expert advice on the Chinese character drawings that appear in this book. Pam Chambers, many thanks for all your professional support over the years and for being a great friend.

I am grateful to many family members for all their encouragement and support. I give special thanks to my mother, and I have dedicated this book to her because she has not only transformed her life with natural medicine but has become a powerful force in motivating others to do the same. Special thanks also go to my father, Gloria, U.J., Ann, Carl, Ernie, Ellen, John, Susan, and Bobbie. Thank you, Aunt Patti and Uncle Gavin, for praying for the best outcome for this book and reminding me that it is all part of God's plan.

Other loved ones I want to acknowledge, who are always within arm's reach or a phone call away, include Jean Kenyon, Liz Cerutti, Carla and Al Joaquin, Jean Freeman, Helene and Larry Fournier, Dr. Elizabeth Greimes, Bindu Van Camp, Jennifer Perry, Lynn Garcia, Alyssa Moreau, Terri Alexander, and Kula. There are many others, far too many to mention here, but you know who you are. Thank you all for being in my life and helping to make this book possible.

As with any written work that incorporates medical knowledge, this book is to a great extent the result of countless other people's work. I am grateful to all those I have quoted and referred to, and to many other medical professionals who have painstakingly researched and documented their findings, which have contributed enormously to this book. And I am indebted to my professors at Bastyr University for their dedication to the highest standards in naturopathic and Chinese medicine.

Finally, I want to thank the thousands of patients who have trusted me with their care over the years, and in particular all the women who have shared their personal stories in these pages. I hope this book will be an inspiration for many other women who will follow in your footsteps on their journey to optimal health.

To your health,
Laurie Steelsmith, N.D., L.Ac

Index